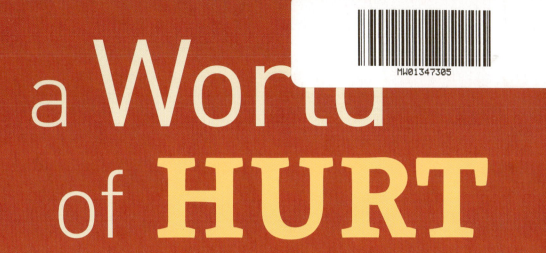

A Guide to Classifying Pain

Melissa C. Kolski • Annie O'Connor

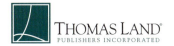
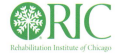

Disclaimer
Every effort has been made to ensure the accuracy of the information presented and to correctly relate generally accepted practice. However, neither the authors nor the publisher is engaged in rendering professional advice or services to the individual reader and shall not be liable or responsible for any loss, injury, or damage allegedly arising from any information or suggestion in this book.

© 2015 Thomas Land Publishers, Inc.

All rights reserved.

Thomas Land Publishers, Inc., 255 Jefferson Road, St. Louis, MO 63119-3627

First printing June 2015

To order: www.thomasland.com

ISBN: 978-0-9853729-0-1

Book design and composition: Kim Scott, Bumpy Design
Illustrations: Nathan Clement

10 9 8 7 6 5 4 3 2 1
Printed in the United States

Table of Contents

Foreword xi

CHAPTER 1
Musculoskeletal Pain: The Big Picture 1
   Complex and Chronic Nature of Musculoskeletal Pain 2
   Factors Correlated with Musculoskeletal Pain 2
      Socioeconomic Status 2
      Age 2
      Gender 3
      Race and Culture 4
      Cognition Level 5
      Other Factors 5
   Current Practice Patterns: Variability in Care 6
      Quality of Care 7
      Defensive Medicine and Routine Practice 7
      The Case for Conservative Care 7
   Better Care via Classification Systems 8
      Pain Mechanism Classification Systems 9
      Mechanical Diagnosis and Therapy 11
   Conclusion 11

CHAPTER 2
Overview of the Pain Mechanism Classification System and Mechanical Diagnosis and Therapy 17
   Brief Review of the Nervous System 18
   Peripheral and Central Factors in Pain 18
   Pain Mechanism Classification System Categories 20
      Nociceptive:Inflammatory 21
      Nociceptive:Ischemia 21
      Peripheral Neurogenic 22
      Central Sensitization 22
      Affective 22
      Motor/Autonomic 23
   Clinical Practice Considerations in the Use of the PMCS 23
      Acute Versus Chronic Pain 23
      Features of the Pain Experience 24
      Clinical Reasoning in Subjective Evaluation 26

    Intervention with CNS Mechanisms 26
    Intervention with PNS Mechanisms 27
        Derangement Syndrome 28
        Dysfunction Syndrome 29
        Posture and Other Syndromes 29
        Restoration of Function in MDT 29

CHAPTER 3
Subjective Evaluation 33
    Review of the Evidence on Musculoskeletal Pain Evaluation and Management 33
    Information Gathered in the PMCS Subjective Evaluation 34
        Pain Location, Description, and Frequency 35
        Onset or Mechanism of Injury 37
        24-Hour Behavior of Symptoms 37
        Aggravating and Alleviating Factors 38
        Thoughts, Beliefs, and Cultural Attitudes Regarding Pain 41
        Past and Current Treatments 44
        Readiness for Treatment 44
    Use of Measurement Tools in the Subjective Evaluation 50
    Use of the Management Plan in the Subjective Evaluation 51
    Use of Patient Education in the Subjective Evaluation 52

CHAPTER 4
Nociceptive Pain Mechanisms: Inflammation and Ischemia 59
    Types of Inflammation 60
        Chemical Inflammation 61
        Mechanical Inflammation 61
    Connective Tissue Healing and Repair 62
        Nociceptive:Inflammatory Pain Mechanism 63
        Nociceptive:Ischemia Pain Mechanism 63
    Healing Processes in Specific Tissue Types 68
        Bone 68
        Ligament 68
        Intervertebral Disc 69
        Tendon 69
        Muscle 72
    Nociceptive Pain Mechanism Evaluation 73
        Subjective Evaluation 74
        Objective Evaluation: Repeated Movement Examination 75
    Intervention for Nociceptive Pain Mechanisms 78
        Guidelines for Establishing the Activity Baseline 79
        Guidelines for Management of Flare-Ups 82

CHAPTER 5
Peripheral Neurogenic Pain Mechanism 105
    Characteristics of Peripheral Neurogenic Pain 106
    Role of Neurodynamics in Classifying Mechanical Problems Related to PNPM ... 107
    Peripheral Nerve Clinical Anatomy 107
        Peripheral Nerve Mobility 108
        Peripheral Nerve Dynamics 109
        Spinal Cord Dynamics 110
        Axoplasm 110
        Peripheral Nerve Conduction 110
    Peripheral Nerve Injury and Impairment 111
        Nerve Conduction Impairment 112
        Abnormal Impulse-Generating Sites 113
    PNPM Connection to Central Sensitization 114
    Nerve Pain Subjective Evaluation 115
        Location 115
        Description 115
        Frequency 116
        Onset or Mechanism of Injury 116
        24-Hour Behavior of Symptoms 117
        Aggravating and Alleviating Factors 117
        Thoughts, Beliefs, and Cultural Responses 118
        Past and Current Treatments 118
    Nerve Pain Objective Evaluation 119
        Nerve Conduction Examination 119
        Neurodynamic Examination 122
        Clinical Reasoning in Neurodynamic Testing 130
    PNPM Mechanical Dysfunction 132
        Container-Dependent Dysfunction 132
        Neural-Dependent Dysfunction 132
        Clinical Reasoning in Differentiating Container-Dependent
        and Neural-Dependent Dysfunction 132
    PNPM Management and Intervention 134
        Intervention Strategies 135
        Management of Container-Dependent Dysfunction 140
        Management of Neural-Dependent Dysfunction 141

CHAPTER 6
Central Sensitization Pain Mechanism 187
    Central Nervous System Sensitizing Processes 188
        Peripheral Sensitization 188
        Plasticity in the Spinal Cord 189
        Supraspinal Modulation 189

Role of the Brain in the Pain Alarm System..................................191
Central Nervous System Pain Mechanisms...................................192
    Health Care Models in Chronic Pain Treatment.........................192
    Psychology in Pain Management......................................194
Pain Evaluation for Central Sensitization.....................................195
    Subjective Evaluation..195
    Maladaptive Pain Behavior..197
    Objective Evaluation...197
Central Sensitization Screening Tools and Tests...............................198
    Waddell's Tests..198
    Fear-Avoidance Beliefs Questionnaire................................198
    Pain Pressure Thresholds...200
    Thermal Pain Thresholds..200
    Light Touch..201
    Diaphragm Breathing Test...201
    Selecting a Screening Tool or Test..................................202
Central Sensitization Management and Intervention...........................203
    Patient Education..204

CHAPTER 7

Affective Pain Mechanism...237
Connection Between Psychosocial Factors and Pain............................238
    Classification of Psychosocial Factors in Health Care Practice.........239
    Identifying the Connection Between Patients' Thoughts
    and Behaviors and Pain...241
Conscious and Unconscious Psychosocial Aspects
of Disabling Musculoskeletal Pain..242
    Affective Characteristics of the Conscious Mind.....................242
    Affective Characteristics of the Unconscious Mind..................250
Clinician Psychology..252
Affective Pain Mechanism Evaluation..255
    Readiness to Change Education and Assessment.....................255
    Use of Psychosocial Screening Tools................................256
    Assessment of Coping Strategies....................................259
Intervention to Address the Affective Pain Mechanism........................261
    Biopsychosocial Approach..261
    Motivational Interviewing..263
    Nonpharmacy Approaches to Pain...................................266
Conclusion..282

CHAPTER 8
Motor/Autonomic Pain Mechanism 317
Complex Regional Pain Syndrome 318
Principles of Neuroplasticity and Cortical Reorganization 322
    Cortical Representation 323
    Mirror Neurons 324
    Facilitation and Disinhibition 325
    Body Matrix 325
Subjective Evaluation for the Motor/Autonomic Pain Mechanism 326
    Location 326
    Frequency of Pain 326
    Descriptors 326
    Onset 327
    24-Hour Behavior 327
    Psychological and Social Status 327
    Thoughts, Beliefs, and Culture 327
Objective Evaluation for the Motor/Autonomic Pain Mechanism 328
    Clinical Examination 328
    Sensory Screening Tools 329
    Motor Screening Tools 332
Intervention for the Motor/Autonomic Pain Mechanism 335
    Patient Education 335
    Training from the Brain to the Periphery 336
    Training from the Periphery to the Brain 339
    Sensorimotor Retraining Programs 342
Conclusion 344

Patient Education Handouts

Figure 4.1	Nociceptive:Inflammatory Pain Mechanism Patient Education Handout	64
Figure 4.4	Nociceptive:Ischemia (Overuse) Pain Mechanism Patient Education Handout	77
Figure 4.6	Baseline Activity Tolerance Tool Patient Education Handout	81
Figure 5.2	Nerve Pain Patient Education Handout	136
Figure 6.7	Persistent Musculoskeletal Pain Patient Education Handout	206
Figure 7.1	Tension Myositis Syndrome Patient Education Handout	253
Figure 7.2	Musculoskeletal Pain Mechanisms Patient Education Handout	264
Figure 7.4	Active Sleep Restoration Strategies Patient Education Handout	269
Figure 8.6	Graded Motor Imagery Patient Education Handout	337
Figure 8.8	Stress Loading Patient Education Handout	340
Figure 8.9	Desensitization Patient Education Handout	341

Foreword

Through our work at the Rehabilitation Institute of Chicago (RIC), we have come in contact with many clinicians from around the world. We are constantly impressed with what these people represent. They are active, hardworking, competent, and caring people dedicated to making a difference. These clinicians consistently tell us of the tremendous struggles they face daily while trying to serve people who suffer from pain.

Why is pain at epidemic proportions? Why is pain becoming the leading disabling condition of mankind? For years we have been given methods, pharmacy techniques, tools, and information on how to manage and control pain. We have been told that if we use this medication, do this procedure, keep working harder, ignore the pain, or use some new device in a particular way, then we will be able to cure pain. So as clinicians, we read a new book, go to a new course, learn a new technique, get a new degree, get a new certification. We learn it, apply it, try harder. And what happens? For most of the people we meet, the result for both the patient and the provider is increased frustration, failure, and guilt. Traditional pain treatments suggest that by focusing on the body, you eventually will gain control of pain and cure it. We disagree. Pain is not a simple experience with simple connections.

Basing pain treatments only on the body is futile. Universal principles exist that allow us to understand the pain system. We cannot control how our patients think and the choices they make, but we can commit to better education and understanding of the principles or lessons pain has taught us. Our experience, which is supported by numerous scientific studies, has taught us four lessons regarding musculoskeletal pain: (1) ignore at your own peril; (2) misinterpret pain and live a life of disability; (3) understand directional preference pain and create miracles; (4) create pain and get your life back.

In this book, we present a different approach to pain. This is a principle-centered approach. It transcends the traditional prescription for pain of pharmacy, procedure, and manual therapy. Rather than offering another technique, this approach provides you with principles carried forward and supported by research in how to educate and guide exercise for your patient who suffers from musculoskeletal pain. In one sense, this approach is new; in another, it's very old. It is deeply rooted in classic, timeless principles that represent a distinct contrast to the quick-fix approach to pain promoted by our modern society. This is not a short cut, but there is a path. The path is based on principles of subgrouping. If there is one message to glean from this wisdom, it is that when you give a man a fish, you feed him for a day; when you teach a man to fish, you feed him for life.

This book presents an interpretation of the nature of musculoskeletal pain, allowing the classification of the dominant pain mechanism to guide patient education and active therapy interventions. Although this book does not advocate passive modalities, medications, and procedures, it does describe a classification system for assessment and treatment of musculoskeletal pain with emphasis on patient education and active exercise. This approach to musculoskeletal pain has grown out of theoretical considerations supported by different levels of research and based on clinical observations at RIC's outpatient facilities for the last 16 years. We synthesized contributions from expert clinicians and present a pain mechanism classification system (PMCS) created for clinical use by Butler and Gifford in collaboration with the McKenzie Method of Mechanical Diagnosis & Therapy as an effectively efficient method with which to subgroup musculoskeletal pain patients. This book brings forward these principles for the purpose of classifying the dominant pain mechanism and discusses their application to patients with musculoskeletal pain and disability along the entire pain continuum. The PMCS offers the evidence-based biopsychosocial approach to musculoskeletal pain and allows better understanding of the dominating mechanism and patient results.

This approach can apply to all who suffer from musculoskeletal pain—from young to old, from disabled to high performance, from women to men. This PMCS is not only invaluable to patient care but also to clinicians. The PMCS is an organized synthesis of clinical reasoning for acute, subacute, and chronic pain patients. It represents all dimensions of pain from chemical, mechanical, structural, to psychological. This book attempts to close the gap between clinicians and patients regarding pain education. By giving patients more detailed information about their pain mechanism, clinicians can help them better understand their pain responses and the path to their healing.

We gratefully acknowledge and express deep appreciation to the many wonderful people who have made this project possible:

- To those RIC Physical and Occupational Therapists from 1998 to present, taking the challenge posed by research, humbling their knowledge and approaches, implementing PMCS into practice, and ultimately proving its effectiveness and changing the standard of practice for musculoskeletal pain at RIC for all patients. Part of the proceeds for this book will go to the Mike Hage Fund, a RIC clinical education philanthropy fund that sparked this clinical innovation for a standard of care for musculoskeletal pain.
- To those RIC patients who accepted the challenge with the clinicians, allowing their beliefs about pain to change and bravely exploring innovative directions.
- To Krista Van DerLaan, Mary Killion (Thomas Land Publishers, Inc.), and RIC senior leadership for their ongoing support to the completion of this book.
- To Katie Rittenberg and Christie Downing for their continued assistance, support, and guidance during the early manuscript.
- To Ed Pierce, the initial caption artist, whose creative wit applied to a serious topic has created a visual representation of each subgroup.
- A special thanks to our families who support our work and our commitment to our patients and this profession. In everything we did in life, they found such enjoyment, pride, and the real meaning to its impact.

—Melissa C. Kolski and Annie O'Connor

CHAPTER 1

Musculoskeletal Pain: The Big Picture

We are first moved by pain, and the whole succeeding course of our lives is but one continuous series of actions with a view to be freed from it.
—Benjamin Franklin

> **POINTS TO DISCUSS**
>
> - High cost of pain and related disability
> - Factors correlated with musculoskeletal pain, including socioeconomic status, age, gender, race and culture, and cognitive level
> - Variability in current practice patterns
> - Role of classification systems in improving treatment of and research on musculoskeletal pain

Pain is a costly problem for both individuals and society. People seek the services of health care practitioners to address pain and its negative effects on their ability to function. Unfortunately, health care costs dedicated to pain management have skyrocketed over the last 15 years, but the ability of pain patients to manage pain and maintain function has not improved. Evidence-based guidelines exist for the rehabilitation of certain conditions; however, these guidelines may not necessarily be generalizable to individual specific needs and have not demonstrated an ability to reduce costs with respect to musculoskeletal pain. Yelin[1] estimated that in 2000, about 2.9% of the gross domestic product, or approximately $240 billion, was spent on medical care for musculoskeletal conditions and related pain. An estimated 70% to 80% of all Americans will have an episode of low back pain in their lifetime,[2] and this pain condition is the fifth leading cause of hospitalizations.[3] The number of people seeking care for spine-related problems increased by 49% from 1997 to 2006,[4] and the number of spine surgeries performed in the United States is roughly double that in most developed countries.[5] Spending for fusions increased from $75 million to $482 million from 1990 to 2003.[6]

So why has spending for pain and conditions such as spinal care increased, but self-reported health status has not changed for the better?[7] Possible explanations include the complexity and chronicity of pain-related conditions, the wide variety of factors correlated with musculoskeletal pain, and high variability in current treatment of these conditions. This chapter describes each of these explanations in turn and then discusses the contribution of classification systems to the treatment of and research on musculoskeletal pain.

Complex and Chronic Nature of Musculoskeletal Pain

If pain level correlated directly with pathophysiology, pain treatment would be straightforward, but this is not the case. Pain is a highly subjective state of being. Evidence shows that degenerative changes in connective tissues bear little relationship to reported pain intensity and sensitivity.[8-11] Musculoskeletal pain has physical, neurological, cognitive, and psychoemotional mechanisms[12-20] and manifests in chronic, highly complex conditions involving multiple body systems, such as the immune, endocrine, musculoskeletal, neurological, and digestive systems. Whereas less involved pain states may require only patient education and a home exercise program, multisystemic pain requires a multifaceted approach that may include biofeedback, occupational and physical therapy, psychology, and pain management. These programs can be highly effective but are also costly and do not guarantee a change. A 2004 study by Proctor et al[21] revealed that 25% of patients with chronic musculoskeletal pain sought additional treatment even after completing a multidisciplinary pain management program. These patients experienced a lower return-to-work rate, a higher level of leaving work after returning, excess health care consumption, and unremitting disability payments.[21] Thus, about a quarter of pain patients consume disproportionate resources over long periods of time. The research suggests that it is crucial to identify these individuals early if care is to be cost-effective.

Factors Correlated with Musculoskeletal Pain

Another reason for the lack of improvement in the health condition of the population experiencing chronic musculoskeletal pain may be the wide variety of factors that have been correlated with pain. Many theories exist as to what predisposes people to pain. Is it genetics, is it life experiences, is it attitude or coping strategies? From a research standpoint, predisposition to pain is difficult to determine because so many factors come into play. In a recent systematic review of persistent pain following traumatic injury, for example, predictive factors for persistent pain included symptoms of anxiety and depression, patient's perception that the injury was attributable to an external source (ie, the patient was not at fault), cognitive avoidance of distressing thoughts, alcohol consumption prior to the trauma, lower educational status, injury at work, eligibility for compensation, pain at initial assessment, and older age[22]—factors that may be a function of biological and physiological vulnerabilities.[22] The sections that follow highlight socioeconomic status, age, gender, race and culture, cognition level, and other factors correlated with pain.

Socioeconomic Status

People of lower socioeconomic status tend to have higher levels of pain.[23] During economic downturns, socioeconomic issues such as job loss affect health care and vice versa, fueling costs. Organizational downsizing has been shown to increase back pain and musculoskeletal problems[24]; downsizing also increases the rate of early retirement on long-term disability and contributes to psychological stress.[25] As organizational structures and work-related stress change, pain statistics change as well.[24]

Age

Pain can happen at any age. The ability to detect and interpret pain is mature at birth.

The public view has often been that older and younger people are capable of feeling less pain than middle-aged people; this is not true.[26] In a 4-year follow-up study, it was shown that widespread pain is common in children, just as in adults.[27] Depression, fatigue and sleep problems, somatic axial pain symptoms, female gender, and older age were predictive of chronic widespread pain among children. However, children were reported to have a "fluctuating course with a more favorable prognosis" compared with many adults with widespread pain.[27]

One age-related difference that relates to pain mechanisms is in patients' affective motivational response to the pain and coping strategies they use. Brain physiology changes with age, especially in the areas of the brain associated with the ability to cope.[28-30] Just as a parent informs a child of the meaning of a sensory input, including pain, health professionals need to inform patients about the meaning of their pain through positive education about pain mechanisms, assessment of the patients' readiness to change behavior, and management individualized to age and learning capability.

Evidence exists of age-related changes in the brain that support the affective and motivational response differences. The older the individual, the less brain activity is noted in these areas. Clinically, children in pain tend to play more aggressively and sleep more compared with adults in pain, who are less active and have difficulty with sleep cycles.[31-34]

A difference in coping also exists in older adults who experience injury. Active coping has been associated with younger age (less than 60 years) and increased disability and passive coping with older age (greater than 60 years).[30] These age-related changes may be best conceptualized as a reduced capacity in the functional reserve of the coping system. Clinically, older adults are especially vulnerable to the negative impacts of pain, the under treatment of pain, functional loss, and pain-associated events.[29,35] Thus it may not be the sensory input of pain that changes, but rather the primary coping mechanism used that influences how pain affects the individual. This can be observed in a study on physical health and psychosocial factors of chronic pain patients in a multidisciplinary retrospective analysis.[36] The investigators found that there were no intrarace differences between younger Black and younger White Americans who reported more depressive symptoms and symptoms related to posttraumatic disorder than their older counterparts. In this sample, both older cohorts reported better coping ability than their younger counterparts from the onset.

Although age-related studies do indicate a maturing of the connective tissues overall, no correlation has been found between age and pain intensity and sensitivity.[8,9,11] There is, however, a direct relationship between functional loss in the elderly and pain intensity, sensitivity, and disability. In the elderly population, it appears that functional loss related to pain motivates the patient to seek treatment, and often restoration of function desensitizes the pain mechanism. In addition to age-related changes, it was commonly thought that wear and tear on the spine may increase the incidence of low back pain with aging. Holmberg et al[37] refuted this concept by demonstrating that aging farmers with elevated physical workloads did not have an increased prevalence of back pain. Focusing on functional improvements and keeping the aging spine active may or may not decrease the incidence of pain depending on whether the brain processes interactions with pain appropriately along the way.

The principles of pain management described in this book are practical for all ages. The education and mode of treatment delivery, however, need to be individualized based on the patient's age and stage of readiness to change.

Gender

Physiological differences exist between the hypothalamus and globus pallidus of men and women between the second and eighth decades of life. Women have 15% more mu opioid receptor binding sites, which have been linked to pain modulation, perhaps related to childbearing.[28] A woman's life cycle may include the hormonal milestones of menarche, pregnancy, contraceptive use, and menopause. Each of these events involves changing levels of sex hormones and may cause a change in frequency and intensity of musculoskeletal pain.[38] Hormonal changes in women have been linked to increased incidence of headaches, osteoarthritis of the knee, and lower back pain, especially during menopause, when there is an imbalance in levels of progesterone, testosterone, and estrogen.[38]

Thus, for women, varying levels of diffuse pain in multiple locations may be a signal of hormonal imbalance as opposed to mechanical symptoms. In women who do not appear to be responding conclusively to mechanically based treatments, clinicians should consider hormonal causes of inflammation. Clinicians should investigate the hormonal milestones in their review of systems with their female patients to understand regularity and pain as it relates to these events. Clinicians may need to refer patients to another professional or recommend further diagnostic testing such as blood levels or a 24-hour urine test to determine whether a hormonal imbalance is present. In addition, some patients may be experiencing a hormone-related inability to cope, depression, or insomnia that may be better addressed psychologically. The clinician should consider multiple triggers other than those related to a direct injury or mechanical effect in the pain differential diagnosis.

Apart from hormonal factors, psychosocial symptoms such as depressive feelings, hypermobility, and waking at night predicted pain reoccurrence in preadolescent and elderly women compared with men.[39,40] Women, as well as people with less education, poorer health, and depression, were found to experience the greatest pain burden[8,38-41] and poorer treatment outcomes.[42]

In a recent critical review of studies on gender and pain, Fillingim et al[43] noted that women are at greater risk for many chronic pain conditions and that pain sensitivity is greater among women than men for most pain modalities, including invasive procedures. They noted, however, that the relationship between gender and pain is not simple. Although pain risk and sensitivity may be greater for women, Fillingim et al[43] noted inconsistencies in pharmacological and nonpharmacological treatments for pain; a tendency was found to undermedicate female pain patients in comparison to male patients. This suggests that health professionals may have underlying sex biases in the treatment of pain in women.[40]

Race and Culture

Culture affects the way people perceive and respond to chronic pain in themselves and in others.[44] Differences in pain thresholds and responses have been found between people of different cultures.[45] Many studies suggest that clinicians should explore the relationship among pain, psychosocial factors, and demographic characteristics when working with patients of different cultures.[46-49] Ethnicity and cultural background are less important factors than the individuals' socioeconomic status and beliefs regarding their ability to improve; regardless of cultural background, lower income, poor self-rated health status, depression symptoms, lower education level, lower functional self-efficacy, and history of smoking predisposed individuals to chronic musculoskeletal pain and disability.[50-53] People in the lowest social class experienced nearly a threefold risk of chronic widespread pain compared with those in the highest social class, and lower social class during childhood was found to be a predictor of regional and widespread chronic pain.[54]

Green et al[49,55] demonstrated that Black Americans of all ages had more depressive symptoms and symptoms consistent with posttraumatic stress disorder than White Americans. Older and younger Black Americans reported more pain and sleep disturbance on initial assessments and more self-identified comorbidities including dizziness, chest pain, and high blood pressure.[49] It has been suggested that Asian Americans may be more reactive to pain than European Americans, but these findings may be more suggestive of acculturation (ie, adaptation to new cultural norms) than true genetic differences.[56]

An understanding of the role a patient's culture plays in his or her health care practices can help the clinician facilitate and advocate for pain control methods that are consistent with the patient's cultural worldview. By recognizing differences in the ways patients of different cultures communicate their perception of the meanings and intensity of pain, researchers can begin to delineate the perspectives on pain of different cultures. It appears that an understanding of how the individual patient feels about the pain is as important as the fact that he or she has pain, regardless of cultural background.[57]

Cognition Level

Pain can be difficult to treat in patients with cognitive or communication deficits. Adults aging with cognitive and physical disabilities experience a variety of pain disorders that affect their functionality and quality of life.[58] Clinical observations of facial expressions and vocalizations are accurate means of assessing the presence but not the intensity of pain in patients who are unable to communicate.[59] Musculoskeletal pain is a common symptom in people with physical disabilities. In general, the more limited a person's function, the more severe the pain. Patients with advanced dementia have a lower reported prevalence of pain and analgesic use,[60,61] but pain may be underreported in patients with dementia because of limitations in awareness and cognition. Patients who had limited communication but awareness of person, place, and time were found to be more at risk for underdetection and undertreatment of pain, indicating that their lack of ability to vocalize their concern led to a discrepancy in their care.[61]

Clinicians relying on the close observation of facial expressions in patients with communicative disorders to infer the presence of pain were found to be correct between 80% and 90% of the time. When facial expressions were integrated into the clinical context of a painful procedure or disease process, the ability of the clinician to detect the presence of pain was even higher.[59] Clinicians caring for patients with cognitive disabilities should be knowledgeable about the prevalence of pain and be able to perform a thorough history and physical examination with respect to the operant pain mechanisms. The classification and intervention strategies presented in this book are appropriate for all levels of mobility and communicative ability. Mode of communication and delivery of education should be patient specific.

Other Factors

Personal contact and emotional support play a big role in coping with life stressors. Social support systems have been found to influence the experience of pain in varied ways. People with few or no social ties who live in less affluent areas are more likely to experience pain that interferes with daily activities.[50,51] In contrast, older adults who have children in more frequent contact have been found to experience greater limitation by pain in daily life,[50] perhaps because their offspring draw attention to their pain. Older chronic pain patients in Sweden were more likely to be divorced, to be blue collar workers, to perceive financial strain, and to use passive coping strategies. They experienced more pain of longer duration with greater disability than their younger cohorts.[50] Current smoking, history of smoking, depression, and insomnia have also been correlated with increased levels of pain and disability.[52,53]

Certain genetic variants may contribute to a predisposition to persistent pain states. Glucocorticoid pathways with genetic variants in *FKBP5* have been identified in patients with traumatic stress exposure who develop persistent pain states.[62] In addition, the catechol-O-methyltransferase (COMT) enzyme degrades catecholamines. A variant of the

COMT gene known as COMT pain vulnerable genotype has been associated with chronic pain. Recently this marker has helped predict which motor vehicle accident patients would take longer to recover physically and emotionally.[63] Therefore, genetic variations may influence psychosocial predispositions to pain and individual processing of pain.

Current Practice Patterns: Variability in Care

The medical community has contributed to the staggering cost to society of the treatment of pain-related disorders.[64] The medical community needs to take responsibility for its management of pain and should focus on positive beliefs and personal potential to enable patients to minimize disability and contribute to society through gainful employment. The high variability in care raises costs without improving outcomes and results from an overreliance on pathoanatomical diagnosis, differences in approach by clinicians of different disciplines, and a tendency to overuse diagnostic tests.

Clinicians often look at the location or structure of the pain symptoms but not at the bigger picture surrounding the pain. The pathoanatomical diagnosis may be of limited help in choosing a treatment unless it is consistent with the physical examination findings of the cause of the pain because the same anatomical structure can be influenced by different pain mechanisms. Some clinicians are convinced that a tissue or structure is creating the patient's pain, whether it is the anterior labrum of the shoulder, the joint capsule itself, an inflammation of the subacromial bursa, or all of these. A diagnosis based on structure or pathology is incomplete; clinicians must be able to identify the stage of a disorder, dictate treatment, and predict outcomes.[65,66] A comprehensive approach to the problem of pain involves not only the location, structure, irritability, and tissue pathology or impairment, but also mechanics and operant pain mechanisms. It is important to consider the patient's history, the biomechanical stress on tissue, and the potential underlying pain mechanisms. Evidence supports the ability to restore patients' function and diminish pain without knowing the pathoanatomic pain generator. According to orthopedic surgeon Ron Donelson, former vice president of the American Back Society, "The only time it really matters where the pain is coming from is if some invasive treatment, like an injection or surgery, is being contemplated."[65(p133)]

Musculoskeletal pain is treated in many different ways by many different disciplines and factions of care, including alternative medicine, conservative care, and surgical care. Clinicians from each discipline frequently provide treatment based on their training and beliefs regarding the clinical problem being treated. A wide variety of treatments may thus be selected for musculoskeletal pain, and a lack of common terminology between physician and nonphysician disciplines hinders a common approach. The evidence suggests that different clinicians come to different conclusions when using different diagnostic and clinical tests.[67,68] Consequently, the various approaches to evaluating and providing a diagnosis for patients are driven by the practitioner's theory of pain production rather than features of the individual patient's clinical presentation.

When arriving at a diagnosis, clinicians too often rely on diagnostic testing that may or may not correlate well with a physical exam. Research by Cherkin et al[69] found a wide variation in tests that physicians commonly ordered for evaluating patients with low back pain. The physician disciplines ordered tests that were more extensive than those recommended by a task force created in the 1980s to study spinal disorders in the workplace.[70] In addition, the diagnostic tests that were ordered depended more on the physician's specialty than on the patient's symptom response. For instance, neurosurgeons and neurologists were twice as likely to order spinal images for patients with acute or chronic low back pain, but physiatrists and neurologists were three times as likely to order an electromyogram.[69]

Quality of Care

Varied definitions of quality of care make it difficult to determine cost-effectiveness. Is quality care the delivery of a desired health outcome on a quality of life measure or joint-specific outcome measure, or is it based on the patient's or payer's satisfaction? Is it important to recognize and diagnose a pain condition appropriately if the outcomes associated with the condition are unknown, subjective, or unmeasurable? Is quality care a responsibility shared among the patient and members of the health care pain team, or does it depend simply on patient compliance with treatment? Campbell et al[71] defined quality care as access and effectiveness. Access involves the ability to obtain the care the patient needs, and effectiveness depends on both clinical care and interpersonal care. The lasting issue of effective outcome measurement for patients with pain remains to be clarified with patient-reported and condition-specific measures.

Defensive Medicine and Routine Practice

To improve outcomes and control costs, it is crucial that clinicians manage musculoskeletal pain with sound clinical reasoning rather than resorting to defensive medicine. For example, despite the fact that imaging is routine in clinical practice for conditions such as low back pain, the American College of Physicians found strong evidence that routine imaging is not associated with any clinically meaningful change in patient outcomes and in fact exposes patients to preventable harm.[72] Chou et al[73] concluded from a meta-analysis that "lumbar imaging for low back pain without indications of serious underlying conditions does not improve clinical outcomes. Therefore, clinicians should refrain from routine, immediate lumbar imaging in patients with acute or subacute low back pain and without features suggesting a serious underlying condition."[(p463)] In addition, although primary care doctors who performed lumbar radiography had higher levels of patient satisfaction, this procedure did not improve outcomes in acute spinal management for function, pain, or overall health status.[74] Although technology has improved and the speed of delivery has increased, using MRIs in place of radiographs for patients with low back pain has produced no significant improvements in outcomes; in addition, Jarvik et al[75] found that substituting rapid MRIs for radiographs "may have increased the costs of care because of the increased spine operations that patients are likely to undergo."[(p2810)]

In addition to the routine practice of imaging, studies comparing costs from 1997 to 2007 found that pharmacy expenditures were more than double those of diagnostic imaging. In contrast, nonphysician services such as physical therapy accounted for less than 30% of direct medical costs.[76]

The Case for Conservative Care

As health care continues to shift and payers demand evidence that procedures are effective, increasing attention will be paid to the cost-effectiveness of conservative (ie, nonoperative) care for certain groups of patients with chronic pain. The evidence indicates that less costly procedures can have a dramatic effect on pain and better enable patients to become active participants in their own care. Clinical examinations conducted with a comprehensive history and an objective look at the patient's movement response and physical performance can guide prescriptive exercises with better accuracy. For example, patients who performed exercises that matched their directional preference showed significantly greater improvements in pain and medication use compared with patients who performed exercises that did not match their directional preference or were nondirectional.[77] Thus, in the lower back, clinical testing and imaging must correlate with patients' symptoms to effectively guide treatment.

Other studies have shown that the treatment of low back pain as a benign, self-limiting condition was more effective in enabling patients to resume activity in contrast to treatment that promoted negative beliefs and unnecessary imaging, which may fuel disability.[64,78] It is thus imperative that clinicians emphasize to patients that they will get better and should return to healthy functional activity as quickly as possible rather than allowing them to adopt a sick role. Moseley et al[79] showed that pain education alone resulted in improvements in physical examination findings, changed beliefs about pain, and normalized catastrophizing thoughts in patients with low back pain. Patient education has far-reaching effects and minimal cost when pain is involved.

Better Care via Classification Systems

Certain aspects of physical examination procedures used in clinical practice for the treatment of musculoskeletal pain have not been validated, and the quality of the research is moderate.[80] At this time, evidence indicates that many palpation techniques are not valid in physical examination and that pain provocation or symptom response methods may be more beneficial.[80,81] Some clinicians rely on physical palpation and imaging studies, but these examinations rarely provide a valid explanation for a patient's pain. Classification systems, in contrast, can help clinicians better understand the nature of the pain and how pain affects each patient's life in order to direct treatment. A meta-analysis showed a statistically significant difference in favor of classification-based treatment over control groups for reduction in pain and disability.[82] Thus, although little evidence is available comparing classification systems, we advocate their use on the basis of available data.[83]

Classification systems contribute to the treatment of many medical conditions. Such systems help create a starting point of common terminology from which to treat and educate patients about musculoskeletal pain. Early identification of the correct mechanism of pain can facilitate the appropriate treatment expectation or promote realistic referrals for patients who may need redirection to services such as nutrition, psychology, or pain management. Classification systems contribute to clinicians' ability to categorize and formulate conclusions based on prior patient experiences, an ability that distinguishes expert from novice clinicians.[84] It is through classification systems that clinical practice can best be structured, measured, and made more efficient.

In addition, classification systems allow clinicians to conduct research in an effective manner by decreasing variation in patient selection and promoting use of a common language to describe prognosis and treatment. Classification systems aid in the accuracy of outcome prediction; studies show that patients whose treatment includes use of a classification system function better[77,85] and that subgroups of patients tend to respond better to one type of intervention than another.[86,87]

It is thus clear that classification systems are an effective means of predicting outcomes, generating effective treatment plans and interventions, and creating efficient use of medical resources on an individual patient basis. This book discusses the use of two classification systems in treatment—the pain mechanism classification system (PMCS) used in our institution and a mechanical classification called mechanical diagnosis and therapy (MDT).

Pain Mechanism Classification Systems

Given the vast health care resources dedicated to the evaluation and treatment of pain, it is important to understand why all patients experiencing pain do not respond to the same interventions in the same way. Just as the mechanical components of musculoskeletal impairments and loss of function can be classified, pain also deserves appropriate classification. Diagnosis and classification systems that lead to erroneous conclusions set the system up for failure. Throughout this book, the argument will be made that a pain mechanism classification system is essential to the proper management of patients with musculoskeletal pain.

In the 1980s, a task force was created to study spinal disorders in the workplace in Quebec. This task force was composed of clinicians, allied health professionals, and methodologists with the goal of identifying a gold standard for the management of spinal disorders. The Quebec Task Force concluded that the effectiveness of low back pain therapies is unproven and that it is very difficult to identify the pain generator and recommended a classification system based on symptom location rather than tissue type.[70] Some may argue that spinal pain differs from pain in the extremities and that one cannot apply the same conclusions to the extremities. Emerging research, however, indicates that extremity joints can behave mechanically similar to the spine in regard to pain provocation, repetitive motions, and classification systems and that this behavior is observable in clinical practice.[88,89] Numerous models of classifying pain have been developed for palliative care in cancer treatment,[90,91] but little evidence addresses the validity or reliability of such systems for generalized musculoskeletal pain.

Because pain is the most common reason that patients seek medical attention, it is imperative that classification systems be used to efficiently evaluate all operant mechanisms and guide patient care. This book presents a musculoskeletal pain classification system that identifies subgroups of musculoskeletal pain mechanisms. These subgroups are based on operant biological pain mechanisms; this simplifies the need to specify anatomical locations and promotes consistency in treatments for various mechanisms of pain production. Diagnosing musculoskeletal pain on the basis of structure or pathoanatomy alone overstates the pathological implications of the disorder[14] and can result in overutilization of resources, inappropriate interventions, and poor outcomes.[21,66,92]

PMCSs have recently become popular as a component of the diagnostic process for pain practitioners such as physical therapists and physicians in pain management.[87,93-95] Problem-based classification systems can improve clinicians' ability to select appropriate interventions, guide communication, and direct care. The use of a PMCS in clinical practice could aid therapists and pain practitioners in identifying patients who are at risk of overutilizing services or who have psychosocial factors that can influence treatment outcomes. This system can also aid clinicians in developing screening and measuring tools and creating potential treatment effect modifiers or prediction rules.[66]

Although the literature has described theoretical support for PMCSs, little empirical evidence indicates that use of such systems will facilitate consistency in decision making. A preliminary reliability study by Smart et al,[95] however, concluded that a PMCS should be investigated using a large sample of patients and multiple independent examiners. Later, the researchers established discriminative validity for the categories of nociceptive, peripheral neuropathic, and central sensitization with 464 patients.[94]

To foster better clinical reasoning among outpatient physical therapists at the Rehabilitation Institute of Chicago, the musculoskeletal practice implemented a pain classification system. Using categories of clinical criteria similar to those of Smart et al,[95] we sought to provide further clinical validation of a mechanisms-based classification system by testing the hypothesis that therapists trained in the use of the system would demonstrate accuracy compared with a computer-driven statistical model in classifying patients who had signs and symptoms of musculoskeletal pain. The classification system consists of six mechanisms: three were related to the peripheral nervous system (ie, mechanical)—nociceptive:inflammatory, nociceptive:ischemia, and peripheral neurogenic; and three were related to the central nervous system (ie, psychosocial)—central sensitization, affective, and motor/autonomic (see **Figure 1.1**). The 24 participants demonstrated good agreement with the computer-generated model, providing empirical support for the use of our PMCS in tandem with therapist education and training.[96] This system is the primary focus of this book. After an overview of the PMCS in Chapter 2, subsequent chapters examine each mechanism in detail.

An important concept in the use of the PMCS with patients suffering from pain is determining when pain is based in the peripheral nervous system and appears related to certain directions or movements versus based in the central nervous system and appears related to cognition, behavior, emotions, and a heightened pain state. One key indicator for a mechanical pain mechanism is known as *centralization*. Centralization is present when pain can be "progressively abolished in a distal to proximal direction with each progressive abolition being retained over time until all symptoms are abolished."[97(p295)] Movements in other directions or the opposite direction potentially cause symptoms or mechanics to worsen. Centralization involves movement of radiating pain from a larger more diffuse area to a more proximal central one; "their intent is very specific: to apply beneficial loads to the

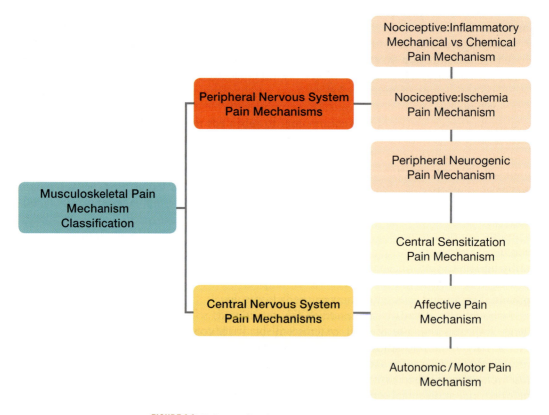

FIGURE 1.1 Pain mechanism classification system.

pain-generating pathology in such a way that the low back and leg symptoms produced by the pathology centralize and abolish and are then prevented from returning"[65(p98)]

It is clinically important to try to identify this phenomenon, but doing so may take several sessions.[97] A careful assessment, patient education, and static loading are critical steps in determining whether a patient is a potential centralizer. Patients who are centralizers have a greater likelihood of good to excellent outcomes, including greater reduction in pain intensity, higher return-to-work rates, greater functional improvement, and less continuous health care use.[98-106] Long et al[100] showed that regardless of pain duration or location, centralizing patients showed decreased pain and improved outcomes with directional preference exercises.

Patients whose symptoms do not correlate well with direction-specific movement may be classified as nonmechanical responders or noncentralizers. Patients initially considered noncentralizers are capable of becoming partial or full centralizers during later therapy sessions, so reassessment of the dominant mechanism is imperative.[107]

Mechanical Diagnosis and Therapy

The McKenzie Method of Mechanical Diagnosis & Therapy is a system for classifying and treating pain in patients with mechanical pain mechanisms. The MDT categories include derangement, dysfunction, posture, and other; these are defined in Chapter 2. Repeated evidence supports intertester and interexaminer reliability and validity in assessment using MDT for evaluation of the spine.[108-112] By using patterns of pain response to repeated end range spinal movements, therapists were able to identify the mechanical syndromes. Classification using this patient response method has shown better outcomes in multiple measures.[113] The MDT syndrome of derangement has been scientifically supported with the concept of centralization as a good prognostic indicator of outcomes with MDT treatment.[97-106] The ability to identify a positive movement in a specific direction often causes symptoms to decrease, abolish, or centralize and typically creates a favorable mechanical response in other directions, altering the patient's function for the better. As with most classification systems, the strength and reliability of the system in clinical practice rely on the training of therapists in its use.[110,111,114,115]

Conclusion

This book looks at all types of musculoskeletal pain in all types of individuals and provides a framework for classification that can enable clinicians to treat patients as people with individual needs, desires, and goals. Rehabilitation is a conceptual process, and all processes requiring change can be difficult. How do clinicians move toward better practice in rehabilitative medicine for their patients with pain? Evidence-based medicine suggests that best practice in pain management merges patient values, clinical practice, and clinical research.

KEY MESSAGES

- Pain is costly, yet health care professionals have not found a way to consistently prevent its reoccurrence or manage it effectively.
- Establishment of a standard of treatment for musculoskeletal pain conditions is elusive. No common rationale exists for spinal surgeries, imaging, or medication use.
- Correlations have been found between age and pain, but it is unclear whether psychology or biology plays the greatest role. Clinicians should provide education appropriate to the patient's age.
- Hormones and psychological symptoms can create gender discrepancies in pain; however, clinicians are cautioned against psychologizing pain in female patients.
- Culture influences the way patients perceive and respond to chronic pain, and clinicians should explore patients' cultural beliefs and attitudes about pain.
- Cognitively impaired patients are capable of communicating pain; assessment requires direct observation of facial expressions and body posture.
- Classification systems provide benefits in both clinical practice and research by providing a common language for discussing prognosis and treatment approaches related to operant pain mechanisms.
- Pain mechanism classification systems have demonstrated discriminative validity and can improve patient outcomes.
- Centralization is a phenomenon in which pain radiates from a larger, more diffuse area to a more proximal central area. The presence or absence of this phenomenon assists clinicians in identifying patients' mechanical pain mechanisms.
- Mechanical diagnosis and therapy has proved highly effective in clinical practice for mechanical pain mechanisms.
- Training for therapists in use of classification systems is critical to their effectiveness.

References

1. Yelin E. Cost of musculoskeletal diseases: Impact of work disability and functional decline. *J Rheumatol Suppl.* 2003;68:8-11.
2. Andersson G. Epidemiology of low back pain. *Acta Orthop Scand Suppl.* 1998;281:28-31.
3. Andersson G. *The Epidemiology of Spinal Disorders.* 2nd ed. Philadelphia, PA: Lippincott-Raven; 1997.
4. Martin BI, Turner JA, Mirza SK, Lee MJ, Comstock BA, Deyo RA. Trends in health care expenditures, utilization, and health status among US adults with spine problems, 1997-2006. *Spine.* 2009;34:2077-2084.
5. Deyo RA, Mirza SK. The case for restraint in spinal surgery: Does quality management have a role to play? *Eur Spine J.* 2009;18(suppl 3):331 337.
6. Weinstein JN, Lurie JD, Olson PR, Bronner KK, Fisher ES. United States' trends and regional variations in lumbar spine surgery: 1992-2003. *Spine.* 2006;31:2707-2714.
7. Martin BI, Deyo RA, Mirza SK, et al. Expenditures and health status among adults with back and neck problems. *JAMA.* 2008;299:656-664.
8. Linton SJ. A review of psychological risk factors in back and neck pain. *Spine.* 2000;25:1148-1156.
9. Lawrence RC, Helmick CG, Arnett FC, et al. Estimates of the prevalence of arthritis and selected musculoskeletal disorders in the United States. *Arthritis Rheum.* 1998;41:778-799.
10. Dahaghin S, Bierma-Zeinstra SM, Reijman M, Pols HA, Hazes JM, Koes BW. Prevalence and determinants of one month hand pain and hand related disability in the elderly (Rotterdam study). *Ann Rheum Dis.* 2005;64:99-104.
11. Lautenbacher S, Kunz M, Strate P, Nielsen J, Arendt-Nielsen L. Age effects on pain thresholds, temporal summation and spatial summation of heat and pressure pain. *Pain.* 2005;115:410-418.

12. Dworkin RH. An overview of neuropathic pain: Syndromes, symptoms, signs, and several mechanisms. *Clin J Pain.* 2002;18:343-349.
13. Melzack R. From the gate to the neuromatrix. *Pain.* 1999;Aug(suppl 6):S121-S126.
14. Dieppe PA, Lohmander LS. Pathogenesis and management of pain in osteoarthritis. *Lancet.* 2005;365:965-973.
15. Johansson E, Lindberg P. Low back pain patients in primary care: Subgroups based on the Multidimensional Pain Inventory. *Int J Behav Med.* 2000;7:340-352.
16. Gallagher RM. Rational integration of pharmacologic, behavioral, and rehabilitation strategies in the treatment of chronic pain. *Am J Phys Med Rehabil.* 2005;84:S64-S76.
17. Turk DC. Understanding pain sufferers: The role of cognitive processes. *Spine.* 2004;4:1-7.
18. Gifford LS, Butler DS. The integration of pain sciences into clinical practice. *J Hand Ther.* 1997;10:86-95.
19. Woolf CJ. Towards a mechanism-based classification of pain? *Pain.* 1998;77:227-229.
20. Cherkin DC. Primary care research on low back pain. *Spine.* 1998;28:1997-2002.
21. Proctor TJ, Mayer TG, Gatchel RJ, McGeary DD. Unremitting health-care-utilization outcomes of tertiary rehabilitation of patients with chronic musculoskeletal disorders. *J Bone Joint Surg Am.* 2004;86:62-69.
22. Rosenbloom BN, Khan S, McCartney C, Katz J. Systematic review of persistent pain and psychological outcomes following traumatic musculoskeletal injury. *J Pain Res.* 2013;6:39-51.
23. Holmes A, Williamson O, Hogg M, Arnold C, O'Donnell ML. Determinants of chronic pain 3 years after moderate or serious injury. *Pain Med.* 2013;14:336-344.
24. Kivimaki M, Vahtera J, Elovainio M, Pentti J, Virtanen M. Human costs of organizational downsizing: Comparing health trends between leavers and stayers. *Am J Community Psychol.* 2003;32:57-67.
25. Vahtera J, Kivimaki M, Forma P, et al. Organisational downsizing as a predictor of disability pension: The 10-town prospective cohort study. *J Epidemiol Community Health.* 2005;59:238-242.
26. Benbow S, Cossins L, Bowsher D. A comparison of young and elderly patients attending a regional pain center. *Pain Clinic.* 1995;8:323-332.
27. Mikkelsson M, El-Metwally A, Kautiainen H, Auvinen A, Macfarlane GJ, Salminen JJ. Onset, prognosis and risk factors for widespread pain in schoolchildren: A prospective 4-year follow-up study. *Pain.* 2008;138:681-687.
28. Ravert HT, Bencherif B, Madar I, Frost JJ. PET imaging of opioid receptors in pain: Progress and new directions. *Curr Pharm Des.* 2004;10:759-768.
29. Gibson SJ, Farrell M. A review of age differences in the neurophysiology of nociception and the perceptual experience of pain. *Clin J Pain.* 2004;20:227-239.
30. Soares JJ, Sundin O, Grossi G. The stress of musculoskeletal pain: A comparison between primary care patients in various ages. *J Psychosom Res.* 2004;56:297-305.
31. Ayearst L, Harsanyi Z, Michalko KJ. The Pain and Sleep Questionnaire three-item index (PSQ-3): A reliable and valid measure of the impact of pain on sleep in chronic nonmalignant pain of various etiologies. *Pain Res Manag.* 2012;17(4):281-290.
32. Cole JC, Dubois D, Kosinski M. Use of patient-reported sleep measures in clinical trials of pain treatment: A literature review and synthesis of current sleep measures and a conceptual model of sleep disturbance in pain. *Clin Ther.* 2007;29(suppl 2):580-588.
33. Sampaio RA, Sewo Sampaio PY, Yamada M, Tsuboyama T, Arai H. Self-reported quality of sleep is associated with bodily pain, vitality and cognitive impairment in Japanese older adults [published online ahead of print September 30, 2013]. *Geriatr Gerontol Int.* doi: 10.111/ggi.12149.
34. Finley GA, Chorney JM, Campbell L. Not small adults: The emerging role of pediatric pain services. *Can J Anaesth.* 2014;61(2):180-187.
35. Brennan TA, Leape LL, Laird NM, et al. Incidence of adverse events and negligence in hospitalized patients: Results of the Harvard Medical Practice Study I. *Qual Saf Health Care.* 2004;13(2):145-151.
36. Baker TA, Green CR. Intrarace differences among black and white Americans presenting for chronic pain management: The influence of age, physical health, and psychosocial factors. *Pain Med.* 2005;6:29-38.
37. Holmberg S, Thelin A, Stiernstrom E, Svardsudd K. The impact of physical work exposure on musculoskeletal symptoms among farmers and rural non-farmers. *Ann Agric Environ Med.* 2003;10:179-184.
38. Rousseau ME, Gottlieb SF. Pain at midlife. *J Midwifery Womens Health.* 2004;49:529-538.
39. Vogt MT, Simonsick EM, Harris TB, et al. Neck and shoulder pain in 70- to 79-year-old men and women: Findings from the Health, Aging and Body Composition Study. *Spine.* 2003;3:435-441.
40. El-Metwally A, Salminen JJ, Auvinen A, Kautiainen H, Mikkelsson M. Prognosis of non-specific musculoskeletal pain in preadolescents: A prospective 4-year follow-up study till adolescence. *Pain.* 2004;110:550-559.
41. Unruh A. Pain across the lifespan. In: Strong J, et al, eds. *Pain. A Textbook for Therapists.* Edinburgh, Scotland: Churchill Livingstone; 2002.

42. Deutscher D, Horn SD, Dickstein R, et al. Associations between treatment processes, patient characteristics, and outcomes in outpatient physical therapy practice. *Arch Phys Med Rehabil.* 2009;90:1349-1363.
43. Fillingim RB, King CD, Ribeiro-Dasilva MC, Rahim-Williams B, Riley JL, 3rd. Sex, gender, and pain: A review of recent clinical and experimental findings. *J Pain.* 2009;10:447-485.
44. Bates MS, Rankin-Hill L, Sanchez-Ayendez M. The effects of the cultural context of health care on treatment of and response to chronic pain and illness. *Soc Sci Med.* 1997;45:1433-1447.
45. Bates MS, Edwards WT, Anderson KO. Ethnocultural influences on variation in chronic pain perception. *Pain.* 1993;52:101-112.
46. Khatun M, Ahlgren C, Hammarstrom A. The influence of factors identified in adolescence and early adulthood on social class inequities of musculoskeletal disorders at age 30: A prospective population-based cohort study. *Int J Epidemiol.* 2004;33:1353-1360.
47. Baker TA. Arthritis symptoms as indicators of pain in older African Americans. *Ethn Dis.* 2003;13:513-520.
48. Miu DK, Chan TY, Chan MH. Pain and disability in a group of Chinese elderly outpatients in Hong Kong. *Hong Kong Med J.* 2004;10(3):160-165.
49. Green CR, Baker TA, Smith EM, Sato Y. The effect of race in older adults presenting for chronic pain management: A comparative study of black and white Americans. *J Pain.* 2003;4:82-90.
50. Peat G, Thomas E, Handy J, Croft P. Social networks and pain interference with daily activities in middle and old age. *Pain.* 2004;112:397-405.
51. Brekke M, Hjortdahl P, Kvien TK. Severity of musculoskeletal pain: Relations to socioeconomic inequality. *Soc Sci Med.* 2002;54:221-228.
52. Palmer KT, Syddall H, Cooper C, Coggon D. Smoking and musculoskeletal disorders: Findings from a British national survey. *Ann Rheum Dis.* 2003;62:33-36.
53. Wilson KG, Eriksson MY, D'Eon JL, Mikail SF, Emery PC. Major depression and insomnia in chronic pain. *Clin J Pain.* 2002;18:77-83.
54. Macfarlane GJ, Norrie G, Atherton K, Power C, Jones GT. The influence of socioeconomic status on the reporting of regional and widespread musculoskeletal pain: Results from the 1958 British Birth Cohort Study. *Ann Rheum Dis.* 2009;68:1591-1595.
55. Green CR, Baker TA, Sato Y, Washington TL, Smith EM. Race and chronic pain: A comparative study of young black and white Americans presenting for management. *J Pain.* 2003;4:176-183.
56. Chan MY, Hamamura T, Janschewitz K. Ethnic differences in physical pain sensitivity: Role of acculturation. *Pain.* 2013;154:119-123.
57. Dickson GL, Kim JI. Reconstructing a meaning of pain: Older Korean American women's experiences with the pain of osteoarthritis. *Qual Health Res.* 2003;13:675-688.
58. Cristian A, Thomas J, Nisenbaum M, Jeu L. Practical considerations in the assessment and treatment of pain in adults with physical disabilities. *Phys Med Rehabil Clin N Am.* 2005;16:57-90.
59. Manfredi PL, Breuer B, Meier DE, Libow L. Pain assessment in elderly patients with severe dementia. *J Pain Symptom Manage.* 2003;25:48-52.
60. Scherder EJ, Oosterman JM, Ooms ME, Ribbe MW, Swaab DF. [Chronic pain in dementia and in disorders with a high risk for congnitive impairment]. *Tijdschr Gerontol Geriatr.* 2005;36:116-121.
61. Mantyselka P, Hartikainen S, Louhivuori-Laako K, Sulkava R. Effects of dementia on perceived daily pain in home-dwelling elderly people: A population-based study. *Age Ageing.* 2004;33:496-499.
62. Bortsov AV, Smith JE, Diatchenko L, et al. Polymorphisms in the glucocorticoid receptor co-chaperone *FKBP5* predict persistent musculoskeletal pain after traumatic stress exposure. *Pain.* 2013;154:1419-1426.
63. McLean SA, Diatchenko L, Lee YM, et al. Catechol O-methyltransferase haplotype predicts immediate musculoskeletal neck pain and psychological symptoms after motor vehicle collision. *J Pain.* 2011;12:101-107.
64. Lin IB, O'Sullivan PB, Coffin JA, Mak DB, Toussaint S, Straker LM. Disabling chronic low back pain as an iatrogenic disorder: A qualitative study in Aboriginal Australians. *BMJ Open.* 2013;3.
65. Donelson R. *Rapidly Reversible Low Back Pain.* Hanover, NH: SelfCare First; 2007.
66. Hill JC, Fritz JM. Psychosocial influences on low back pain, disability, and response to treatment. *Phys Ther.* 2011;91:712-721.
67. Cushnaghan J, Cooper C, Dieppe P, Kirwan J, McAlindon T, McCrae F. Clinical assessment of osteoarthritis of the knee. *Ann Rheum Dis.* 1990;49:768-770.
68. Liesdek C, Van der Windt D, Koes B, Bouter L. Soft-tissue disorders of the shoulder: A study of inter-observer agreement between general practitioners and physiotherapists and an overview of physiotherapeutic treatment. *Physiotherapy.* 1997;83:12-17.
69. Cherkin DC, Deyo RA, Wheeler K, Ciol MA. Physician variation in diagnostic testing for low back pain: Who you see is what you get. *Arthritis Rheum.* 1994;37:15-22.

70. Spitzer EA. Scientific approach to the assessment and management of activity-related spinal disorders: S monograph for clinicians. Report of the Quebec Task Force on Spinal Disorders. *Spine*. 1987;12(7 suppl):S1-S59.
71. Campbell SM, Roland MO, Buetow SA. Defining quality of care. *Soc Sci Med*. 2000;51:1611-1625.
72. Chou R, Qaseem A, Owens DK, Shekelle P. Diagnostic imaging for low back pain: Advice for high-value health care from the American College of Physicians. *Ann Intern Med*. 2011;154:181-189.
73. Chou R, Fu R, Carrino JA, Deyo RA. Imaging strategies for low-back pain: Systematic review and meta-analysis. *Lancet*. 2009;373:463-472.
74. Kendrick D, Fielding K, Bentley E, Kerslake R, Miller P, Pringle M. Radiography of the lumbar spine in primary care patients with low back pain: Randomised controlled trial. *BMJ*. 2001;322:400-405.
75. Jarvik JG, Hollingworth W, Martin B, et al. Rapid magnetic resonance imaging vs radiographs for patients with low back pain: A randomized controlled trial. *JAMA*. 2003;289:2810-2818.
76. Dagenais S, Caro J, Haldeman S. A systematic review of low back pain cost of illness studies in the United States and internationally. *Spine*. 2008;8:8-20.
77. Long A, Donelson R, Fung T. Does it matter which exercise? A randomized control trial of exercise for low back pain. *Spine*. 2004;29:2593-2602.
78. Indahl A, Velund L, Reikeraas O. Good prognosis for low back pain when left untampered: A randomized clinical trial. *Spine*. 1995;20:473-477.
79. Moseley GL, Nicholas MK, Hodges PW. A randomized controlled trial of intensive neurophysiology education in chronic low back pain. *Clin J Pain*. 2004;20:324-330.
80. May S, Littlewood C, Bishop A. Reliability of procedures used in the physical examination of non-specific low back pain: A systematic review. *Aust J Physiother*. 2006;52:91-102.
81. Seffinger MA, Najm WI, Mishra SI, et al. Reliability of spinal palpation for diagnosis of back and neck pain: A systematic review of the literature. *Spine*. 2004;29:E413-E425.
82. Fersum KV, Dankaerts W, O'Sullivan PB, et al. Integration of subclassification strategies in randomised controlled clinical trials evaluating manual therapy treatment and exercise therapy for non-specific chronic low back pain: A systematic review. *Br J Sports Med*. 2010;44:1054-1062.
83. Werneke MW, Hart D, Oliver D, et al. Prevalence of classification methods for patients with lumbar impairments using the McKenzie syndromes, pain pattern, manipulation, and stabilization clinical prediction rules. *J Man Manip Ther*. 2010;18:197-204.
84. Jones M. Clinical reasoning in manual therapy. *Phys Ther*. 1992;72:875-884.
85. Fritz JM, Delitto A, Erhard RE. Comparison of classification-based physical therapy with therapy based on clinical practice guidelines for patients with acute low back pain: A randomized clinical trial. *Spine*. 2003;28:1363-1371; discussion 1372.
86. Childs JD, Fritz JM, Piva SR, Erhard RE. Clinical decision making in the identification of patients likely to benefit from spinal manipulation: A traditional versus an evidence-based approach. *J Orthop Sports Phys Ther*. 2003;33:259-272.
87. Childs JD, Fritz JM, Flynn TW, et al. A clinical prediction rule to identify patients with low back pain most likely to benefit from spinal manipulation: A validation study. *Ann Intern Med*. 2004;141:920-928.
88. Mercer SR, Bogduk N. Intra-articular inclusions of the elbow joint complex. *Clin Anat*. 2007;20:668-676.
89. May S, Ross J. The McKenzie classification system in the extremities: A reliability study using McKenzie assessment forms and experienced clinicians. *J Manip Physiol Ther*. 2009;32:556-563.
90. Knudsen AK, Aass N, Fainsinger R, et al. Classification of pain in cancer patients—A systematic literature review. *Palliat Med*. 2009;23:295-308.
91. Bruera E, Schoeller T, Wenk R, et al. A prospective multicenter assessment of the Edmonton staging system for cancer pain. *J Pain Symptom Manage*. 1995;10:348-355.
92. Deyo RA, Mirza SK, Martin BI. Back pain prevalence and visit rates: Estimates from U.S. national surveys, 2002. *Spine*. 2006;31:2724-2727.
93. Smart KM, Blake C, Staines A, Doody C. Clinical indicators of "nociceptive," "peripheral neuropathic" and "central" mechanisms of musculoskeletal pain: A Delphi survey of expert clinicians. *Man Ther*. 2010;15:80-87.
94. Smart KM, Blake C, Staines A, Doody C. The discriminative validity of "nociceptive," "peripheral neuropathic," and "central sensitization" as mechanisms-based classifications of musculoskeletal pain. *Clin J Pain*. 2011;27:655-663.
95. Smart KM, Curley A, Blake C, Staines A, Doody C. The reliability of clinical judgments and criteria associated with mechanisms-based classifications of pain in patients with low back pain disorders: A preliminary reliability study. *J Man Manip Ther*. 2010;18:102-110.
96. Kolski M, VanDerLaan K, O'Connor A, Jungwha J, Koslowski A, Deutch, A. Validation of a musculoskeletal pain classification system in clinical physical therapy practice [published online ahead of print September 8, 2014]. *J Man Manip Ther*. doi: 10.1179/2042618614Y.0000000090

97. McKenzie RA, May S. *The Lumbar Spine: Mechanical Diagnosis and Therapy.* Waikanae, New Zealand: Spinal Publications; 2003.
98. Werneke M, Hart DL, Cook D. A descriptive study of the centralization phenomenon: A prospective analysis. *Spine.* 1999;24:676-683.
99. Donelson R, Silva G, Murphy K. Centralization phenomenon: Its usefulness in evaluating and treating referred pain. *Spine.* 1990;15:211-213.
100. Long AL. The centralization phenomenon: Its usefulness as a predictor or outcome in conservative treatment of chronic law back pain (a pilot study). *Spine.* 1995;20:2513-2520; discussion 2521.
101. May S, Aina A. Centralization and directional preference: A systematic review. *Man Ther.* 2012;17:497-506.
102. Aina A, May S, Clare H. The centralization phenomenon of spinal symptoms—A systematic review. *Man Ther.* 2004;9:134-143.
103. Skytte L, May S, Petersen P. Centralization: Its prognostic value in patients with referred symptoms and sciatica. *Spine.* 2005;30:E293-E299.
104. Werneke M, Hart DL. Centralization phenomenon as a prognostic factor for chronic low back pain and disability. *Spine.* 2001;26:758-764; discussion 765.
105. Werneke MW, Hart DL, Resnik L, Stratford PW, Reyes A. Centralization: Prevalence and effect on treatment outcomes using a standardized operational definition and measurement method. *J Orthop Sports Phys Ther.* 2008;38:116-125.
106. Werneke MW, Hart DL, Cutrone G, et al. Association between directional preference and centralization in patients with low back pain. *J Orthop Sports Phys Ther.* 2011;41:22-31.
107. Werneke M, Hart DL. Discriminant validity and relative precision for classifying patients with nonspecific neck and back pain by anatomic pain patterns. *Spine.* 2003;28:161-166.
108. May S. Classification by McKenzie mechanical syndromes: A survey of McKenzie-trained faculty. *J Manip Physiol Ther.* 2006;29:637-642.
109. Wilson L, Hall H, McIntosh G, Melles T. Intertester reliability of a low back pain classification system. *Spine.* 1999;24:248-254.
110. Clare H, Adams R, Maher CG. Reliability of McKenzie classisfication of patients with cervical or lumbar pain. *J Manip Physiol Ther.* 2005;28:122-127.
111. Kilpikoski S, Airaksinen O, Kankaanpaa M, Leminen P, Videman T, Alen M. Interexaminer reliability of low back pain assessment using the McKenzie method. *Spine.* 2002;27:E207-E214.
112. Clare HA, Adams R, Maher CG. A systematic review of efficacy of McKenzie therapy for spinal pain. *Aust J Physiother.* 2004;50:209-216.
113. Cook C, Hegedus EJ, Ramey K. Physical therapy exercise intervention based on classification using the patient response method: A systematic review of the literature. *J Man Manip Ther.* 2005;13:152-162.
114. Bybee RF, Dionne CP. Interrater agreement on assessment, diagnosis, and treatment for neck pain by trained physical therapist students. *J Phys Ther Educ.* 2007;21:39-47.
115. Dionne C, Bybee RF, Tomaka J. Correspondence of diagnosis to initial treatment for neck pain. *Physiotherapy.* 2007;93:62-68.

CHAPTER 2

Overview of the Pain Mechanism Classification System and Mechanical Diagnosis and Therapy

All truth passes through three stages.
First, it is ridiculed.
Second, it is violently opposed.
Third, it is accepted as being self-evident.
—Arthur Schopenhauer

POINTS TO DISCUSS

- Brief review of the nervous system
- Peripheral nervous system (PNS) physiological factors and central nervous system (CNS) psychological factors in pain
- Pain mechanism classification system (PMCS) categories of pain: nociceptive: inflammatory, nociceptive:ischemia, peripheral neurogenic, central sensitization, affective, and motor/autonomic
- Role of PMCS in supporting clinical practice through consideration of multiple dimensions of the pain experience
- Intervention with PNS and CNS mechanisms
- Mechanical diagnosis and therapy syndromes: derangement, dysfunction, posture, and other

---

Everyone experiences pain; it is part of the body's normal protective mechanism. Pain is a complex sensory, cognitive, and emotional experience that is influenced by psychological and physiological factors, including chemical, hormonal, mechanical, emotional, social, nutritional, spiritual, and cultural factors. Psychological factors, which are governed by the central nervous system (CNS), influence the physiological changes, which are governed by the peripheral nervous system (PNS), that occur during healing. Everyone is going to have painful conditions. Nortin M. Hadler, a researcher and physician who has studied the experience of low back pain in people who are otherwise healthy, refers to painful conditions as "just a window on the predicament of life."[1(p342)] Each type of factor has the ability to activate the brain's protective response, and pain may be the output. All dimensions of pain are essential to the pain experience, and they interact differently in patients to produce altered physiological outputs and behaviors. Most pain scientists recommend that clinicians address all dimensions.[2-4] This chapter reviews the role of the PNS and CNS in pain and explains the pain mechanism classification system (PMCS) used at the Rehabilitation Institute of Chicago to assist clinicians in recognizing dominant psychological and physiological factors to aid in the interpretation of the patient's prognosis and selection of interventions and to maximize outcomes.

Brief Review of the Nervous System

The CNS consists of the brain and spinal cord. The PNS involves the cranial and peripheral nerves and consists of the autonomic nervous system (ANS). The ANS helps regulate the basic organ functions required for living and visceral function (eg, respiration, digestion, cardiac function, body fluid production). Most of the time, the ANS functions unconsciously, but at times it provides conscious control over respiration and breathing patterns. The ANS encompasses the sympathetic and parasympathetic nervous systems. ANS functions include motor (efferent) and sensory (afferent) subsystems.

The sympathetic nervous system (SNS) functions under extreme stress and controls the "fight-or-flight" response. The parasympathetic system controls bodily functions, including the "feed and breed" or "rest and digest" functions as compared to the sympathetic system. The two systems balance each other out. The SNS is more active during day when a person is active, and the parasympathetic nervous system is more operational when a person is at rest. Both systems should be a focus of attention in patient education. The parasympathetic system is the healing and helping system directly related to sleep health, relaxation ability, and coping. The sympathetic system has preganglionic motor neurons that arise in the spinal cord. Specifically, the cell bodies of the first (preganglionic) neuron are located in the thoracic and lumbar spinal cord (T1-L2). Two chains run parallel to the spinal cord, and these preganglionic neurons pass into sympathetic ganglia. In the parasympathetic system, the cell bodies are located in the sacral region of the spinal cord and in the medulla from preganglionic parasympathetic fibers of cranial nerves 3, 7, 9, and 10. The preganglionic fiber is very close to the target organ it synapses on. In the sympathetic system, the fibers can be longer. In some cases these fibers synapse with neurons known as postganglionic neurons, pass up or down the sympathetic chain, and finally synapse with postganglionic neurons in a higher or lower ganglion or leave the ganglion by way of a cord leading to special ganglia in the viscera. Here it may synapse with postganglionic sympathetic neurons running to the smooth muscular walls of the viscera. The SNS and pain interact through descending inhibition in the spinal cord and in the control of peripheral inflammation and nociceptive activation.[5]

Peripheral and Central Factors in Pain

Pain is governed by the PNS and CNS. PNS factors are related to the body in a physiological or movement sense, and CNS factors are related to the brain in a psychological sense. Saper[6] recognized that psychological factors can be a major contributor to disability that is related to pain and that the "largely neglected central nervous pain system may be more important than the neospinothalamic [peripheral] system in generating the disability and medical consequences of chronic pain."[(p238)] Saper divided pain into two distinct tracts: the psychological and the physiological tracts (see **Figure 2.1**). In the physiological tract, detailed information about pain location, quality, frequency, aggravating and alleviating activities, and intensity

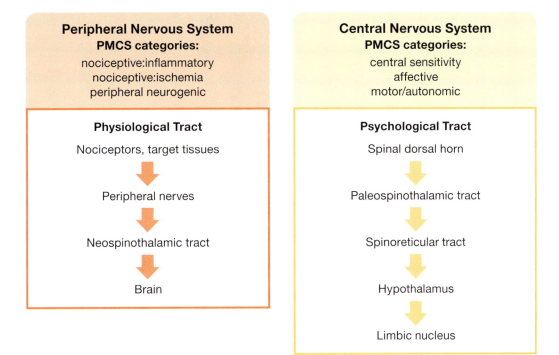

FIGURE 2.1 Physiological and psychological pain tracts. PMCS = pain mechanism classification system.

are projected to the brain via the neospinothalamic tracts. The psychological tract, a large projection system, courses from the spinal dorsal horn to hypothalamic and limbic nuclei via the paleospinothalamic and spinoreticular tracts. Thus, musculoskeletal pain can be analyzed anatomically, and the recognition of each tract's contribution to the pain experience allows for better understanding of which tract is dominating. The subjective pain evaluation, discussed in detail in Chapter 3, can be guided to screen the physiological and psychological factors that dominate the pain experience and better target the objective exam.

The physiological (neospinothalamic) tract is present throughout the body, with receptors present in all connective tissues and peripheral nerves. This pathway transmits two of three pain sensations. The first is fast pain, consisting of a sharp, pricking sensation that is accurately localized and results from activation of A-δ fibers, which are myelinated.[7] Myelinated refers to the presence of a myelin sheath around the nerve. The second pain sensation is slow pain, consisting of a burning sensation that has a slower onset, greater persistence, and less clear location. Slow pain results from activation of C fibers, which are unmyelinated.[7] **Figure 2.2** illustrates the interaction that occurs when an injury to the muscle connective tissue activates pain receptors, called *nociceptors*, which communicate the message to the spinal cord; the spinal cord reflexively increases motor activity as a response to protect the area and begins inflammation, the first stage of healing.

The third type of pain sensation is described as aching pain, sometimes with a burning sensation, and results from stimulation of visceral and deep somatic receptors. These receptors are connected with nerve fibers running largely in sympathetic and somatic pathways consisting of both unmyelinated and A-δ myelinated afferent fibers.[7] This pain sensation is attributable to the CNS pain mechanisms transmitted via the psychological (paleospinothalamic and spinoreticular) tract. The paleospinothalamic and spinoreticular pathways

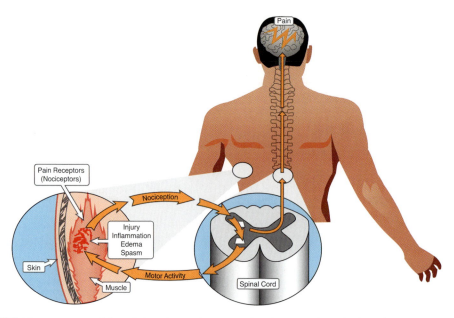

FIGURE 2.2 Messages travel from injured muscle connective tissue to the spinal cord via nociceptors; the spinal cord signals an increase in motor activity to protect the tissue and begins inflammation. The sensation of pain is perceived when the brain interprets these messages as a threat.

mediate the autonomic and reflexive responses to painful input and the emotional and affective components of pain.[7]

The CNS pain mechanism involves the patient's interpretation of what the nociceptive signal means and represents the cognitive and motivational dimension of pain, commonly referred to as *neuropathic pain*. Neuropathic pain is a lesion of the somatosensory processing system that exists in the CNS from the spinal cord dorsal horn to the hypothalamus and limbic nuclei of the brain. **Figure 2.2** illustrates the CNS mechanisms, highlighting the spinal cord and brain involvement in pain. Note the label "pain" located in the brain; this placement indicates that the sensation of pain is not perceived until the brain interprets the message as a threat. In other words, pain is an output of the patient's brain perception of threat. Pain researchers[8,9] have concluded that "not all pain experiences result from noxious stimuli, nor do all noxious stimuli lead to the experience of pain through the neurological process of pain."[9(404)]

Pain Mechanism Classification System Categories

Butler[10] and Gifford and Butler[11] presented a pain classification system distinguishing six common pain mechanisms. We adopted this classification system in our practice and training program at the Rehabilitation Institute of Chicago, where we investigate use of the system in relation to patient outcomes and resource utilization. The PMCS categories are as follows:

1. Nociceptive:inflammatory
2. Nociceptive:ischemia
3. Peripheral neurogenic

4. Central sensitization
5. Affective
6. Motor/autonomic

This classification system addresses both the physiological and the pathophysiological processes of pain in the sensory, cognitive, and emotional dimensions. Regardless of the location of musculoskeletal pain, any or all of these mechanisms may contribute to the patient's pain experience. A brief overview of each mechanism is provided in the sections that follow. In addition, Chapters 4 through 8 detail each mechanism and provide case examples and patient education materials.

Nociceptive:Inflammatory

The PMCS category *nociceptive:inflammatory* is described in detail in Chapter 4. Connective tissue (eg, muscle, ligament, bone, tendon, fascia, cartilage) has neurons that detect irritations to target tissue. This mechanism occurs at the neuron level in response to specific irritation from inflammation. Three mechanisms that activate nociceptors are thermal, mechanical, and chemical.[12,13] McKenzie and May[14(p53)] offered a simple example of mechanical articular pain:

> Bend your left forefinger backwards, using your right forefinger to apply overpressure. Keep applying this pressure until the nociceptive receptor system indicates its enhanced active state by the arrival of pain. This is simple mechanical deformation of pain sensitive structures. If you bend the finger backwards further, the intensity of the pain will increase; and if you maintain the painful position longer, the pain will become more diffuse, widespread and difficult to define. Thus, pain alters with increasing and prolonged mechanical deformation. If you now slowly return the finger to its normal resting position, the pain will disappear.

This mechanical pain mechanism quality is intermittent and normally occurs at end range. No chemical treatment will rectify or prevent the pain caused by mechanical deformation. Clinicians should explain to patients that this mechanical pain is normal when tissues approach end range. Nociceptive pain is related primarily to acute and subacute pain. The initial phases of healing are chemical processes that occur at the tissue level and involve inflammatory mediators that react differently to movement. Because of the chemical and mechanical processes, the symptoms are local to the target tissue. Repeated movement and special tests affect the pain in most, all, or one direction.

Nociceptive:Ischemia

The PMCS category *nociceptive:ischemia* is also described in detail in Chapter 4. Ischemia, like inflammation, is a type of target tissue irritation at the neuronal level. Inflammation can be thought of as excessive fluid and ischemia as insufficient blood flow and oxygen. Ischemia originates in target tissues as a result of mechanical and physiological processes of injured tissues that stimulate high threshold primary afferent C and A-δ fibers.[15,16] The tissues become more acidic, hypoxic, and rich in chemicals such as bradykinin, potassium ions, and prostaglandins. Essential circulation is deprived as a result of continuous stretching, compression, sustained positioning, or poor repair and remodeling phases of connective tissue healing.[17]

For example, the cumulative positional stress with repeated typing and the cumulative overpronation stress in running restrict blood flow, which can activate mechanical nociceptors registering as local pain during prolonged activity. Remodeling healing stages of connective tissue repair depend on movement to finish healing and return to full function. If movement is too much for repair, then chemical inflammation is triggered; if movement is too weak in remodeling, a weak scar continues to be sensitized to movement. All these situations require a similar approach in managing the ischemic pain mechanism; however, the movement prescription would vary depending on the actual tissue.

Peripheral Neurogenic

The PMCS category *peripheral neurogenic* is described in detail in Chapter 5. This pain mechanism is related to neural tissue outside the dorsal and medullary horns, such as nerve root, trunk, and axon and their connective tissues. Neuropathic and neurogenic pain result from alterations in nerve structure, function, and dynamics that cause neural dysfunction. It may also involve the nerve's interface with other tissues in its anatomical path, as in neural entrapment. Pain associated with trauma or disease of the peripheral nerves is associated with a nociceptive process of inflammation and ischemia occurring simultaneously or in isolation. This relationship among pain production, neurodynamics, and neural tissue versus muscle or tendon entrapment is why peripheral neurogenic pain has become a unique category of the PNS mechanisms.[18]

Central Sensitization

The PMCS category *central sensitization* is described in detail in Chapter 6. This pain mechanism is related to altered cognition and interpretation of the nociceptive signal occurring in the CNS. The patient's pain alarm system is in an overprotective mode. The altered CNS circuitry and processing are dominated by the patient's thoughts, beliefs, fears, worries, and concerns related to the pain experience and the potential threat of the injury, unhealed tissue, or pathology. Evidence indicates that pain states become imprinted in unique CNS pathways like those that produce memory.[19] Therefore, some musculoskeletal pain, especially in chronic conditions, has central mechanisms that dominate the maintenance of symptoms to a greater extent than peripheral nociception.[10] The descending inhibitory tracts are sensitized to all nociception based on the cognitive misinterpretations of nociceptive signals.

Affective

The PMCS category *affective* is described in detail in Chapter 7. This pain mechanism involves central pathways and circuits and is related to negative emotions and their perception. The way people think and feel has vast repercussions on brain processing, especially from a metaphysical standpoint.[4] Emotion or affect is a dimension of the pain experience, as well as a possible mechanism contributing to it. In other words, pain can manifest as the result of emotional turmoil.[20] The affective pain mechanism includes anxiety, depression, psychological stress disorders, anger, blame, and significant life-changing events such as severe trauma, abuse, or neglect and is influenced by the patient's coping relative to the changes these circumstances bring to his or her life and pain experience. Growing evidence has shown that psychosomatic (mind-body) disorders may develop as a result of repressed negative emotions in the unconscious mind related to life pressures, childhood experiences, and relationships.

Motor/Autonomic

The PMCS category *motor/autonomic* is described in detail in Chapter 8. This mechanism involves pain related to various output systems of the brain. The motor/autonomic pain mechanism involves the involuntary sympathetic and parasympathetic systems. Symptoms are heavily influenced by the somatic, motor, and autonomic nervous systems, and neuroendocrine and immune system symptoms are also common.[21] General malaise, lymphedema, spasticity, tone, and hypersensitivity are common symptoms when this pain mechanism is dominating. These symptoms indicate multisystem involvement, with each system needing direct attention.[22] The central focus in care should be on the dominating systems and mechanisms.

Clinical Practice Considerations in the Use of the PMCS

Acute Versus Chronic Pain

Clinicians use time as a reference point for determining the treatment of musculoskeletal pain based on the concept of healing stages for connective tissues. All tissues have an initial phase of healing that may be complicated by inflammation. As inflammation is controlled, a balance between proinflammatory cytokines and anti-inflammatory cytokines is established, and pain appears to decline. The term *acute pain* refers to pain that has been present for less than 3 months. The acute stage involves the nociceptive mechanism of chemical inflammation and healing stages progressing to repair and remodeling.[23,24] Pain that lasts 3 months or longer is *chronic*.[25] Often chronic pain is described as having the following characteristics:

- Persists longer than the normal tissue healing time frames
- Recurs with less activity
- Results in dissatisfaction with work and life
- Decreases self-efficacy

When musculoskeletal pain persists longer than 3 months, it is likely related to small, cumulative changes in lifestyle and behavior that the patient has made in order to cope with acute musculoskeletal pain.[26] Lifestyle changes that result in behaviors such as stopping or lessening activity cause tissue disuse, decrease the patient's tolerance for function, and sensitize the tissues to activity. Recurring acute inflammatory tissue mechanisms may be involved in chronic deconditioning, increasing the sensitivity of tissues to activity. In addition, physiological factors may predispose certain patients to chronic pain conditions.

The intensity, duration, and perception of pain can influence a patient's psychosocial response and behavior toward pain. This response can create a vicious cycle of life imbalance; acute pain may transition to chronic pain and back to acute pain if proper treatment does not occur. A combination of behaviors, beliefs, and emotions may be involved in these transitions.[26] Because these transitions are fluid, vary among individuals, and appear to dominate at different times during the pain experience, the clinician must reassess the dominating mechanisms at each session to confirm the musculoskeletal pain classification and care plan. As with any classification system, ongoing reassessment is critical.

It is essential to identify patients with acute pain who are at risk of developing chronic pain characteristics. It may be best to refer to levels of irritability in a tissue as high or low, so the clinician can determine what pain mechanism is dominating at each reassessment. Through a detailed subjective history, the clinician uses the PMCS to assess whether the patient is at risk of developing disability related to pain. The subjective history addresses the cognitive and motivational dimensions that govern pain interpretation and action. Clinicians must be able to identify acute adaptive and chronic maladaptive behaviors in patients to effectively diagnose, manage, and treat pain.

Acute adaptive behaviors are normal and useful for healing injured tissues. These behaviors, which include stopping activity, splinting an extremity, or modifying postures or load, activate protective reactions and the healing systems of the body. As pain decreases, restoration of movement and social activities naturally return. Maladaptive pain behavior (MPB), in contrast, is the refusal to resume activities of daily living (lifting, dressing, self-care, and work/play-related tasks) and household, social, and recreational and leisure functions until all pain is abolished. MPB provides no biological advantage to the patient's healing. It is regarded as a neurological disease state in which impulses from the nerve tissue are normal and the pain is attributed to an altered interpretation of threat that occurs in the CNS.[27,28] Many patients with MPB present with tender joints, tendons, and muscles and abnormally reactive peripheral nerves. These tissue changes result from remote submicroscopic aberrations and altered interpretations in the CNS rather than a local tissue disruption.[29]

The PMCS categorizes chronic maladaptive behaviors as manifestations in central sensitization, affective, or autonomic/motor pain mechanisms. Simple screening questions geared toward understanding the patient's beliefs about the relationships among activity, pain, and the ability to improve can help clinicians identify even the most subtle MPB. Screening questions may include the following:

- Help me understand why you have not returned to work, sport, or life activities as a result of this pain.
- Do you believe you can get back to those functions?
- Do you believe that the pain has to be gone before you can return to those functions, or is that not the case?
- Do you believe you can recover from this episode of pain?

Features of the Pain Experience

The foundation for effective diagnosis and treatment of pain is the analytical process of history taking from the patient's perspective. The clinician should explore the sensory-discriminative dimension of pain, which includes the intensity, location, quality, and behavior of pain; the cognitive-evaluative dimension of pain, which is related to thoughts about the problem and is influenced by past and present experiences and previous knowledge or beliefs about the pain; and the motivational-affective dimension of pain, which is related to the emotional response that governs or motivates responses to pain and may include fear, anxiety, anger, blame, or inability to function. When using the PMCS to identify a patient's dominant pain mechanism, clinicians should bear in mind three features of the pain experience:

1. Multiple pain mechanisms may be involved at one time. The treatment focus should be on the dominating mechanism.
2. Pain mechanisms can alter and shift with time.
3. Pain is based on the patient's brain perception of threat.

Focus on the Dominating Mechanism

For a patient who presents with pain lasting longer than 4 months, the injury or stress to the connective tissues is likely to have healed over time. To some extent, connective tissue repair and remodeling have occurred. Nociceptive signals at the tissue level may continue to be a mix of inflammatory and ischemic mechanisms depending on the amount of movement the patient undertakes. Continued tissue irritation may be the result of deconditioning, immobilization, or a change in lifestyle. In addition to tissue inflammation or ischemia, the patient may demonstrate negative emotions because of the changes in his or her life due to the pain. Common emotions such as fear, blame, anger, frustration, hopelessness, and sadness may be the patient's response to how the pain has changed his or her lifestyle.

The clinician needs to decide whether the tissue irritation mechanism or the negative coping mechanism is the dominant mechanism of persistent symptoms. PNS (tissue irritation) and CNS (negative coping) involvement is expected, so the question becomes which mechanism is dominating the present treatment session. Possible peripheral mechanisms include inflammation from too much activity or ischemia from not enough activity and poor remodeling after initial injury; possible CNS mechanisms include poor coping, adjustments in lifestyle, and negative emotions that result as pain persists. The clinician needs to address the dominant mechanism for that day to enable continued progress. The PMCS aids clinicians in selecting the dominant mechanism in patients who present with multiple mechanisms.

Alteration of Pain Mechanisms with Time

For a patient with an acute wrist problem that is 2 weeks old for whom the initial physical exam and diagnostic imaging reveal no gross boney or soft tissue damage, the dominant pain mechanism most likely is nociceptive pain from peripheral tissue irritation. If the same patient returns 1 year later with continued complaints of pain and significant loss of function related to the same wrist, the structures in the hand likely have healed by virtue of time. Therefore, it is unlikely that the pain and loss of function are attributable solely to a nociceptive mechanism; rather, the patient's pain likely resides deeper in the circuitry and processing of the CNS, and affective mechanisms may play a dominating part in the presentation as pain persists.

At 1-year follow-up, the clinician should consider the cognitive and emotional dimensions of the patient's pain. Predictive factors for persistent pain following traumatic injury include symptoms of anxiety and depression, patient's perception that the injury was attributable to an external source (ie, that the patient was not at fault), and affective symptoms such as avoidance behaviors related to distressing thoughts and beliefs.[8] Whereas the initial subjective history for the patient with acute wrist pain goes relatively quickly, the evaluation of a patient whose wrist problem continues a year later requires lengthy discussions. The clinician must ascertain how ongoing pain states affect the patient, especially if the problem has not been validated or successfully managed by other clinicians.[30]

Brain Perception of Threat

Painful experiences are not limited to those involving the firing of high threshold A-δ or C fibers. The purpose of a general anesthetic is to take away the awareness of pain; these high threshold fibers, however, continue to fire. The excitatory and inhibitory currents of higher level neurons in operation at the time of the stimulation influence whether the brain perceives this pain as a threat. Patients with severe pain often say the injury did not hurt at the time of occurrence, demonstrating the power of the CNS in suppressing pain when the threat is high. One study found that chronic low back pain was accompanied by brain atrophy and suggested that the physiology of chronic pain includes thalamocortical processes of the brain.[31] Through use of the PMCS, clinicians may discover that a brain-down approach may be more important than a body-up approach (these approaches are explained in Chapter 3).[32]

Clinical Reasoning in Subjective Evaluation

PMCS use in practice relies on the clinician's clinical reasoning.[33] The PMCS provides a critical thinking structure that is influenced by all dimensions of pain to guide decisions and prognosis. Clinicians can use the PMCS to demonstrate the uniqueness of each patient's pain experience and to help patients think of and react to their pain differently.

In the subjective evaluation, the clinician asks questions to expose the patient's pain mechanisms based on the patient's behavior and emotional, social, and mechanical symptoms. A patient's pain experience is defined by how pain limits the performance of daily life functions and how the intensity of pain changes. Once the interview is completed, the clinician uses the PMCS and clinical reasoning to determine the dominating pain mechanism, which forms the basis for the objective evaluation and allows for patient education, an active care plan, a palliative care plan, and a prognosis.

Consider a patient whose injury occurred with no diagnostic findings 6 months previously. The patient's negative thoughts about this injury and pain aroused negative emotions that affected the autonomic and neuroendocrine response systems and contributed to an increase in inflammatory chemicals. This reaction affected the sensory system a second time, maintaining a chemical inflammatory nociceptive presentation. Simultaneously, the patient altered activity levels and movement patterns under the influence of subconscious reflex activity and conscious processing of the pain experience. Use of the PMCS guides the clinician in diagnosing and treating not only the inflammatory response in the local tissue, but also the negative thoughts that contributed to the sustained negative chemical reactions. Chapter 3 describes the use of the PMCS in subjective evaluation.

Intervention with CNS Mechanisms

Table 2.1 provides guidelines on the order of interventions for PNS and CNS pain mechanisms.[34] When the dominating pain mechanisms involve the CNS, the first approach after assessing the patient's readiness for change is patient education about pain. Education should cover the different pain mechanisms and their treatment, reinforce the patient's understanding of pain as an alarm system, and explain how the system works and what the signals mean to the patient's life. Activity and pain analysis are taught to enable the patient to identify when pain symptoms related to activity or movements are safe and necessary for improvement. Finally, education includes instruction in journaling to increase the patient's skill in identifying the social, emotional, and psychological triggers of pain symptoms and awareness of the positive coping strategies necessary for improvement; journaling and other educational techniques are described in Chapter 3.

Along with education, the clinician establishes activity and movement guidelines and a healthy pace of progression for the patient. All de-conditioned tissues require stress to improve. The activities chosen should provide meaning to the patient's life, bring happiness, and restore the patient's faith and confidence in his or her ability to recover. Recommending activities that patients do not like will result in noncompliance. Various forms of exercise, from isolated weight circuits to organized movement protocols (eg, Feldenkrais yoga, Tai Chi) to functional exercise, have been successful starting points for function restoration when CNS pain mechanisms dominate. The key is for the patient to like the activity.

Assessment and treatment of yellow flags (psychological factors) contributing to and dominating a patient's disability related to pain need to be part of the care plan for CNS mechanisms. Yellow flags are likely relevant and dominating in CNS pain mechanisms. Often the pain is a protective symptom arising from imbalance in the emotional and/or

TABLE 2.1 Treatment Guidelines for Peripheral Nervous System and Central Nervous System Pain Mechanisms

Type of Pain Mechanism	Treatment Interventions
Central nervous system	Establishment of readiness to change behavior
	Pain mechanism education
	Healthy body movement guidelines
	Pacing and graded exposure to activity
	Assessment and treatment of yellow flags
	Referral to psychology for cognitive-behavioral therapy
	Mechanical diagnosis and therapy
	Wheelchair seating and positioning
Peripheral nervous system	Mechanical diagnosis and therapy
	Healing: repair and remodeling guidelines
	Wheelchair seating and positioning
	Assessment of yellow flags
	Progression of forces
	Remodeling for function
	Skill development

social aspects of the patient's life. Patients may demonstrate poor active coping strategies, anger, blame, catastrophizing, and many other personality traits and behaviors that warrant a referral to a behavioral psychologist to manage these emotional and behavioral components. Chapter 7 will discuss recommended psychometric outcome measures to aid the discussion and referral when yellow flags dominate. The last intervention with CNS pain types is mechanical diagnosis and therapy (MDT) and potential seating and positioning adaptations if the patient uses a wheelchair to address PNS pain mechanisms that may now be dominating. As the patient gains control over his or her emotions and social environment and becomes less limited by pain, the clinician addresses any relevant PNS pain mechanisms using this approach.

Intervention with PNS Mechanisms

As shown in **Table 2.1**, when the dominating mechanisms are governed by the PNS, the first step in management is to perform a repeated movement assessment to identify the patient's MDT syndrome. The MDT syndrome classifications of *derangement, dysfunction, posture,* and *other* are defined by pain location changes and mechanical response to repeated or sustained end range movements (see **Figure 2.3**[34]). The syndrome selection of MDT determines the specific active care exercise prescription. The clinician needs to subgroup the mechanical problem further and identify whether the mechanical pain mechanism is related to alteration of normal joint mechanics or weakened and shortened connective tissue or whether this is a quality of position or function problem. Dominating PNS pain mechanisms require a screen for yellow flags. When screening for the involvement of yellow flags with PNS mechanisms, the most important characteristic is the patient's belief in his or her ability to recover, also known as self-efficacy.

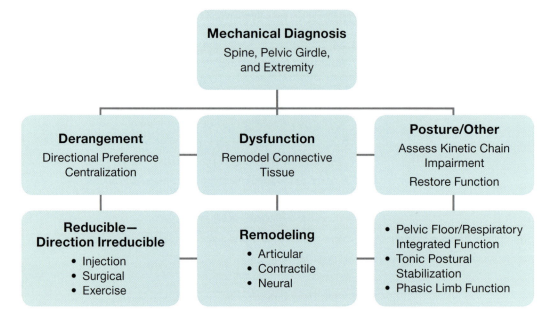

FIGURE 2.3 Modified McKenzie Method of Mechanical Diagnosis & Therapy. Patient has a peripheral nervous system pain mechanism that requires mechanical subgrouping.

MDT is an approach created by Robin McKenzie, a New Zealand physiotherapist, to classify spine, pelvis, jaw, and extremity disorders based on the patient history and repeated movement examination for the purpose of providing active treatment, education, and prevention of mechanical pain mechanisms. The MDT syndromes of derangement, dysfunction, posture, and other provide a universal language for approaching mechanical pain mechanisms. The extensive literature supporting the use of this system in musculoskeletal pain has shown good reliability and validity.[35-39] We recommend the use of MDT as an evidence-supported method for identifying mechanical pain mechanisms. It complements the PMCS and strengthens the clinician's ability to use the PMCS in patient education and active care planning when the patient is dominated by PNS mechanisms. The following definitions of MDT syndromes will assist the readers' understanding of the case studies described in the following chapters. MDT comprises three syndromes and the category of "other."

Derangement Syndrome

Derangement syndrome is an internal disturbance of the normal resting position of affected joint surfaces or disc material. The surrounding tissues are slightly off the axis of rotation, which causes positional asymmetry and allows faulty movement patterns, resulting in deformation of the capsule, periarticular, and annular ligaments.[14] This syndrome's hallmark sign of direction sensitivity dictates the specific directions and loading strategies needed in an active care plan and the predictability of a rapid outcome.

The derangement syndrome is either reducible or irreducible. A *reducible derangement* presents with a directional preference. The direction that reduces, centralizes, or abolishes symptoms in the spine or reduces, localizes, or abolishes symptoms in the periphery, pelvic girdle, and jaw is called the *preferred direction*. An *irreducible derangement* does not have a directional preference and is unaffected by movement in a positive way. Directions may worsen or produce no effect on the symptoms and the function. If the result of repeated movement assessment is an irreducible derangement, other interventions, such as an injection or surgical consult, are recommended. The focus of care from this point forward, regardless of impending procedures, is on restoration of function.

Dysfunction Syndrome

Dysfunction syndrome is a mechanical deformation of impaired soft tissues that may be the product of previous trauma or an inflammatory or degenerative process that results in contraction, scarring, adherence, adaptive shortening, and weakness.[14] Tight, weak contractile, articular, and neural tissue need remodeling to desensitize the ischemic pain mechanism. Remodeling includes progressive repeated end range movements when the problem is articular or neural in nature. Progressive resisted remodeling movements should be performed into the target zone, or point of pain, in a contractile tissue dysfunction without tissue irritability as a result. With this syndrome, the exercise prescription is tissue dominant.

Posture and Other Syndromes

Posture syndrome is a mechanical deformation of soft tissues from prolonged postures or positions of end range that deprive vascular transmission and create normal sustained end range forces. Soft tissues that are affected can be joints, muscles, tendons, periosteal insertions, spinal discs, and peripheral nerves.[14] Poor postural alignments can be related to spinal, extremity, pelvic, or jaw pain. Education and modification against sustained end range positioning deactivates the ischemic pain mechanism involved. In the posture syndrome, pathology has not had time to develop or occur in most cases.

The *other syndrome* applies to entities that do not fit the pattern of previously described syndromes; a couple of examples are the pathology of stenosis and rheumatoid arthritis.[14] Any mechanically inconclusive symptom that is affected by loading strategies in an unrecognizable or inconsistent pattern can be classified as other as well. For the other syndrome, the clinician can use a movement approach that focuses on restoring function rather than targeting a specific direction or tissue.

The posture and other syndromes do not respond in the patterns identified with derangement or dysfunction syndromes (eg, problems caused by prolonged poor positional stress, cumulative stress, or poor quality motor activation strategies). The exercise prescription focus includes restoring quality positions, modifying cumulative stress, and restoring quality kinetic chain movement strategies for desired individualized functions. Quality kinetic chain function focuses directly on restoring a diaphragm breath stereotype, pelvic floor function, static and dynamic tonic postural muscle endurance, and phasic limb function and performance. The exercise prescription should focus on self-directed very specific activation maneuvers and patient empowerment before palliative procedures. If the local tissue problem is specific to an injury or surgery, the clinician needs to understand tissue healing time frames, repair and remodeling guidelines, and the mechanical diagnosis.

Restoration of Function in MDT

Rehabilitation is focused on establishing the patient's faith and confidence in his or her ability to improve further. In a restoration of function program, the clinician applies the appropriate progression of forces to ensure the patient's functional independence. The clinician breaks down the function into exercises that are within the patient's capability and establishes opportunities for the patient to practice regularly during the day. This regularity encourages the reprogramming and remodeling process of connective tissue. A restoration of function program needs to provide the necessary force to the tissues involved in the functional limitations for the patient to resume the desired functional task. Progression of forces begins with active self-driven movements; if a plateau prevents patient progress, the clinician progresses to manual therapy procedures. The ability to use function, gravity, and ground reaction forces before manual therapy reinforces to the patient that he or she can improve with minimal to no external assistance and enhances self-efficacy and positive outcome.

Quality of movement approaches can guide restoration of function interventions. One approach involves the use of kinetic chain tests aimed at assessing faulty movement patterns to guide exercise prescriptions specific to certain functions. Enhancing quality kinetic chain movement patterns improves the cumulative nature of the nociceptive:ischemic pain mechanism involved with the faulty pattern. Kinetic chain tests break down function, allowing identification of movement faults distally and proximally from the involved area that contribute to the overuse or underuse precipitating the pain. Evaluating the painful function and selecting exercises to restore efficient kinematics and kinetics can have profound effects on how patients feel and move. In this situation, the clinician manages and treats the function using task-specific exercise or activation.

Table 2.2 lists treatment guidelines for each MDT syndrome. For further information on MDT, refer to *The Lumbar Spine Mechanical Diagnosis and Therapy*[14] and *Rapidly Reversible Low Back Pain*.[40]

TABLE 2.2 Treatment Guidelines for the Mechanical Diagnosis and Therapy Syndromes

Syndrome	Treatment Interventions
Derangement	Identify directional preference and reduce derangement
	Establish ability to centralize and maintain reduction
	Restore function and reduce medication
Reducible	Identify direction that reduces and abolishes symptoms and promotes centralization
Irreducible	Refer for injection, then reassess mechanical syndrome
	Refer for surgical consult
	Recommend exercise that maximizes function and leaves patient feeling no worse
Dysfunction	Remodel articular, contractile, and neural connective tissue
	Restore function
Posture	Educate regarding faulty posture
	• Perform slouch overcorrect frequently during day
	• Use of lumbar roll for prolonged sitting
	Restore function
Other	Assess kinetic chain impairment with a focus on the following:
	• Pelvic floor and respiratory integrated function
	• Tonic postural stabilization
	• Phasic limb function
	Restore specific function

KEY MESSAGES

- Pain is a symptom of the neurological system. Both the PNS and CNS have contributing mechanisms.
- The PMCS is a tool for identifying both physiological (PNS) and psychological (CNS) factors contributing to pain.
- The PMCS guides assessment of the transition from acute to chronic pain.
- The clinician identifies all operant musculoskeletal pain mechanisms using PMCS and focuses each care session on the dominant mechanism, keeping in mind the following:
  - Multiple pain mechanisms may be involved at one time.
  - Pain mechanisms alter and shift with time.
  - Pain is based on the brain's perceptions of threat.
- The PMCS has six categories:
  1. Nociceptive:inflammatory
  2. Nociceptive:ischemia
  3. Peripheral neurogenic
  4. Central sensitization
  5. Affective
  6. Motor/autonomic
- Nociceptive and peripheral neurogenic pain correlate with movement or function. MDT further aids diagnosis and prescription of exercise for these mechanical pain mechanisms.
- MDT is a classification system for mechanical pain mechanisms:
  1. Derangement syndrome is characterized by directional preference. Patient education regarding centralization and localization and direction-specific exercise are imperative in reducing and eliminating this syndrome.
  2. Dysfunction syndrome is related to specific connective tissues (contractile and inert) that may be weakened and shortened, poorly healed and remodeled, or degenerative. Patient education addressing remodeling pain and movement expectations and tissue-specific progressive exercise are imperative in eliminating this syndrome.
  3. Posture syndrome is related to prolonged poor postures or positions at end ranges. Patient education and modification of pain-producing postures applied to function are required to eliminate this syndrome.
  4. Other is related to poor quality function causing repetitive cumulative stress over time with prolonged activity. Patient education regarding quality kinematics and kinetics and very specific activation functional exercise to learn new patterns of movement are imperative in eliminating this syndrome.

References

1. Hadler NM. Workers with disabling back pain. *N Engl J Med*. 1997;337:341-343.
2. Melzack R, Casey KL. Sensory, motivational, and central control determinants of pain: A new conceptual model. In: Kenshalo DR, ed. *The Skin Senses*. Springfield, IL: Charles C Thomas; 1968:423-443.
3. Melzack R. Pain measurement in people in pain. In: Wall PD, Melzack R, eds. *Textbook of Pain*. 3rd ed. Edinburgh, Scotland: Churchill Livingstone; 1994.
4. Chapman CR. *The Affective Dimension of Pain: A Model*. New York: Raven Press; 1995.
5. Schereth T, Birklein F. The sympathetic nervous system and pain. *Neuromolecular Med*. 2008;10(3):141-147.
6. Saper CB. Pain as a visceral sensation. *Prog Brain Res*. 2000;122:237-243.
7. Gilman S, Winans S. *Essentials of Clinical Neuroanatomy and Neurophysiology*. 6th ed. Philadelphia, PA: F. A. Davis; 1982.

8. Janssen SA. Negative affect and sensitization to pain. *Scand J Psychol.* 2002;43:131-137.
9. Lundeberg T, Ekholm J. Pain—From periphery to brain. *Disabil Rehabil.* 2002;24:402-406.
10. Butler DS. *The Sensitive Nervous System.* Adelaide, Australia: Noigroup; 2000.
11. Gifford LS, Butler DS. The integration of pain sciences into clinical practice. *J Hand Ther.* 1997;10:86-95.
12. Cavanaugh JM. Neural mechanisms of lumbar pain. *Spine.* 1995;20:1804-1809.
13. Bogduk N. *The Anatomy and Physiology of Nociception.* Oxford, England: Butterworth-Heinemann, 1993.
14. McKenzie R, May S. *The Lumbar Spine: Mechanical Diagnosis & Therapy.* Waikanae, New Zealand: Spinal Publications; 2003.
15. Meyer RA, Campbell JN, Raja SN. Peripheral neural mechanisms of nociception. In: Wall PD, Melzack R, eds. *Textbook of Pain.* 3rd ed. Edinburgh, Scotland: Churchill Livingston; 1994.
16. Treede RD, Meyer RA, Raja SN, Campbell JN. Peripheral and central mechanisms of cutaneous hyperalgesia. *Prog Neurobiol.* 1992;38:397-421.
17. Sanderson RA, Foley RK, McIvor GW, Kirkaldy-Willis WH. Histological response on skeletal muscle to ischemia. *Clin Orthop Relat Res.* 1975;113:27-35.
18. Bloodworth D, Calvillo O, Smith K, et al. Chronic pain syndromes: Evaluation and treatment. In: Braddom RL, ed. *Physical Medicine and Rehabilitation.* 2nd ed. Philadelphia, PA: Saunders; 2001:913-933.
19. Basbaum AI. Memories of pain. *Sci Med.* 1996;3(6):22-31.
20. Gamsa A. Is emotional disturbance a precipitator or a consequence of chronic pain? *Pain.* 1990;42:183-195.
21. Ohrbach R, McCall WD Jr. The stress-hyperactivity-pain theory of myogenic pain: Proposal for a revised theory. *Pain Forum* 1996;5:51-66.
22. Janig W, Stanton-Hicks M. *Reflex Sympathetic Dystrophy.* Seattle, WA: IASP Press; 1996.
23. Merskey H. Pain terms: A list with definitions and notes on usage recommended by the IASP Subcommittee on Taxonomy. *Pain.* 1979;6:249-252.
24. Bonica JJ. *The Management of Pain.* Philadelphia, PA: Lea and Febiger; 1953.
25. Merskey H, Bogduk N. *Classification of Chronic Pain: Descriptions of Chronic Pain Syndromes and Definitions of Pain Terms.* 2nd ed. Seattle, WA: IASP Press; 1994.
26. Linton SJ. *Why Does Chronic Pain Develop? A Behavioral Approach.* Amsterdam: Elsevier Science; 2002.
27. Edwards CL, Fillingim RB, Keefe F. Race, ethnicity and pain. *Pain.* 2001;94:133-137.
28. Hagen KB, Bjorndal A, Uhlig T, Kvien TK. A population study of factors associated with general practitioner consultation for non-inflammatory musculoskeletal pain. *Ann Rheum Dis.* 2000;59:788-793.
29. Melzack RW, Wall PD. *The Challenge of Pain.* London: Penguin; 1996.
30. Hadler NM. If you have to prove you are ill, you can't get well: The object lesson of fibromyalgia. *Spine.* 1996;21:2397-2400.
31. Apkarian AV, Sosa Y, Sonty S, et al. Chronic back pain is associated with decreased prefrontal and thalamic gray matter density. *J Neurosci.* 2004;24:10410-10415.
32. Backonja MM. Primary somatosensory cortex and pain perception: Yes sir, your pain is in you head (Part 1). *Pain Forum.* 1996;5:171-180.
33. Higgs J, Jones MA. *Clinical Reasoning in the Health Professions.* London, England: Butterworth-Heinemann; 1995.
34. Rehabilitation Institute of Chicago Musculoskeletal Pain Committee. *Allied Health Musculoskeletal Pain Course Manual.* Chicago, IL: Rehabilitation Institute of Chicago; 2006.
35. May S. Classification by McKenzie mechanical syndromes: A survey of McKenzie-trained faculty. *J Manip Physiol Ther.* 2006;29:637-642.
36. Wilson L, Hall H, McIntosh G, Melles T. Intertester reliability of a low back pain classification system. *Spine.* 1999;24:248-254.
37. Clare H, Adams R, Maher CG. Reliability of McKenzie classisfication of patients with cervical or lumbar pain. *J Manip Physiol Ther.* 2005;28:122-127.
38. Clare HA, Adams R, Maher CG. A systematic review of efficacy of McKenzie therapy for spinal pain. *Aust J Physiother.* 2004;50:209-216.
39. Kilpikoski S, Airaksinen O, Kankaanpaa M, Leminen P, Videman T, Alen M. Interexaminer reliability of low back pain assessment using the McKenzie method. *Spine.* 2002;27:E207-E214.
40. Donelson R. *Rapidly Reversible Low Back Pain.* Hanover, NH: SelfCare First; 2007.

CHAPTER 3

Subjective Evaluation

Painful things are not the enemy, but the signal—announcing that it's time to change, to improve, to heal, and to embrace life.
    —Mike Hage, *The Back Pain Book*

> **POINTS TO DISCUSS**
>
> - Guidelines for evaluation and management of patients with musculoskeletal pain
> - Categories of information gathered in the pain mechanism classification system subjective evaluation:
>   - Pain location, description, and frequency
>   - Onset or mechanism of injury
>   - 24-hour behavior of symptoms
> - Aggravating and alleviating factors
> - Thoughts, beliefs, and cultural attitudes regarding pain
> - Past and current treatments
> - Readiness for treatment
> - Role of measurement tools
> - Role of management plan
> - Role of patient education

Pain is a message from the brain that there is a state of imbalance in certain body systems. Where is the imbalance? Is it in one or all body systems? Which ones can be identified? Musculoskeletal pain originates from imbalances in the chemical, mechanical, visceral, cognitive, emotional, social, hormonal, nutritional, spiritual, and cultural realms. In the subjective evaluation for musculoskeletal pain, the clinician screens these realms to best identify which system or systems require deeper investigation. This chapter describes how to conduct an in-depth subjective evaluation that will enable the clinician to determine a provisional dominant pain mechanism and to establish a relationship with the patient based on respect and trust.

Review of the Evidence on Musculoskeletal Pain Evaluation and Management

Research indicates that successful evaluation and management of patients with musculoskeletal pain include the following steps[1-4]:

- Identify red flags (serious conditions) and yellow flags (psychosocial factors) and any other social, biological, psychological, and emotional inputs to the pain experience.
- Provide early management of acute pain.

- Decrease fear, manage catastrophizing thoughts, and promote activity as soon as possible.
- Educate patients regarding pain mechanisms, mechanical diagnosis, and restoration of function when appropriate.
- Perform a skilled physical evaluation; use diagnostic testing to back up the physical examination as needed.
- Focus the intervention on education and active care first. Use pharmacology, manual therapy, and interventional procedures judiciously as the last interventions if needed.
- Adapt interventions on the basis of the pain mechanism and mechanical diagnosis classification.
- Promote and encourage self-care.
- Provide a prognosis related to function, activity, and pain that minimizes the detriments to quality of life.
- Coordinate care by helping the patient own the next steps, and enlist additional team members based on the number of active pain mechanisms.

In 2003, Australia's Acute Musculoskeletal Pain Guidelines Group[5] summarized the evidence for successful pain management. The group made the following recommendations on the basis of the review:

- Clinicians should use a partnership approach with patients.
- Management of acute pain can help prevent chronic pain.
- Even if a specific diagnosis cannot be determined, pain treatment can be effective.
- Imaging and other investigations are not indicated for acute musculoskeletal pain unless features of serious conditions are evident.
- The clinician should provide the patient with information, assurance, and encouragement to remain active. Simple interventions may be sufficient to successfully manage the patient's pain.
- Clinicians should monitor patients to review their progress and check for red and yellow flags that may interfere with recovery.

Use of these guidelines in conducting the subjective evaluation helps clinicians ensure that they are applying evidence-based care when using the pain mechanism classification system (PMCS).

Information Gathered in the PMCS Subjective Evaluation

To apply the PMCS, the clinician organizes patient information gathered during the subjective evaluation to aid in the identification of dominant pain mechanisms and ensures that all aspects of the patient's pain are addressed. After the subjective evaluation, the clinician is able to provisionally diagnose the operant and dominant pain mechanisms. The following history characteristics are supported by evidence[5] as assisting with pain mechanism classification:

- Pain location, description, and frequency
- Onset or mechanism of injury
- 24-hour behavior of symptoms
- Aggravating and alleviating factors
- Thoughts, beliefs, and cultural attitudes regarding pain
- Past and current treatments
- Readiness for treatment[6]

These subjective evaluation categories can help clinicians identify features of the patient's pain that may influence recovery and the need for formal treatment. Clinicians who treat pain are in an excellent position to assemble and classify this information because they see patients over many treatment sessions, have time to discuss issues, are able to gather and find patterns in details, and are licensed to educate, move, and touch patients.

Pain Location, Description, and Frequency

Information on pain location, description, and frequency can be collected on a patient intake form that includes body charts to allow patients to shade in all symptom areas for current and past episodes (**Figure 3.1**). Location assists the clinician in understanding the presentation of the pain experience with respect to anatomy. The patient intake form is an efficient tool to gather the information necessary to understand the patient's subjective history and classify his or her pain mechanisms. Clinicians note as they review the intake form how much information the patient has given. Some patients report very little about their pain and other symptoms, and others have diaries with lengthy entries. Filling out a patient intake form allows the patient to prepare for the subjective evaluation interview and identify some key behaviors of the symptoms.

Pain location is especially important for the identification of peripheral nervous system (PNS) versus central nervous system (CNS) mechanisms because multiple parts of the limb in a dermatome path or generalized body pains characterize different pain mechanisms. When one part of the limb presents as more painful than another and becomes the focus of investigation, the clinician needs to probe further whether other areas in that limb are symptomatic. For example, a patient with shoulder pain may also have lateral elbow pain and intermittent forearm pain that he or she has failed to mention. Probing assists the clinician in ruling out the peripheral neurogenic pain mechanism because many patients do not connect the relationship of symptoms in the same limb.

Description and frequency of symptoms are important in identifying pain mechanisms. Showing the patient a list of common descriptors can aid clinicians in their clinical reasoning regarding which pain mechanisms are present and dominating. In addition, this list of written descriptors can prompt patients to use more vivid expressions of pain, such as "raging wildfire," "knife-like pain that is killing me," or "insects crawling," as opposed to general descriptors such as "dull," "achy," and "nagging."

Frequency is typically described as constant or intermittent. Constant means that there is not one minute in the day that the symptoms are not present. Many patients feel that their symptoms are constant because they are present the majority of the day, but because of its ability to not be present or abolish, pain during most of the day is considered intermittent. Frequency is important in differentiating the PNS pain types because it helps identify a potential mechanical syndrome. CNS pain mechanisms often have constant symptoms, so the quality of intermittency may help rule this mechanism out.

Red flags are clinical characteristics that may be associated with the presence of serious conditions requiring urgent evaluation. Such conditions include tumors, infections, fractures, and neurological damage. Screening for serious conditions is part of the history and physical examination and should occur at the initial assessment and at every follow-up visit. Most patients do not recognize subtle signs from their bodies. Although many patient medical history intake forms request this information, subtle signs are often overlooked. Clinicians must take the time to ensure that patients understand the questions on the patient intake form by discussing the information they have written. The earlier red flags are addressed by the appropriate disciplines, the greater the chances of patient recovery and prevention of

Medical History Intake Form

Today's date: _____ Referred by: _____

Patient name: _____ Age: _____

What problem/issue brings you here today?
How and when did it start?
List 3 activities you are now unable to do:
What makes it *worse*?
What makes it *better*?
What do you want to accomplish from today's visit?
Is this a worker's compensation claim or is there litigation pending? ☐ Yes ☐ No
What diagnostic tests have you had for this problem? ☐ X-ray ☐ MRI ☐ CT scan ☐ EMG ☐ Bone scan
What treatments have you had? ☐ Massage ☐ Injections ☐ Physical therapy ☐ Psychotherapy ☐ Chiropractic

Please make a *mark on the line* below to indicate the level of discomfort you have today.
No pain _____ Worst pain ever
         0 1 2 3 4 5 6 7 8 9 10

Please describe what the pain feels like: Dull, Achy, Burning, Stabbing, Numbness, Tingling, Pulling, Cramping, Tightness
Please describe the course of your pain: Constant, Comes and goes, Getting worse, Getting better, Staying about the same

Medications (current): List *all* medications including prescription, over-the-counter (ie, ibuprofen), supplements, vitamins	**Please shade all locations you have pain or discomfort**
Medical/surgical history: List *all* surgeries, diabetes, cancer, high blood pressure, heart attack, pacemaker, arthritis, fractures, accidents, osteoporosis	
Allergies to medicines:	
Family history: Cancer, heart disease, stroke, arthritis, osteoporosis	

What do you do for exercise?
Tobacco use (cigarette, cigar, pipe, chew): ☐ Current ☐ Quit ☐ Never
Number of alcoholic beverages per week?
Number of caffeinated beverages per day?
Occupation:
Physical requirements: ☐ Prolonged sitting ☐ Prolonged standing ☐ Lifting ☐ Travel ☐ Driving ☐ Computer
                            ☐ Phone ☐ Child care
Employment status: ☐ Full-time ☐ Part-Time ☐ Light duty ☐ Off duty due to injury ☐ Full-time parent
                        ☐ Not working ☐ Retired

• Night pain, fevers, unintentional weight change?	☐ Yes ☐ No	Review of Systems (ROS) comments:
• Vision change, double vision?	☐ Yes ☐ No	
• Difficulty swallowing, headaches?	☐ Yes ☐ No	
• Chest pain, palpatations?	☐ Yes ☐ No	
• Shortness of breath, wheezing, cough after exercise?	☐ Yes ☐ No	
• Nausea, vomiting, black stools, loss of control of stools?	☐ Yes ☐ No	
• New rashes or psoriasis?	☐ Yes ☐ No	
• Dizziness, weakness, numbness, tingling?	☐ Yes ☐ No	
• Depressed mood, sleep problems, anxiety?	☐ Yes ☐ No	Patient's Signature: _____
• Current low back pain, other joint swelling or muscle pain?	☐ Yes ☐ No	☐ ROS Reviewed / Recommendations:
♀ Are you pregnant, trying to get pregnant, or breastfeeding?	☐ Yes ☐ No	
♀ Last menstrual period date: _____ Periods regular?	☐ Yes ☐ No	MD / Therapist Initials / Date:

FIGURE 3.1 Sample patient intake form.

life-threatening problems. The more red flags, the greater the need to follow up the physical examination with necessary diagnostics. The following is a list of potential red flags:

- Age <20 or >50 years
- Trauma
- Cancer history
- Unrelenting night pain that does not change with movement
- Fevers
- Unexplained weight loss
- Pain at rest that does not change
- Immune suppression (eg, with corticosteroid use)
- Recent or recurring infection
- Generalized systemic disease (eg, diabetes)
- Failure after 4 weeks of conservative treatment
- Signs of cauda equina syndrome
- Saddle anesthesia
- Sphincter disturbance
- Motor weakness of the lower or upper limbs

Cauda equina and neurological disorders may cause symptoms of bladder dysfunction, saddle anesthesia, and loss of anal sphincter tone, progressive major motor weakness, gait disorders, and perianal or perineal sensory loss. Patients may be uncomfortable mentioning these symptoms, so it is best to ask them specific questions—for example, "Have you noticed any subtle issues with your bowels or bladder, such as leakage of urine in your underwear or increased flatulence, in the past 1 to 2 weeks, or is that not the case?"

Inflammatory disorders may be indicated by gradual-onset symptoms such as morning stiffness, peripheral and spinal joint stiffness in all directions, persistent severe restriction of lumbar flexion, skin rashes, colitis, and a family history of such disorders. Patients rarely connect issues of gradual onset. The clinician needs to ask about and screen for areas of the body that provoke complaints. These areas may be relevant to more systemic inflammatory conditions or mind-body disorders, and the clinician should rule out such mechanisms.

Onset or Mechanism of Injury

Information about the onset or mechanism of injury can be collected on the patient intake form. The clinician should review with the patient any information provided about the onset of injury. Many patients state initially that their pain symptoms have been ongoing, but with prompting they can recall a time when the pain symptoms were not present. This review helps the clinician differentiate a recurring pain mechanism from a new injury. Injury dates help the clinician identify the healing stage of the tissue as well; time since injury dictates the tissue loading exam and guides decisions regarding the strength of the repair tissue. Many patients have problems that occur for no apparent reason, which may indicate a positional or cumulative mechanical problem or a nonmechanical mechanism. If on further questioning the clinician finds that the recent pain onset was related to an anniversary of a stressful or injury event, a CNS pain mechanism may be dominating.

24-Hour Behavior of Symptoms

The 24-hour behavior of symptoms is a summary of the patient's symptoms in the morning, throughout the day, in the evening, and during sleep. This description guides the clinician's clinical reasoning in choosing between the nociceptive:inflammatory and nociceptive:ischemia pain mechanisms. Many patients are dealing with both mechanisms, so a reevaluation of the 24-hour behavior of symptoms at each visit allows the clinician to understand which mechanism is dominating that session and should be the focus of the visit. Nociceptive mechanisms in particular may change in presentation from initial interview to follow-up visits.

The presence of a diurnal pattern of pain indicates a chemical inflammatory pain mechanism (see Chapter 4). In a diurnal pain pattern, the pain worsens as the day progresses and either progressively worsens or remains constant throughout the night. The worsening of symptoms overnight and into the next morning confirms that the pain is chemical inflammation. It is also useful to note whether too much activity, too much time spent in one position, or catastrophic thoughts related to the condition presented with the chemical inflammation and symptoms flare-up.

Aggravating and Alleviating Factors

Aggravating and alleviating factors can be collected on the patient intake form. These factors may provide clues about possible mechanical influences. It may also help the clinician determine whether the patient is using more passive means of management such as medications or modalities such as ice, heat, and electrical devices or alternative therapies like acupuncture. It is useful for the clinician to understand how patients perceive their symptoms. For example, a patient may write under aggravating factors "everything" and under alleviating factors "nothing"; in this situation, it is crucial for the clinician to probe during the interview for details on how the symptoms become better or worse. The clinician also gains insight into the patients' coping strategies; patients who are passive copers indicate using medication, modalities, rest, and massage as ways to alleviate their symptoms, and active copers identify positions, movements, activities, relaxation, and meditation. Further questioning is best done by focusing the interview on three dimensions of pain:

1. The *mechanical dimension* is related to the postures, movements, positions, or activities that change the pain location, description, and frequency.
2. The *social dimension* is related to the social circumstances that trigger or initiate the pain, such as the patient's job, school, marital relationship, and interpersonal functioning.
3. The *psychological* or *emotional dimension* is related to the effects of life pressures, stress, thoughts, behaviors, fears, worries, anxieties, and depression on pain. Screening tools for depression and anxiety can confirm that CNS pain mechanisms are dominating, and they are needed for psychological referral.

Patients often are initially unaware of or unwilling to admit the connection between their pain and the social and psychological dimensions of their lives. A pain journal can increase the patients' awareness of these dimensions of pain and can be a screen for their readiness for treatment. The pain journal allows self-discovery of triggers to symptoms and the patients' degree of willingness to participate in care planning. This information can provide the clinician with insight into pain-related disability risk characteristics that may need to be formally measured. Evidence suggests that fear avoidance and distress are important factors in the development of a pain-related disability.[7]

When the subjective evaluation indicates that CNS pain mechanisms are dominating, the pain journal can help patients understand the connections between their symptoms and the mechanical, emotional, and social dimensions of pain. Keeping a pain journal may also help them discover their level of readiness to change and take action.[8] The clinician asks the patients to record intolerable pain experiences (ie, pain at an unacceptable level) in a journal. Patients write down three types of information about their pain both at the moment and 3 hours before: (1) what they were doing physically (eg, sitting, standing, gardening), which identifies the mechanical dimension; (2) where they were and whom they were with (eg, daughter's school, mother-in-law's home, work, with an ex-spouse), which identifies the social dimension; and (3) what emotions they were feeling (eg, happy, angry, anxious, blameful, fearful, helpless), which identifies the psychological dimension. Together with the patients, the clinician can identify trends in each dimension, help develop active strategies to cope, and promote awareness of ways to modify the pain experience. In addition, using this exercise when the patients' pain is at an acceptable level can identify dimensions that may help them control their pain. **Figure 3.2** provides instructions for patients on keeping a pain journal.

FIGURE 3.2 Instructions for Keeping a Pain Journal

Keeping a journal describing when your pain is at its worst (least tolerable) or best (most tolerable) will help you and your clinician understand factors connected to your pain and other symptoms. In each entry in your journal, include the following information related to your activities both at the moment and 3 hours before:

- **Mechanical**—What are you doing? Examples: sitting, standing, walking, going up or down stairs, gardening, watching a movie
- **Social**—Where are you, and whom are you with? Examples: at the grocery store with your sister, driving to your son's practice, visiting your mother at the nursing home
- **Emotional**—How are you feeling? Use the descriptors below to represent your feelings as accurately as possible:

Happy	Excited	Tender	Scared	Angry	Sad
Delighted	Aroused	Affectionate	Worried	Uptight	Discouraged
Elated	Nervous	Loving	Nervous	Hot tempered	Depressed
Jolly	Thrilled	Compassionate	Frightened	Bitter	Dissatisfied
Complete	Spirited	Warmhearted	Apprehensive	Infuriated	Down
Satisfied	Chipper	Kind	Horrified	Mad	Heartbroken
Optimistic	Enthusiastic	Sensitive	Anxious	Irritated	Dejected
Pleased	Frenzied	Congenial	Jittery	Outraged	Troubled
Upbeat	Antsy	Sympathetic	Intimidated	Resentful	Blue

(continues on next page)

> **FIGURE 3.2** Instructions for Keeping a Pain Journal
>
> *(continued from previous page)*
>
> Use the following template to be sure you include all the necessary information:
>
> **What are you doing at the moment?** _____
> _____
>
> **Date:** _____ **Time:** _____
>
> **Pain:** ☐ At its worst   ☐ At its best
>
> **Mechanical:**
> What are you doing? _____
> _____
>
> **Social:**
> Where are you? _____
>
> Whom are you with? _____
>
> **Emotional:**
> How are you feeling?   happy / excited / tender / scared / angry / sad
>
>
> **What were you doing 3 hours before?** _____
> _____
>
> **Date:** _____ **Time:** _____
>
> **Pain:** ☐ At its worst   ☐ At its best
>
> **Mechanical:**
> What are you doing? _____
> _____
>
> **Social:**
> Where are you? _____
>
> Whom are you with? _____
>
> **Emotional:**
> How are you feeling?   happy / excited / tender / scared / angry / sad

Thoughts, Beliefs, and Cultural Attitudes Regarding Pain

Thoughts, beliefs, and cultural attitudes that may influence patients' ability to recover and cope are best assessed through interview. Denison et al[9] found that self-efficacy beliefs were a more important determinant of disability than fear avoidance beliefs in patients with musculoskeletal pain and that both qualities were better predictors of disability than pain intensity and duration. Thought processes are powerful enough to maintain a pain state and even to maintain inflammation in the tissue believed to be the area of the problem.[10] Maladaptive cognitive and evaluative processes in patients with pain can cause education and active programs to fail. For example, the common belief that pain means something harmful is happening may lead patients to avoid participating in exercise in order to prevent further harm, thus triggering the brain to protect and maintain a pain state.

Research by Cairns et al[11] demonstrated that distress associated with low back pain is very common. In fact, one-third of patients referred to physical therapy for low back pain experienced some form of distress, which was found to increase their risk for poor outcomes three- to fourfold.[11] Common distress signals that can increase the risk for poor outcomes include maladaptive beliefs, expectations, and pain-related behavior; reinforcement of pain-related behavior by family; heightened emotional activity; job dissatisfaction; poor social support; and compensation issues. Yellow flags are psychological, social, emotional, and occupational factors that increase the risk of transition to disability related to pain. **Table 3.1** provides examples of common yellow flags.[8] Clinicians should screen initially for these factors and reassess them often, particularly when the patients' progress is slower than expected. The presence of such characteristics is a prompt for further detailed assessment and early intervention. Kendall and Watson[1] identified the following interview topics for identifying yellow flags:

- Attitudes and beliefs about the pain experience
- Behaviors related to the pain experience
- Compensation issues regarding the pain experience
- Diagnostic and treatment issues with respect to the pain experience
- Emotions related to the pain experience
- Family support with respect to the pain experience
- Work-related support and issues related to the pain experience[12]

Many patients do not express their thoughts and beliefs without being asked. It is important for the clinician to ask patients what they believe is happening or what they do when the pain occurs. The answers can give the clinician insight into the patients' rehabilitation potential. While assessing for yellow flags, clinicians should ask themselves what can be done to help these patients experience less distress and disability. What are the patients' methods to cope with their pain? Are their methods effective in helping minimize distress? The yellow flag assessment occurs over several visits as patients and clinician establish a respectful relationship that enables the clinician to ask questions and understand more fully the impact of the situation, especially when CNS mechanisms are dominating the pain experience. As the subjective evaluation process proceeds, further yellow flags may become apparent.

Butler and Moseley,[13(p80)] in their book *Explain Pain*, identified the following common thoughts, beliefs, and fears regarding persistent pain:

- I'm in pain, so there must be something harmful happening to my body.
- I'm staying at home; I'm keeping quiet and out of things.
- I've got tons of scarring from my surgery—the worst my doc has ever seen.
- My surgeon told me I can never go back to that job.
- Why can't someone just fix this pain for me?

TABLE 3.1 Common Yellow Flags

Category	Examples
Attitudes and beliefs about pain	Belief that pain is harmful or disabling, resulting in avoidance behaviors (eg, guarding, fear of movement)
	Belief that all pain must be abolished before attempting to return to work or normal activity
	Expectation of increased pain with activity or work; lack of ability to predict capability
	Catastrophizing, thinking the worst, misinterpreting bodily symptoms
	Belief that pain is uncontrollable
	Passive attitude toward rehabilitation
Behaviors	Use of extended rest, disproportionate downtime
	Reduced activity level, with significant withdrawal from activities; boom-bust cycle of activity
	Avoidance of normal activity, progressive substitution of lifestyle away from productive activity
	Report of extremely high intensity of pain (eg, "above 10" on a 0–10 scale)
	Excessive reliance on use of aids or appliances
	Reduction in sleep quality since onset of pain
	High intake of alcohol or other substances (possibly as self-medication), with an increase since onset of pain
	Smoking
Compensation issues	Lack of financial incentive to return to work
	Delay in accessing income support and treatment cost, disputes over eligibility
	History of claims due to other injuries or pain problems
	History of extended time off work due to injury or other pain problems (eg, >12 weeks)
	Previous experience of ineffective case management (eg, absence of interest, perception of being treated punitively)
Diagnosis and treatment	Experience with a health professional who sanctioned disability or did not provide interventions to improve function
	Experience of conflicting diagnoses or explanations for pain, resulting in confusion
	Catastrophizing and fear (eg, of "ending up in a wheelchair") caused by diagnostic language
	Dramatization of pain by a health professional resulting in dependency on treatments and continuation of passive treatment
	Frequent visits to a health professional in the past year (excluding the present episode of pain)
	Expectation of a "techno-fix" (eg, view of body as a machine)
	Lack of satisfaction with previous treatment for pain
	Acceptance of advice to withdraw from job

Category	Examples
Emotions	Fear of increased pain with activity or work
	Depression, especially long-term low mood, loss of sense of enjoyment
	Increased irritability
	Anxiety about heightened awareness of body sensations, including sympathetic nervous system arousal
	Feeling of being under stress and unable to maintain a sense of control
	Presence of social anxiety or disinterest in social activity
	Feeling of being useless and not needed
Family	Overprotective partner or spouse (usually well intentioned) who emphasizes fear of harm or catastrophizes
	Solicitous behaviors from spouse (eg, taking over tasks)
	Socially punitive responses from spouse (eg, ignoring, expressing frustration)
	Lack of support by family members for an attempt to return to work
	Lack of available support person with whom to talk about problems
Work	History of manual work in industries such as fishing, forestry, farming, construction, nursing, trucking, migrant or contract labor
	Pattern of frequent job changes, experience of stress at work, job dissatisfaction, poor relationships with peers or supervisors, lack of vocational direction
	Belief that work is harmful, will do damage, or is dangerous
	Unsupportive current work environment
	Low educational background, low socioeconomic status
	Job that involves significant biomechanical demands such as lifting; manual handling of heavy items; extended sitting, standing, driving, or vibration; maintenance of sustained postures or movements; inflexible work schedule without breaks
	Minimal availability of selected duties and graduated return-to-work pathways with poor implementation
	Absence of interest of supervisor, peers, employer

Common fears associated with persistent pain include the following[13(p100)]:

- Fear of the pain itself and of not knowing the seriousness of the cause
- Fear of not being believed, not being compensated, or not receiving help
- Fear of certain movements or any movement
- Fear of being reinjured, making it worse, or slowing the healing
- Fear of ending up in a wheelchair
- Fear of not being able to work and having no income
- Fear of therapy, injections, surgery, and botched surgery
- Fear of drug addiction

Many patients will not bring this information forward; the clinician can ask the following questions to ascertain whether these common beliefs and fears are present and persist:

- What do you think and do regarding your pain?
- What would someone in your culture or family do in response to this pain?
- What do you think is happening to the tissues when pain occurs?
- What does the pain message mean to you?
- Do you believe you can get better and have less pain?
- What do you believe will help you get rid of this pain?
- Do you believe the pain has to leave before you start returning to your functions and activities?

Answers to these questions can help the clinician understand whether the patients' thoughts and beliefs are maladaptive, catastrophic, self-limiting, or limited by culture and whether PNS or CNS pain mechanisms are dominating.

Past and Current Treatments

Data on past and current treatments can be collected on the patient intake form. The clinician should probe further with respect to the type of treatment and who provided it. The vast number of clinicians treating musculoskeletal pain offer patients many types of approaches. It is important for patients to understand that some palliative care approaches provide temporary benefits without changing the underlying problem over the long term. Patients need education to accept an active approach that is based on education and exercise when passive treatments have failed to end the need for rehabilitative and medical care. Reasons why certain types of treatment have not changed the patients' underlying problem or ability to manage it can be discussed in the interview. The PMCS is valuable in guiding education that enables patients to understand their dominant pain mechanism and the relative effectiveness of past and proposed treatments.

Readiness for Treatment

The patients' readiness for treatment is often not assessed, but it may have an important effect on treatment outcomes. Readiness refers to patients' willingness to change their behavior toward the pain—in other words, their willingness to be helped. It is acceptable not to be ready to make changes. Clinicians, however, should not continue to provide care for patients who are not ready to help themselves. People who are not ready to change consume disproportionate health care resources and realize unsatisfactory outcomes. Burns et al[14] studied patients' action readiness before and after treatment and found that those who were ready to change experienced decreased pain and increased functional outcome measurements and satisfaction with services. Those who were not ready or unsure had the worst outcomes, some even worse than when they started.

An important dimension of motivation with respect to musculoskeletal pain is the patients' self-efficacy and level of confidence in their ability to recover and heal. Some patients are overly confident and consider themselves to be accelerated healers, whereas others feel hopeless and put the clinician in the position of healer. In addition, motivation is not a binary state of being motivated versus not motivated. Rather, motivation levels occupy a continuum and can vary rapidly, sometimes day to day. Depending on the patient's level of readiness or change stage, different motivational intervention strategies will be more or less effective.

Prochaska et al's[15] stages of change have inspired the creation of instruments for assessing patients' motivational change state. One such tool, the Readiness Ruler (see **Figure 3.3**), is

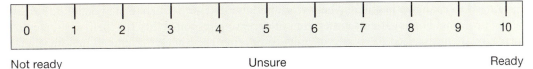

FIGURE 3.3 Readiness Ruler: "On a scale of 0 to 10, how ready are you to make the changes necessary to control your pain?"

a visual analog scale developed by Rollnick that is used extensively in general medical settings.[16] The clinician asks the patient, "On a scale from 0 to 10, where 0 = *not ready* and 10 = *ready,* how ready are you to make the changes necessary to control your pain?" The question can be modified to specific aspects of recommended treatments. The lower numbers indicate less readiness and the higher numbers indicate greater readiness for change and responsibility. For patients who rate themselves as not ready (0–3), clinicians can respond by expressing concern, offering information, providing support, and committing to following up. Ongoing treatment at this level is not effective. For patients who rate themselves as unsure (4–7), clinicians should explore the positive and negative aspects of treatment. For patients who rate themselves as ready (8–10), clinicians should help them plan action and continue with treatment.

The clinician can use the Readiness Ruler periodically to monitor patients' changes in motivation as treatment progresses. Patients' readiness levels can move up and down. Also, it is an acceptable outcome for the clinician to help patients move toward higher readiness scores, even if they never reach a decision-making or action stage. Most patients cycle through the change stages several times, sometimes up and sometimes down, before they settle into treatment or a stable recovery. One significant feature of the Readiness Ruler is that patients assess their own readiness by marking the ruler or voicing a number. The clinician can pose the question, "What would it take to move from a 3 to a 5?" and can recognize movement along the continuum by asking, "Where did you rate yourself last month [or last year] compared with now?"

When pain is the result of occupational injury, the clinician needs to screen job satisfaction and avoidance behaviors, as they influence readiness to engage in treatment with the goal of returning to work. Soares and Jabionska[17] found that workers who experienced greater job strain and burnout had a higher degree of disability due to pain. Workers' compensation cases may benefit from the use of a screening tool (eg, Fear-Avoidance Beliefs Questionnaire[7,18]) to assess patients' job satisfaction, desire to return to the same job, and desire to work in general. The tool should also address anger, blame, and, most importantly, the worker's beliefs about pain and return to activity.[6]

Prochaska et al[15] identified six stages in readiness for behavioral change: precontemplation, contemplation, preparation, action, maintenance, and termination. A clinician needs to be aware of what stage the patients are in. Just because patients present in the therapy session does not mean they are ready to change; many patients are receiving care because their doctor sent them, and they have yet to accept the notion that some of their behaviors must change for their treatment to be successful.

Stage 1: Precontemplation

Resistance to recognizing or modifying a problem is the hallmark of the precontemplation stage. Sixty percent of the patients that clinicians encounter are in this stage.[15] Patients in this stage have no intention of changing their behavior in the foreseeable future. They may have tried to change a particular behavior and have given up, or they may deny the reality of the problem. These patients either are not accepting responsibility for their well-being or are unaware of the need to change in order to improve their lives. Patients in this stage may express a hollow wish to improve their quality of life. They may be demoralized and may dismiss the possibility of ever changing.

Patients in the precontemplation stage perceive the clinician's training and evaluative activities as a waste of time and typically do not volunteer to participate. They may resist cooperating and vocalize their resistance. They may feel coerced to participate and may express the belief that if other people changed, everything would be fine. Patients in the precontemplation stage may

- Show no intention of changing their behavior and deny having a problem
- Note that other people see the problem and are putting pressure on them to change
- Prefer that others change rather than think about changing themselves
- Engage in denial, evidenced in failure to obtain information about their problem, attempts to maintain ignorance, and placement of responsibility for their problems on factors such as genetic makeup, family, and society
- Feel demoralized, seeing the situation as hopeless
- Readily use the words "yes, but" to explain why something will not work.

Even people in this stage will progress toward change if the proper interventions are given at the proper time. Clinicians can help patients create an environment for success by committing to follow-up and reevaluating patient readiness. Clinicians can respond in the following ways to patients in the precontemplation stage:

- Encourage patients to establish a good working relationship with someone who will support their desire for change or with someone who has a similar problem who is actively working on changing.
- Suggest a good book for patients to read, for example, *Changing for Good* by Prochaska.[15]
- Raise patients' consciousness by providing education to the public using mass media or small groups.
- Encourage patients to accept that they are responsible for improving their quality of life and that negative energy regarding precontemplation affects the positive energy associated with change.

Stage 2: Contemplation

Patients in the contemplation stage acknowledge that they have a problem, are aware of a need to improve the quality of their life, and are willing to think about their need to change because they desire something better. Patients begin to take their core values seriously and realize that they have not made a true commitment to embrace the discipline required to change. Patients are open to information and feedback, although they may remain in the contemplation stage for years, realizing they have a problem but unable to generate the energy to change. Some people express resistance to a process to improve their personal lives because they are undecided about what needs to be improved or about the most effective way to proceed. They may also question the benefits they can achieve by taking their life more seriously. Patients in the contemplation stage may

- Acknowledge they have a problem and begin to think seriously about solving it
- Struggle to understand their problem, explore its causes, and wonder about possible solutions

- Make indefinite plans to take action within the next 6 months or so
- Know their destination and even how to get there but not be ready to go
- Become a chronic contemplator, eternally substituting thinking for action
- Engage in two types of thinking that signal readiness to move to the next stage: (1) focusing on the solution rather than the problem and (2) thinking more about the future than the past.

The end of the contemplation stage is a time of anticipation, activity, anxiety, and excitement—these are foreign emotions for a contemplator who needs nurturing. Clinicians can respond in the following ways to patients in the contemplation stage:

- Explain how to prepare for action.
- Encourage them to express past failures and accept the failures as a learning research project.
- Acknowledge their frustration and emphasize the disadvantages of the present situation.
- Review with them difficult situations or problems and the solutions and point out that the benefits they will receive from the energy derived from living a values-based life will exceed the disadvantages associated with remaining the same.
- Encourage contact and discussion with role models.
- Engage in guided imagery in which they imagine themselves in the new situation or create the image they want (eg, commitment to moderation or to regular movement).
- Encourage their self-examination, considering pros and cons in a nonthreatening and supportive manner and inspiring them to take responsibility for their situation.

The Readiness Ruler (**Figure 3.3**) is useful when working with a contemplator and can be adapted to address readiness to engage in specific activities related to the care solutions, such as drinking eight glasses of water a day, attending an exercise class three times per week, or performing deep breathing when pain or negative emotion increases. Likewise, the clinician can use the Readiness Ruler to understand the patient's perceived readiness to commit to a daily exercise habit to support the management of pain and return to meaningful function. For example, the clinician can ask the question, "How ready are you to apply diaphragm breathing and meditation when your pain is above level 5 on the 0 to 10 pain scale?" A patient in the contemplation stage usually selects 5, indicating that he or she is unsure. Even though the clinician has discussed the importance of and demonstrated these skills and the patient has demonstrated competency in using them, the patient's uncertainty and lack of action could continue for weeks or years.

Internal motivation comes from seeing the change as important and having the confidence that it can be accomplished. The clinician can provide contemplators with encouragement by using a visual analog scale such as the Importance Scale or the Confidence Scale to help them recognize deeper areas to change. The Importance Scale,[16] like the Readiness Ruler, has gradations from 0 to 10 (see **Figure 3.4**). The clinician asks the patient, "How important would you say it is for you to use diaphragm breathing for pain control? On a scale from 0 to 10, where 0 is *not important at all* and 10 is *extremely important*, how important do you feel this behavior is?" Likewise, the Confidence Scale[16] uses a ruler with gradations from 0 to 10 (see **Figure 3.5**), and the clinician asks the patient, "How confident are you in your ability to use diaphragm breathing for pain control, where 0 is *not at all confident* and 10 is *extremely confident*?"

The contemplation stage of readiness is vitally important to the patients' progress and success. The clinician can use the Readiness Ruler and the Importance and Confidence Scales to monitor the daily changes that occur in their patients who are contemplators as

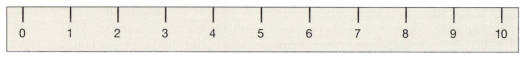

Not important at all — Extremely important

FIGURE 3.4 Importance Scale: "On a scale from 0 to 10, where 0 is *not important at all* and 10 is *extremely important*, which number indicates how important you feel this pain control behavior is?"

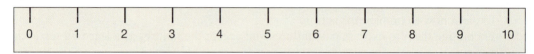

Not at all confident — Extremely confident

FIGURE 3.5 Confidence Scale: "On a scale from 0 to 10, where 0 is *not at all confident* and 10 is *extremely confident*, how confident are you in your ability to use this pain control behavior?"

a nonconfrontational way of discussing a very important but tough topic and guiding the treatment focus for that visit.

Stage 3: Preparation

Patients in the preparation stage are on the verge of action. They may still be questioning how to improve, but they are developing an action plan and may even have made small changes with successes and relapses. Patients in this stage are in the process of defining their core values and may even have taken small steps toward change, but they have not committed to the behavior change. In spite of slight improvements, these patients have not reached the final decision to make a full effort to change. Patients in the preparation stage may

- Plan to take action within the very next month and be making the final adjustments before they begin to change their behavior
- Make their intended change public
- Still be somewhat ambivalent, needing to convince themselves that taking this action is what is best for them
- Already have instituted a number of small behavior changes
- Develop a firm, detailed scheme for action and make sure that they have learned the change processes they need.

Clinicians can respond in the following ways to patients in the preparation stage:

- Encourage them to believe that they can change and can create the social conditions needed for change.
- Emphasize the advantages and personal benefits to be achieved by defining and living their core values.
- Be a life coach, mentor, and friend instead of an expert.
- Work with them to develop an action plan that has goals that are realistic, attainable, and measureable and that has specific, practical manageable steps.
- Encourage them to commit to time frames for re-measuring progress toward goals.

Stage 4: Action

Patients in the action stage are executing the action plan they have developed. They recognize that the work they did in the contemplation and preparation stages will contribute to their success and that, as important as it is, this stage is neither the first nor the last stage of change. Patients in the action stage may

- Make the overt changes in their behavior and surroundings for which they have been preparing
- Be very busy and make the greatest commitment of time and energy of all the stages
- Receive the most recognition and encouragement from others.

Clinicians can respond in the following ways to patients in the action stage:

- Reinforce positive steps toward desired behaviors and commit to giving praise, encouragement, and recognition.
- Emphasize the importance of substituting healthy behaviors for problem behaviors to improve self-efficacy.
- Encourage patients in an empathic, caring style to adjust and reset goals so they are realistic, attainable, and measureable.
- Encourage them to outline specific, practical, and manageable steps toward their goals
- Encourage them to commit to time frames to remeasure progress toward goals.

Stage 5: Maintenance

Patients in the maintenance stage have been continuously engaged in their change process for at least 6 months. They are actively involved in living life to the fullest and making a positive impact on the lives they touch. These patients have discovered their life purpose and core values. Although "just doing it" feels more natural at this stage, overconfidence and life pressures can lead to relapse. Patients in the maintenance stage may

- Consolidate the gains attained during the action and other stages
- Struggle to prevent lapses and relapse
- Remain in this stage for as little as 6 months to as long as a lifetime.

Clinicians can respond in the following ways to patients in the maintenance stage:

- Continue positive reinforcement and social support and consider recommending community opportunities for rewards and recognition such as community races, health fairs, running support groups.
- Encourage patients to avoid triggers for unhealthy behaviors and strive for solutions of healthy behaviors.
- Encourage them to maintain self-efficacy by adjusting and resetting goals; outlining specific, practical, and manageable steps; and committing to time frames to remeasure progress toward goals for themselves.
- Discharge them with biannual wellness appointments.

Stage 6: Termination

In the termination stage, the patients' new behavior has become so much an integral part of daily life that the likelihood of relapse is essentially nonexistent. Some professionals question whether people ever reach this stage; Prochaska and colleagues[15] consider it possible for a small percentage of people. Patients are committed to doing whatever it takes to be the best that they can be and volunteer to participate in any activity that will improve the process of living. They serve as leaders by encouraging others to participate in and benefit from the process of maximizing one's potential. Patients in the termination stage may

- Feel assured that their former problems no longer present any temptation or threat
- Have complete confidence that they can cope without fear of relapse.

Clinicians can respond in the same ways as in the maintenance stage because these patients have accepted the challenge to make the changes necessary to get the most out of treatment and out of their lives.

Use of Measurement Tools in the Subjective Evaluation

During the initial subjective evaluation and at each subsequent visit, the clinician can use measurement tools to identify the patients' pain and function levels. Measuring progress in relation to a baseline helps patients own their outcomes and provides direction for care. In addition, these tools can be used to identify the functions (eg, activities of daily living, occupational and household activities, and recreational and leisure pursuits) that are most limited by pain. Many tools and scales are available for use in measuring changes in pain and function. The clinician can select baseline measurement tools that either have fixed properties (eg, Five Times Sit to Stand Test, 6-Minute Walk Test) or are self-administered by the patient, who selects responses that reflect personal importance.[19] Case reports described in Chapters 4 through 8 use both region-specific and patient-specific measures to represent change from initial session to discharge.

Region-specific measures standardize the questions related to pain and function and are best suited for research when the intent is to compare large groups of people over long periods of time or to test the validity of one intervention versus another. A region-specific measure assesses a particular area of the body and provides an objective way to measure symptoms. In the clinic, standardized region-specific tools are best used with all patients especially if they are in cognitive-behavioral pain management or work-hardening programs, because the questions allow for repeated measures to reflect relevant changes. Region-specific tools should be administered repeatedly every month from the start to the end of care to allow for continued assessment and care plan adjustment. The following region-specific measures are recommended and are discussed further in Chapter 7:

- **Lower Extremity Functional Scale.**[20] The LEFS was developed as an outcome measure to be used in place of a number of condition-specific measures and to yield reliable and valid measurements for a patient's ability to perform specific functional tasks related to his/her lower extremity orthopedic injury.
- **Disabilities of the Arm, Shoulder and Hand Questionnaire.**[21] Patients assess their symptoms and function resulting from musculoskeletal disorders of the upper extremity.
- **Neck Disability Index.**[22] NDI was developed as a self-report condition-specific outcome measure to determine level of disability of a patient with neck pain.
- **Oswestry Disability Index.**[23] This index is used to determine the level of disability of a patient with lower back pain.

Patient-reported measures are best used to compare changes within an individual patient's status from visit to visit and throughout initiation to discharge of care using functional activities specific to the patient. Patient-reported outcomes involve outcomes directly reported from the patient, as opposed to a clinician-reported outcome, which assesses the patient from the clinician's perspective. Monitoring progress at each visit informs the clinician as to whether a patient's status is changing as expected, enabling him or her to progress treatments as rapidly as appropriate. Patient-reported measures are valid for monitoring change within one patient but are not recommended for comparing treatment groups. Recommended patient-reported measurement tools are the Patient-Specific Functional Scale (PSFS) and other visual analog scales such as the Readiness Ruler (**Figure 3.3**). The PSFS is appropriate for use with a variety of clinical presentations, both neuromuscular and musculoskeletal. The developers of the PSFS found moderate to excellent reliability, validity, and sensitivity to change.[24] In studies on pain and disability in patients with orthopedic conditions (eg, neck pain, anterior cruciate ligament reconstruction), the PSFS was found to be reliable, with good construct validity and sensitivity to change.[25,26] The tool is sensitive to change in individual patients and applicable in clinical use as well.[27]

The PSFS asks patients to rate three specific areas: function limitation, pain limitation, and pain intensity:

1. The function limitation section asks patients to identify three to five specific activities they are not able to do or have difficulty doing as a result of their problem. The patients rate each activity from 0 = *unable to perform the activity* to 10 = *able to perform at prior level*.
2. The pain limitation section asks the patients to rate how much the pain has limited them from performing normal daily activities over the past 24 hours from 0 = *severely limited* to 10 = *no limitation*.
3. The pain intensity section asks the patients to rate how bad the pain has been over the past 24 hours from 0 = *no pain* to 10 = *worst pain ever*.

The responsiveness of a measure is an indication of how well it detects clinically relevant change over time.[28] The PSFS developers found the minimal detectable important change (MDIC) to be 3 points on the 11-point scale for any single activity. Understanding the MDIC assists the clinician in creating short- and long-term measureable goals.

The clinician should discuss with patients their goals related to activity, explain the intervention by describing the pain mechanisms, and identify potential outcomes. Use of an outcome measure is an effective way to include patients in goal setting and active care planning and promotes a partnership between the patient and clinician toward recovery.

Use of the Management Plan in the Subjective Evaluation

A management plan for musculoskeletal pain is designed to help the patients get through the episode of pain and regain normal function and is reviewed at each treatment session. Chapters 4 through 8 discuss elements of management plans specific to each PMCS category; this section provides some general guidelines. To develop an evidence-supported plan,[5] the clinician

- Develops the plan in conjunction with the patients, fostering a cooperative, supportive environment
- Tailors the plan to meet the patients' needs, accounting for their preferences and abilities
- Includes actions that patients and clinician may take in the event of an exacerbation or recurrence of pain (flare-up plan) to continue progress toward recovery
- Facilitates participation by keeping the plan simple, reviewing it at follow-up visits using outcome tools to show reliable and valid change

- Enables the patients to take responsibility for their care, bearing in mind that some patients require greater levels of assistance and support
- Takes responsibility for modifying the plan to promote the patients' success.

The plan should include reasonable activity levels, nonpharmacological (active, passive, and behavioral) interventions, and pharmacological interventions to be used as needed to enable patients to return to normal activity. The plan should be developed in partnership with the patients, giving due consideration to the potential risks and benefits of various treatment options. It is important that patients have realistic expectations of the interventions and goals for the outcomes of interventions.

At each patient visit, the clinician can inquire whether the plan has been satisfactory and explore questions, concerns, and possible alternatives as required. Ongoing reassessment using the PMCS provides an important opportunity to identify pain mechanisms and red or yellow flags that may not have been evident on previous visits. By reviewing goals and outcome tools, the clinician demonstrates his or her concern about the patients' progress. The need for further visits should be discussed at each visit with a focus on the continued need for therapy rather than how many visits the insurance provider will cover. The use of outcome measures allows the clinician and patients to see progress, validates the management plan, and identifies the continued need for therapy.

Use of Patient Education in the Subjective Evaluation

The use of a preventive approach to shape behavior is best begun at the initial visit. This approach is particularly important with patients with dominant PNS pain mechanisms to prevent a transition to CNS pain mechanisms. Patient education should be seen as the first line of effective treatment, and it starts at the initial evaluation.

All patients need information from their health care professionals; at a minimum, they require an explanation of their disorder and an indication of how it contributes to their pain.[29,30] Clinicians' failure to provide adequate information is a common cause of dissatisfaction among patients, especially those with musculoskeletal problems.[31,32] Patients desire the following information[31]:

- An understandable explanation of the disorder and dominant pain mechanism
- What they can do to help themselves
- Applicable tests, diagnoses, and interventions
- Their prognosis, with reassurance if appropriate
- Outcome measurements to be used to show improvement
- Reassurance that they will be taken seriously (ie, be seen, heard, and believed), will receive patient-centered communication, and will have their perspectives and preferences addressed

Specific requirements for information vary among individuals. The depth and detail of information should be appropriate for the patients' learning style and level but cover the essentials necessary to enable them to self-manage the problem to the extent possible, alleviate their fear, and enable them to focus on preventing disability from pain by returning to activities as soon as possible.[33] A clinician who places more emphasis on education and who has better communication skills can be more effective at enhancing empowerment.[34] Empowerment of the patients promotes self-efficacy, self-esteem, reflexive thought, and active participation in shared decision making and goal setting. Active patient participation is associated with better outcomes.[35,36]

After completing the subjective and objective evaluation, the clinician should end each session with a summary of the data collected. Presenting the data to patients in a consistent, organized format will save time during each visit and reduce the need for follow-up communication. The clinician should also provide simple, concise written information to help patients understand and apply the new knowledge gathered at each session.[37]

Gifford and Butler[2] and Butler[4] recommended using a seven-step clinical reasoning summary to educate patients:

1. Pathobiological pain mechanisms
2. Specific tissue dysfunction
3. Sources of pain
4. Contributing factors
5. Prognosis for pain and function
6. Precautions
7. Management and intervention

Discussion of pathobiological mechanisms includes a description of the connective tissue healing stage and tissue health. In addition, musculoskeletal pain mechanisms are identified, with an emphasis on the dominating mechanism.

The summary of specific tissue dysfunction addresses general, specific, and psychological or mental dysfunction. General dysfunction is related to activities or specific functional tasks that the patient has identified. The clinician can use the PSFS to quantify the limitation. The specific dysfunction is identified through the results of objective evaluation and may address directional preference, stiff joints, weak or tight contractile or neural tissues, and poor quality positions or movement patterns contributing to the general dysfunction. The clinician highlights the specific tests and measures used to show change each visit and correlates these findings to the PSFS findings. Discussion of psychological and mental dysfunction centers around the yellow flags identified, including the patients' maladaptive thoughts, beliefs, motivation, and emotions with respect to pain, activity, and work.

The summary of sources of pain consists of descriptions of the tissue site where the intervention should be targeted in the body or brain. Patients need to understand the body-up versus brain-down approach to pain treatment. In a body-up approach, a PNS pain mechanism is dominating, and the source of the symptoms may be certain body connective tissue that needs direct stress to continue healing. In a brain-down approach, a CNS pain mechanism is dominating, and the source of symptoms may be processes in the CNS responsible for central sensitization, such as the dorsal horn of the spinal cord or the reticular formation or cerebrum of the brain. The more complex and diverse the CNS pain mechanisms, the more futile it is to direct intervention at a specific body connective tissue; a brain-down approach built on pain mechanism education and graded exposure to meaningful activity will be more effective.

Review of contributing factors addresses yellow flags such as anxiety, life and job dissatisfaction, and fear of pain, activity, and work. Klenerman et al[38] advised clinicians to provide patients with not only an explanation of their therapy, but also attention to the contributing factors that place them at risk for poor outcomes of therapeutic interventions for pain in any location.

In the summary of the prognosis for pain and function, the clinician reviews the results of outcome measures so the patients can see change over time. Central pain mechanisms may be unalterable in intensity, but the patients' suffering and disability may change dramatically. The clinician can use the PSFS to set goals and expectations from visit to visit, focusing on function and pain management (as described in Chapters 4 through 8), and can use region-specific tools monthly to guide and adjust PSFS goals.

The clinician should review precautions related to red flags identified during the interview. This is an opportunity for the clinician to convey to the patients any critical decisions made on the basis of the history and examination.

In the summary of management and intervention, the clinician reviews the management plan, addressing all dimensions and mechanisms of the patients' pain. The PMCS approach sets the stage for specific patient education topics and active care recommendations to address the dominating mechanism. Education occurs by understanding the learning style of each patient.

Learning is not only the receiving of information but is also the application of it. The learning styles of each patient are crucial to the success of the rehabilitation outcomes. Learning takes time and requires mutual respect and readiness between the teacher and the student.

Mazzuca demonstrated how patient education has a proven impact on health outcomes, including reducing morbidity and even mortality.[39] Patient education needs to be age appropriate to ensure the patient understands and then follows advice.[40] Clinicians should consider the age and the culture of the patients when choosing teaching aids and tactics. Many authors support using functional movement patterns and addressing the social and emotional dimensions of pain to achieve the greatest outcome with elderly people in musculoskeletal pain.[41,42] In children, researchers suggest the use of imagery, virtual reality, drawing, and coloring as effective ways to communicate regarding musculoskeletal pain. This is especially effective with children with the fewest abilities and the most pain.[43,44]

Certain cultures, for example, urban American Indian, responded better when education was performed in support groups and education topics of self-care, pain management, and communication of symptoms to physicians were covered.[45] In working with people of a different culture, the clinician should determine the patients' knowledge regarding their culture's practice with musculoskeletal pain. Tapping into patients' cultural beliefs and patients' solutions has been shown to have long-lasting benefits.[46]

Medical terminology or jargon is often as incomprehensible as a foreign language to patients. Studies have shown that physicians use jargon without realizing it.[47] Inappropriate words can create unnecessary stress for patients. For example, medicalizing the condition by using terminology that connotes structural pathology or damage promotes concern in most patients. Describing the cause of the pain as an abnormality or deformity causes patients to fixate on the structure. Words used in education that promote fear include "herniation," "sciatica," "degenerative disc disease," "arthritis," and "fibromyalgia." Other statements that produce fear include "I totally disagree with your doctor or therapist" and "They don't know what they are talking about." The blanket statement "If it hurts, stop it or do not do it" should be avoided unless it is accompanied by specific information conveying the clinician's clinical reasoning and providing specific time frames for stopping the activity.

Open-ended questions such as "What brings you in here?" tend to allay fear. They allow the patient to decide what direction to take with the conversation, but the clinician should use professional reasoning to redirect the patient when appropriate. The clinician should confirm to the patient that he or she was heard by repeating what the patient said in a summary statement at the conclusion of the subjective evaluation. Depending on the patient, different words communicate different messages. The clinician can use metaphors, analogies, and humor when appropriate to promote learning and understanding. Whenever possible, the clinician should reassure the patients about the positive course of their prognosis and the behaviors and actions they are taking to get there.

Learning about pain physiology is a great pain liberator. The role of rehabilitation is to help patients apply their new knowledge and restore their faith that their condition will improve by their actions. Moseley[46,48] showed that patients of all education levels were able to benefit from education about pain physiology and that education reduced the threat value of pain, lessened protective systems, and restored normal immune system function. When Moseley[49] combined education about pain physiology with movement approaches, participants achieved additional benefits of increased physical capacity and improved quality of life. The PMCS is a great guide to helping patients understand their pain physiology and active care needs.

KEY MESSAGES

- The subjective evaluation takes place within evidence-based guidelines for the evaluation and management of musculoskeletal pain.
- The categories of information gathered in the PMCS subjective evaluation are pain location, description, and frequency; onset or mechanism of injury; 24-hour behavior of symptoms; aggravating and alleviating factors; thoughts, beliefs, and cultural attitudes regarding pain; past and current treatments; and readiness for treatment. These characteristics of the patient's pain are required for pain mechanism classification.
- Use of a patient intake form can assist in the collection of information before the subjective evaluation interview. During the interview, the clinician asks more detailed questions to clarify information and rule out red flags and yellow flags.
- Keeping a pain journal and reviewing it with the clinician can help patients identify the social and psychological dimensions of their pain symptoms.
- The six stages of behavior change are precontemplation, contemplation, preparation, action, maintenance, and termination. Awareness of patients' stage of readiness to make the changes required in treatment helps clinicians tailor their communication and interventions to maximize patient outcomes.

- Measurement tools can be used in evaluating the patients' pain and function levels and in showing change from visit to visit and from the start to the end of therapy. The Patient-Specific Functional Scale (PSFS) can assist the clinician in setting goals and identifying prognosis.
- The clinician should review the patients' management plan for musculoskeletal pain at each treatment session. This plan is developed in collaboration with the patients. It is designed to help them progress through the episode of pain and regain normal function.
- The subjective evaluation should conclude with a summary of the clinician's clinical reasoning that addresses seven topics:
  1. Pathobiological pain mechanisms
  2. Specific tissue dysfunction
  3. Sources of pain
  4. Contributing factors
  5. Prognosis for pain and function
  6. Precautions
  7. Management and intervention
- A successful subjective evaluation takes place in an environment of listening and learning. Clinicians must present information to each patient on the basis of his or her personal characteristics, taking into consideration evidence-based guidelines for effective patient education.

References

1. Kendall N, Watson P. Identifying psychosocial yellow flags and modifying management: A case study. In: Gifford L, ed. *Topical Issues in Pain 2*. Falmouth, England: CNS Press; 2000:131-139.
2. Gifford LS, Butler DS. The integration of pain sciences into clinical practice. *J Hand Ther.* 1997;10:86-95.
3. Linton SJ. The socioeconomic impact of chronic back pain: Is anyone benefiting? *Pain.* 1998;75:163-168.
4. Butler DS. *The Sensitive Nervous System*. Adelaide, Australia: Noigroup; 2000.
5. Australian Acute Musculoskeletal Pain Guidelines Group. *Evidence Based Management of Acute Musculoskeletal Pain*. Brisbane, Australia: Australian Academic Press; 2003.
6. Fouquet B. Clinical examination as a tool for identifying the origin of regional musculoskeletal pain. *Best Pract Res Clin Rheumatol.* 2003;17:1-15.
7. Boersma K, Linton SJ. Screening to identify patients at risk: Profiles of psychological risk factors for early intervention. *Clin J Pain.* 2005;21:38-43.
8. Rehabilitation Institute of Chicago Musculoskeletal Pain Committee. *Allied Health Musculoskeletal Pain Course Manual*. Chicago, IL: Rehabilitation Institute of Chicago; 2006.
9. Denison E, Asenlof P, Lindberg P. Self-efficacy, fear avoidance, and pain intensity as predictors of disability in subacute and chronic musculoskeletal pain patients in primary health care. *Pain.* 2004;111:245-252.
10. Price DD. *Psychological Mechanisms of Pain and Analgesia (Progress in Pain Research Vol. 15)*. Washington, DC: International Association for the Study of Pain Press; 1999.
11. Cairns MC, Foster NE, Wright CC, Pennington D. Level of distress in a recurrent low back pain population referred for physical therapy. *Spine.* 2003;28:953-959.
12. National Advisory Committee on Health and Disability and Accident Compensation Corporation. *Guide to Assessing Psychosocial Yellow Flags in Acute Low Back Pain: Risk Factors for Long-Term Disability and Work Loss*. Wellington, New Zealand: Author; 1997.
13. Butler D, Moseley GL. *Explain Pain*. Adelaide, Australia: Noigroup Publications; 2003.
14. Burns JW, Glenn B, Lofland K, Bruehl S, Harden RN. Stages of change in readiness to adopt a self management approach to chronic pain: The moderating role of early treatment stage progression in predicting outcome. *Pain.* 2005;115:322-331.
15. Prochaska J, Norcross J, DiClemente C. *Changing for Good*. New York: Morrow; 1994.
16. Ehrlich-Jones L, Zeigler M. *Course Handouts for Beginning Motivational Interviewing*. Chicago, IL: Feinberg School of Medicine, Northwestern University; 2011.
17. Soares JJ, Jabionska B. Psychosocial experiences among primary care patients with and without musculoskeletal pain. *Eur J Pain.* 2004;8:79-89.
18. Waddell G, Newton M, Henderson I, Somerville D, Main CJ. A Fear-Avoidance Beliefs Questionnaire (FABQ) and the role of fear-avoidance beliefs in chronic low back pain and disability. *Pain.* 1993;52:157-168.
19. Jolles BM, Buchbinder R, Beaton DE. A study compared nine patient-specific indices for musculoskeletal disorders. *J Clin Epidemiol.* 2005;58:791-801.
20. Binkley J, Stratford P, Lott S, Riddle D. The Lower Extremity Functional Scale (LEFS): Scale development, measurement properties, and clinical application. *Phys Ther.* 1999;79:371-383.
21. Hudak P, Amadio PC, Bombadier C; Upper Extremity Collaborative Group. Development of an upper extremity outcome measure: The DASH (Disabilities of the Arm, Shoulder and Hand). *Am J Industr Med.* 1996;29:602-608.
22. Vernon H, Mior S. The Neck Disability Index: A study of reliability and validity. *J Manip Physiol Ther.* 1991;14(7):409-415.
23. Fairbank J, Couper J, Davies J, et al. The Oswestry Low Back Pain Questionnaire. *Physiotherapy.* 1980;66:271-273.
24. Stratford P, Gill C, Westaway M, Binkley J. Assessing disability and change on individual patients: A report of a patient specific measure. *Physiother Can.* 1995;47:258-263.
25. Westaway MD, Stratford PW, Binkley JM. The Patient-Specific Functional Scale: Validation of its use in persons with neck dysfunction. *J Orthop Sports Phys Ther.* 1998;27:331-338.
26. Cooper RL, Taylor NF, Feller JA. A randomized controlled trial of proprioceptive and balance training after surgical reconstruction of the anterior cruciate ligament. *Res Sports Med.* 2005;13: 217-230.
27. Pietrobon R, Coeytaux RR, Carey TS, et al. Standard scales for measurement of functional outcome for cervical pain or dysfunction: A systematic review. *Spine.* 2002;27:515-522.
28. Guyatt G, Walter S, Norman G. Measuring change over time: Assessing the usefulness of evaluative instruments. *J Chron Dis.* 1987;40:171-178.
29. Charles C, Gafni A, Whelan T. Shared decision making in the medical encounter: What does it mean? *Soc Sci Med.* 1997;44:681-692.

30. Williams S, Weinman J, Dale J, Newman S. Patient expectations: What do primary care patients want from their GP and how far does meeting expectations affect patient satisfaction? *Fam Pract.* 1995;12:193-201.
31. Ong LML, de Haes CJM, Hoos AM, Lammes FB. Doctor-patient communication: A review of the literature. *Soc Sci Med.* 1995;40:903-918.
32. Laerum E, Indahl A, Skouen J. What is "the good back-consultation"? A combined qualitative and quantitative study of chronic low back pain patients' interaction with and perceptions of consultations with specialists. *J Rehabil Med.* 2006;38:255-262.
33. Main CJ. Concept of treatment and prevention in musculoskeletal disorders. In: Linton SJ, ed. *Pain Research and Clinical Management.* Vol. 12. Amsterdam: Elsevier Science; 2002.
34. Resnik J, Jensen GM. Using clinical outcomes to explore the theory of expert practice in physical therapy. *Phys Ther.* 2003;83:1090-1106.
35. Roberts KJ. Patient empowerment in the United States: A critical commentary. *Health Expect.* 1999;2:82-92.
36. Brennan P, Safran C. Report of conference track 3: Patient empowerment. *Int J Med Inform.* 2003;69:301-304.
37. Becker MH. Patient adherence to prescribed therapies. *Med Care.* 1985;23:539-555.
38. Klenerman L, Slade PD, Stanley IM. The prediction of chronicity in patients with an acute attack of LBP in a general practice setting. *Spine.* 1995;20:478-484.
39. Mazzuca, SA. Does patient education in chronic disease have therapeutic value? *J Chron Dis.* 1982;35:521-529.
40. Carter WB, Inui TS, Kukull WA, Haigh VH. Outcome-based doctor-patient interaction analysis: II. Identifying effective provider and patient behavior. *Med Care.* 1982;20:550-566.
41. Sofaer B, Moore AP, Holloway I, et al. Chronic pain as perceived by older people: A qualitative study. *Age Ageing.* 2005;34:462-466.
42. Turner J, Ersek M, Kemp C. Self-efficacy for managing pain is associated with disability, depression, and pain coping among retirement community residents with chronic pain. *J Pain.* 2005;6:471-479.
43. Steele E, Grimmer K, Thomas B, et al. Virtual reality as a pediatric pain modulation technique: A case study. *Cyberpsychol Behav.* 2003;6:633-638.
44. Breau LM, Camfield CS, McGrath PJ, Finley GA. The incidence of pain in children with severe cognitive impairments. *Arch Pediatr Adolesc Med.* 2003;157:1219-1226.
45. Kramer J, Harker J, Wong AL. Arthritis beliefs and self care in an urban American Indian population. *Arthritis Rheum.* 2002;47:588-594.
46. Moseley GL, Nicholas MK, Hodges PW. A randomized controlled trial of intensive neurophysiology education in chronic low back pain. *Clin J Pain.* 2004;20:324-330.
47. Korsch BM, Negrete VF. Doctor-patient communication. *Sci Am.* 1972;227:66-74.
48. Moseley GL. Unraveling the barriers to reconceptualization of the problem in chronic pain: The actual and perceived ability of patients and health professionals to understand the neurophysiology. *J Pain.* 2003;4:184-189.
49. Moseley GL. Physiotherapy is effective for chronic LBP. *Austr J Physiother.* 2002;48:297-302.

CHAPTER 4

Nociceptive Pain Mechanisms: Inflammation and Ischemia

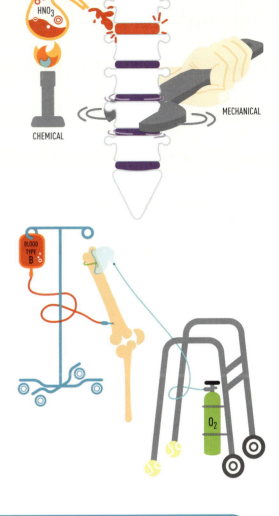

Pain (any pain—emotional, physical, mental) has a message. The information it has about our life can be remarkably specific, but it usually falls into one of two categories: "We would be more alive if we did more of this," and, "Life would be lovelier if we did less of that." Once we get the pain's message, and follow its advice, the pain goes away.

—Peter McWilliams, *Life 101*

POINTS TO DISCUSS

- Processes in nociceptive:inflammatory and nociceptive:ischemia pain mechanisms
- Chemical vs mechanical inflammatory pain
- Stages of connective tissue healing and repair—inflammation, proliferation, and remodeling—and corresponding pain mechanisms
- Healing processes in bone, ligament, intervertebral disc, tendon, and muscle
- Characteristics of subjective and objective evaluations for the nociceptive pain mechanisms
- Guidelines for intervention using baseline activity levels
- Strategies for preventing and managing flare-ups

The first fundamental mechanism that originates from the peripheral nervous system is the nociceptive pain mechanism. Nociceptive pain can be considered either inflammatory or ischemic. It presents as an actual or potential lesion of the musculoskeletal system. Both processes, inflammation and ischemia, result from the deformation of connective tissues (eg, muscle, ligament, bone, tendon, fascia, cartilage), inflammation of innervated structures, and/or stimulation of high-threshold primary afferent C and A-δ fibers.[1,2] Nociception is transmitted along A-δ fibers, which are thinly myelinated fibers that generate a signal with acute, sharp characteristics as a first line of defense. C fibers are unmyelinated and transmit a slower, secondary response over time, resulting in a symptomatic dull and achy response. Damage to the body's tissues is transferred to the brain via protective body systems. Pain, as an output of the brain, teaches the patient's system to react to unpleasant stimuli, resulting in the stimulation of nerve endings that are sensitive to mechanical, chemical, or thermal irritants. Mechanoreceptors detect mechanical displacement of the tissues, chemoreceptors detect chemicals, and thermoreceptors detect temperature changes. Nociceptors are sensory neurons that respond to threats, and the response is then interpreted by the brain and is perceived as pain.

For somatosensation to occur, the body must recognize where it is in space proprioceptively and account for surrounding sensory changes (pain, touch, temperature) using the body's receptors for sensation. Examples of proprioceptive mechanoreceptors include Golgi tendon organs, muscle spindles, and joint receptors. Examples of cutaneous receptors include Pacinian corpuscles, Ruffini corpuscles, Meissner's corpuscles, Merkel disks, and free nerve endings.

The type of nociceptive pain (inflammation or ischemia) patients present with depends in part on their daily activities and habits. Ischemic pain typically involves tissues that become more acidic, hypoxic, and rich in chemicals such as bradykinin, potassium, and prostaglandins,[3] whereas inflammatory pain originates in target tissues as a result of mechanical and physiological processes of tissue injury or abnormal stimulation caused by a physical, chemical, or biological agent.[4] An inflammatory cascade results and generates a traditional pain response. Typically, inflammatory pain results in an abundance of fluid to the tissues generated by the inflammatory response, whereas ischemic pain is a mechanism of insufficient fluid (or lack of oxygenation, nutrition, or blood flow to the tissues). Ischemic pain requires movement, easily and often, to help targeted tissues recover from their hypoxic state. Inflammation requires controlled motion and identification of inflammatory triggers while establishing baseline activity levels to help targeted tissues proceed to a reparative state.

When using the pain mechanism classification system (PMCS), it is crucial to do a subjective evaluation, provisionally classify the pain mechanism, and then perform a thorough repeated movement examination to validate or refute the provisional classification. Once the provisional classification has been confirmed, the clinician can develop a treatment plan and home exercise programs that are individualized to the patient.

Types of Inflammation

Chemical pain is the cascade that results when tissues undergo inflammation or are under constant irritation, whereas *mechanical pain* is pain that originates from a sustained or intermittent deformation of the tissues. **Table 4.1** highlights the differences between chemical and mechanical inflammation.

TABLE 4.1 Chemical Versus Mechanical Inflammation

Characteristic	Chemical Inflammation	Mechanical Inflammation
Cause	Cascade from tissue inflammatory process	Sustained or intermittent deformation of the tissues
		Signs of directional preference and centralization
Frequency of symptoms	Constant	Intermittent or constant
Modalities	May be helpful	Typically no effect
Medication	May be helpful	May have no effect

Chemical Inflammation

Chemical pain is unrelenting; it is constant. There is not a moment when the patient does not feel pain because of the chemical state of the tissues. Chemical inflammation may be activated because of infection (bacterial, viral, fungal, parasitic, toxin), presence of foreign bodies, trauma (blunt or penetrating), presence of physical or chemical agents (eg, burn, frostbite, irradiation, pressure, vibration), or autoimmune or allergic response at the tissue level. The clinician attempting to treat a chemical inflammatory state must use the patient's pain as a guide. Modalities may assist in decreasing edema or reducing the inflammatory response in the tissues. A repeated movement examination of most directions makes the pain worse.

Mechanical Inflammation

It is possible to sensitize a joint and create musculoskeletal pain via local irritants. In cats, a knee joint that originally presents with no mechanosensitivity becomes sensitive to experimental arthritis induced in low- and high-threshold units.[5] A similar sensitivity can occur in humans if a peripheral joint becomes mechanically irritated. The sensitization of unmyelinated C fibers can result in mechanical hypersensitivity through the actions of proinflammatory cytokines such as interleukin 6 (IL-6), which lowers the activation thresholds of the high-threshold nociceptors and increases the responsiveness of low-threshold fibers.[6] Osteoarthritic mechanisms include the release of these mediators from synovial structures or bone and the instigation of pain from sensory fiber innervations from periosteum, subchondral, and marrow bone.[7] The repeated movement examination in the objective evaluation assists the clinician in determining what mechanical irritant and mechanism are dominating.

Mechanical pain in a nociceptive:inflammatory state becomes evident as the patient's repeated movement examination reveals a connection with movements or positions. Mechanical pain is intermittent. It comes and goes and is dependent on movement positions or activities. Bogduk[8] observed, "There are no drugs available that can inhibit the transduction of mechanical nociception. It is therefore futile to attempt to treat mechanical nociception with peripherally-acting drugs. Mechanical transduction can only be treated by correcting the mechanical abnormality triggering nociception."(p80)

During the movement examination, pain that changes from constant to intermittent indicates a mechanical component because chemical pain typically worsens rather than improves with repeated movement testing. If improvement occurs with movement, the clinician has likely found a directional preference. *Directional preference* occurs when positioning or repetitive movements in one direction decrease or abolish pain and cause a patient's symptoms to move proximal, or closer to midline, and to improve as a result.[9] If the movement examination does not improve the pain outright, the clinician may consider several diagnostic possibilities. The exam may reveal the mechanical diagnosis and therapy (MDT) syndrome of derangement (see Chapter 2) if a preferred direction is established after more repetition of movement. The history may reveal another classification—a contractile or articular dysfunction—that may be currently inflamed because of significant stress to the tissues. The patient may present as mechanically inconclusive or as having an irreducible derangement, meaning that no direction of movement creates a lasting improvement in the patient's symptoms. Pain that changes from intermittent to constant during a movement examination can result from irritation to the tissues and the creation of a local mechanical inflammatory response.

True nociceptive back pain typically presents as a dull aching in the back. It is evoked by stimulation of noxious lumbar spine structures. In turn, somatic referred pain typically shares the same segmental innervations as the source of spinal discomfort, and this pain can spread in a way that is difficult to localize.[10] Radicular pain, in contrast, results from a discharge from the dorsal nerve root or its ganglion and from the affected nerve. Bogduk[10] differentiated radicular pain from radiculopathy, which is a neurological state in which sensory and motor fiber damage can result in objective neurological signs of sensory or motor loss. We consider the nociceptive pain mechanisms to operate in much the same way as radiculopathy, and radicular pain is referred to in this book as the peripheral neurogenic pain mechanism (discussed in Chapter 5).

Connective Tissue Healing and Repair

The human body is composed of cells and a connective tissue matrix within the mechanical system. Each component plays diverse roles in resisting mechanical forces. The extracellular matrix consists of fibers, proteoglycans, and glycoproteins. Fibers or fibrous components such as elastin and collagen aid the body in resisting tensile loads and form the tendons and ligaments. Proteoglycans resist compressive forces, provide hydration and stabilization to the tissues, form parts of the interstitial spaces and basement membranes, and function as receptors (eg, articular cartilage). Glycoproteins aid in linkage of the extracellular matrix and creation of the body's mechanical system.[11] Culav et al[11] provided an in-depth review of the connective tissue matrix. When connective tissue experiences a traumatic event, its function may be altered, but it follows a predictable pattern of healing, and exercise has a beneficial effect on restoring the tissues to optimal health.

Healing has three phases, each requiring very specific rehabilitation goals: inflammation, proliferation, and remodeling. **Table 4.2** summarizes the phases of healing and identifies the principle pain mechanism in each phase.

TABLE 4.2 Phases of Healing and Potential Pain Mechanism in Each Phase

Phase of Healing	Time Frame	Potential Pain Mechanism
Inflammation	0–7 days	Nociceptive:inflammatory
Proliferation	5–21 days	Nociceptive:ischemia
Remodeling	21+ days	Nociceptive:ischemia

Nociceptive:Inflammatory Pain Mechanism

The first phase of healing, the inflammation phase, can take up to 7 days for mild sprains and strains and longer, up to 6 weeks, if the health of the tissues is poor or the sprain, strain, or rupture is serious. At the cellular level, the initial onset of inflammation begins with a transient vasoconstriction to protect the body against blood loss, followed by microvascular dilatation with leukocyte infiltration, which causes redness and swelling at the arteriole level.[12] During the acute cellular response, granulocytes appear, typically neutrophils and then monocytes, which mature into inflammatory macrophages and proliferate.[13] The resulting action of inflammatory mediators can produce hypersensitivity in the tissues via sensory neurons. Overexcitability through depolarization can occur, with a resultant lowered firing threshold and then delayed repolarization.[14] Biosynthesis occurs during the initial acute inflammatory process, and apoptosis results in a shortened period of neutrophil infiltration. Subsequently neutrophils are phagocytized by macrophages present at the site. Reparative cytokines such as transforming growth factor β1 clear neutrophils from the area as a result.[13] Macrophages can be reprogrammed by ingesting apoptotic cells and thereby promote repair or emigration into the lymphatic system. The body's lymphatic system helps stop the inflammatory process through removal of macrophages.[13]

During the inflammation phase of healing, therapeutic treatment must take into account the newly injured tissues, and the practitioner should work the patient in the middle of his or her available range of motion using pain as a guide. The MICE algorithm—motion, ice, compression, and elevation—should be applied in this phase. A gradual reduction of inflammation and inflammatory mediators occurs over 3 to 6 weeks, so midrange motion should progress to full range of motion by 4 to 6 weeks in healthy patients. Patients should be considered on a case-by-case basis, however, based on their stage of healing. During this period, the clinician should rule out a directional preference through the patient's movements using pain and mechanical response to motion as a guide.[12,15-17]

All tissue traumas begin with a chemical process, and the mechanical properties of pain gradually become more evident as time progresses. It is critical during early management not to introduce too much motion too quickly in a range of motion program. Overstressing the tissues could affect tissue repair and consequently facilitate the production of chemical mediators. The inflammation phase of healing is the one time during musculoskeletal rehabilitation when the clinician should educate patients not to reproduce or increase their symptoms too frequently because doing so can delay the reparative process that will follow. **Figure 4.1** is a patient education handout on the nociceptive:inflammatory pain mechanism. **Appendix 4.A** describes a patient with nociceptive:inflammatory pain who is in the inflammatory phase of healing.

Nociceptive:Ischemia Pain Mechanism

The nociceptive:inflammatory pain mechanism encompasses only the first phase of tissue healing. The next two phases of healing, proliferation and remodeling, can involve the nociceptive:ischemia pain mechanism as the patient transitions into a reparative stage. If a new stressor occurs, or if the patient encounters a new trauma during the proliferation or remodeling phases, the nociceptive:inflammatory pain mechanism can become the dominant pain mechanism once again. For example, if a patient with a new surgical repair of the rotator cuff uses the surgical extremity at 4 to 6 weeks and overshoots his or her surgical precautions with excessive activity, the patient may find that the area becomes warm, red, swollen, and irritated and that he or she is unable to sleep or rest comfortably in the immobilization device.

FIGURE 4.1 Nociceptive:Inflammatory Pain Mechanism Patient Education Handout

Inflammation Pain

WHAT IS INFLAMMATION?

Inflammation is the body's response to injury or flare-up. A *flare-up* is increased pain (at least 2 points on a scale of 0 = *no pain* to 10 = *worst pain ever*) that lasts more than a day. Symptoms can include any of the following: redness, pain, warmth, swelling, loss of movement, and loss of function. Inflammation is a sign that your body is starting the repair process after a flare-up or injury. The body's cells release chemicals to alert the nervous system, which in turn alerts you by creating pain! Once this chain begins, you have entered the healing stages.

WHAT ARE THE CAUSES?

Injuries that may cause inflammatory pain include

- Tissue damage or trauma, including surgery, bone fracture, or ligament or cartilage tear
- Overactivity or repetitive movements or flare-up, such as muscle sprain, joint strain, bursitis, or arthritis.

WHAT DOES INFLAMMATION FEEL LIKE?

If you have inflammatory pain, you might describe it as follows:

- Your pain will be in a specific, pinpointed location, and you might tell the clinician, "It hurts right here" and point to the location of the pain.
- You might have muscular or joint tightness and tell the clinician, "I feel stiff."
- You might have swelling or edema and tell the clinician, "I see swelling."
- If you've had joint trauma, you might tell the clinician, "I hear crackling."

WHAT CAN YOU DO?

First, it is important to recognize the type of pain you have and to seek the attention of a medical professional for proper diagnosis. As you progress through your healing, you can expect to work through the following stages:

1. Inflammatory stage: 1 to 2 weeks after injury
   - For the first 72 hours, it is important to use MICE (comfortable range of motion, ice, compression, and elevation).
   - Movement is recommended within tolerance. Remember, pain is your guide! Recognize your baseline or level of tolerance for daily activity. Try to move only in the midranges, that is, don't try to overdo or overstretch the muscles or do too much activity.
   - Refer to your flare-up plan for additional strategies.

2. Proliferation stage: 2 to 4 weeks after injury
   - Your body is starting to build scar tissue. It is important to work through mid-ranges or in a pain-free range to stretch and strengthen this scar tissue.
   - Remember, "no worse" is your guide. It is important not to increase your pain level after any activity, again recognizing your baseline or tolerance level for tasks and exercise. *No worse* is defined as having the same or lesser level of pain after you complete your daily tasks and activities than when you started. If your pain increases but then diminishes by the end of the day, you are performing in a good range. If your pain lasts until the next day or longer, you are having a flare-up, and it is time to review your activity baseline. Your activities may need to be adjusted to keep you within the no-worse range. Work with your clinician to find a good pacing strategy and establish a flare-up plan that will work for you.
   - You can also use heat therapy to reduce pain and promote tissue healing. (Check with your health professional regarding the use and duration of heat.) Heat therapy can include hot packs, water bottles, and over-the-counter low-level heat wraps.

3. Remodeling stage: week 4 and beyond
   - You are in the final stages of healing! It is important to keep a close record of your tolerance of activities and exercise and to look for the potential to increase your activity and function daily.
   - Start working at the end ranges of movement to continue to strengthen scar tissue and reeducate once-injured tissues to tolerate your preexisting activities. Muscles and joints can begin to take heavier challenges to increase strength.
   - Remember, *no worse* is still your guide. To feel pain at the end of movements is good to strengthen tissue and fully heal, but your pain should get no worse as a result.

WHAT ELSE CAN HELP?

Inflammatory pain can respond well to anti-inflammatory pain medications. Talk with your physician to explore your medication options.

Resource
Caudill MA. *Managing Pain Before It Manages You*. Rev ed. New York: Guilford Press; 2002.

Proliferation Phase

The second phase of healing, the proliferation phase, may take between 5 and 21 days, depending on the degree of injury or surgery. Fibroblastic infiltration and collagen formation begin to occur, showing early signs of scar formation. The scar tissue at this stage has less tensile strength than in later stages of healing. Treatment consisting of midrange movement should begin in all three planes of motion (transverse, frontal, and sagittal) with the goal of achieving full range of motion by approximately 4 to 6 weeks. Occasionally there may be a rationale for delaying the achievement of this full range of motion, such as the need to allow tissue stiffness to occur to promote bone or tendon healing or the need to follow surgical repair guidelines. The clinician should use the patient's pain as a guide, and movements should progress into the barrier of stiffness and pain; however, pain should abate on release of the movement. If the pain persists several hours after completion of exercises, the inflammatory process may be retriggered, and healing will be delayed.

An option during the proliferation stage of healing is a trial of continuous low-level heat therapy to maximize blood flow and allow greater active range of tissue motion.[18-20] An adverse reaction to low-level heat may indicate the presence of peripheral sensitization.[21]

The strength of reparative collagen depends on appropriate application of stress to the tissues during the proliferation stage of healing (see **Figure 4.2**). Motion with a low-level tensile load is critical to organize granulation tissue in the lines of stress to restore function in the newly formed scar within the connective tissue. It is easy to overstress and reinitiate the injury and the chemical process of inflammation with too much tensile load too quickly. In spinal disc granulation tissue, studies have shown a difference between the reparative granulation tissue response to stress (pressure created by discography) and the inflammatory granulation tissue response to stress.[22] The inflammatory granulation tissue produces the proinflammatory cytokines and mediators that sensitize the nociceptors, whereas the reparative granulation tissue produces a blood flow reaction with no inflammatory production.[22] This difference explains why a patient's responses to movement act like inflammation on some days and like ischemia on other days.

The clinician should determine whether the tissue is ready for end range stress through the patient's history and a thorough repeated movement exam working toward end range. In

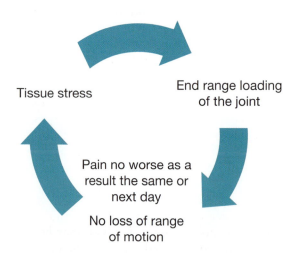

FIGURE 4.2 Cycle of appropriate tissue stress.

the proliferation stage, worsening of symptoms immediately after the activity, later that day, or the next day is an indication that too much stress was placed on the tissues too quickly. When an injury has occurred, the body goes through a natural course of events to ensure proper regeneration and repair of the connective tissue that was traumatized. The clinician can assist this natural course of events by calming the patient's catastrophic thinking and facilitating application of proper, progressive stress to healing tissue to maximize strength of repair and return the tissue to previous levels of function. **Appendix 4.B** describes a patient with nociceptive:inflammatory pain in the proliferation phase of healing.

Remodeling Phase

The remodeling phase of healing can take from 21 days to 1 year or more, depending on initial tissue health and severity of the injury. As remodeling progresses, scar tensile strength increases and vascularity decreases. Pain becomes less of a guide and determinant during this stage. Especially with the MDT syndrome of dysfunction, producing pain becomes the goal for remodeling. Treatment in this phase focuses on increasing stress to the scar tissue to ensure that appropriate tensile stresses are applied to the joint. Specific movements can help load the tissue to improve its capacity to perform at an optimal level for the required functional task. The treatment goal is to provide end range stress to the involved connective tissue to create enough load to transform the involved tissue.

Tissues and structures must be assessed in loaded and unloaded states. Sometimes a tissue can tolerate being loaded (with gravity) better than it can tolerate being unloaded (without gravity). If the tissue is unable to respond positively to an unloaded situation (eg, in which the effect of gravity is eliminated), it may become more appropriate to stress the tissue with some added load or property of increased weightbearing. For example, when a specific patient who has neck radiculopathy lies down (ie, unloads), the pain peripheralizes down the arm and the symptoms increase. When the patient sits up, however, the pain improves, and the patient is able to tolerate neck movements without peripheralization of symptoms. In this example, rehabilitation may proceed by remodeling the tissues in a loaded state and then reassessing in an unloaded state as the patient improves. Another example is a patient who cannot tolerate taking weight through the hip joint while walking but who responds well to extension stretching of the hip. For this patient, it may be desirable to start prone and initiate stretching in that position versus starting in tall kneel (loaded) or with the knee on a chair (semi-loaded).

The clinician can estimate the time needed to remodel on the basis of blood supply to the injured tissue. Clinical experience and research indicate that in healthy adults, mild sprains and strains can take a different amount of time to achieve 95% return of tensile force, indicating that the tissue is ready for advancement of a functional program to a sport-specific level. Muscle requires approximately 2 weeks to achieve 95% of its tensile strength; however, ligament, peripheral nerve, cartilage, and disc can take at least 16 weeks to achieve 95% tensile strength, and with some ligamentous injuries, that level of strength may never return. Tendon, on the other hand, can still gain strength up to 52 weeks post injury. Training of healthy tendon also increases tensile strength and tissue stiffness.[23] In healing states, changes in mechanical properties may be related to the concentration of intermolecular cross-links in the tendon as opposed to an actual increase in collagen concentrations.[23]

Unnecessarily restricting a patient's activities can be a disservice to the patient because the tissue will not be prepared for functional activities and will not be able to properly progress in a restoration of function program. Just as it may be a problem to do too much too soon, it is detrimental to not do enough during the remodeling stage of healing. Appropriate stress to the appropriate tissue is critical. If an injury occurs, the clinician needs to identify the healing stage and the level of activity the patient is performing to accelerate healing. **Appendix 4.C** describes a patient with nociceptive:ischemia pain in the remodeling phase of healing.

Healing Processes in Specific Tissue Types

Bone

Bone serves a mechanical purpose. It protects internal and vital organs from trauma, provides the body its basic shape, facilitates movement, and forms a framework for support. Bone is a dynamic tissue that, like other tissues, is driven by dynamic load. Constant remodeling of bone occurs in response to its mechanical environment via bone cells that adapt to resist the loads experienced during habitual activity. Turner[24] noted that for bone adaptation to occur, only a short duration of loading is necessary; extended loading durations have diminishing adaptive returns. In addition, bone cells accommodate to customary loading, making them less responsive to routine loading signals.

The properties of bone—the integrity of structure, mineralization (stiffness), work to failure (energy required to break), and displacement (inversely related to brittleness)—are important factors to consider in a rehabilitation or exercise program.[25] If energy applied exceeds what bone can absorb, it will break. Stress-strain curves help clinicians determine the amount of energy needed for a bone to break. Strength is independent of the size or shape of the bone.[25] A bone that is more compliant with a large displacement but not well mineralized (eg, in a child) requires more energy to break than a brittle, highly mineralized bone (eg, in an adult who has osteoporosis).[25] Bones that undergo greater trauma experience greater energy of impact, resulting in cracks secondary to the high release of energy.

Bone cells called osteoblasts (formation), osteocytes (communication and homeostasis), and osteoclasts (resorption) help with bone adaptation or modeling and remodeling of bone. Bone forms in areas where it is under the greatest strain. It is not yet known exactly how cells that transduce, or respond to mechanical signals, influence bone formation and resorption to create an anabolic response. Hormones such as parathyroid and estrogen can affect mechanical loading as well.[25] As research sheds more clarity on bone communication, clinicians will have better guidance for targeting bone loading and osteoporosis prevention through strengthening or pharmacological techniques.

Little evidence indicates that exercise can specifically influence disease processes in bone, muscle health, or fractures.[26] To date, not much is known about ways to facilitate bone regeneration and fracture healing other than typical healing guidelines. Although technologies are increasing at a rapid rate, more information is needed for critical analysis of treatments such as gene therapy, tissue engineering, growth factors, osteoconductive agents, and physical forces, which still lack good evidence for use in clinical practice.[27] In addition, research findings on the effect of vitamin D and E supplementation on bone fracture healing remain inconclusive.[28,29] General recommendations for osteoporosis prevention include at least 1000 mg of calcium, 800 IU of vitamin D, and 1 g/kg body weight of protein daily.[29]

Ligament

Unlike other tissues, ligaments never recover their initial resistance to load when injured; however, moderate exercise can aid in promoting optimal function.[30,31] Injured ligaments present with a disorganized collagen network capillary development and randomly oriented scar tissue. Cross-sectional area is reduced, and enlarged collagen fibers are difficult to return to their normal ability to resist tension based on tissue mass and mechanical resistance.[30,31]

Intervertebral Disc

Biomechanical and potential biochemical causes of pain can occur in spinal tissues as well as various joint structures. Disruption of the intervertebral lumbar disc can also be a source of pain through physiological changes to its internal structure,[32] which can induce changes in innervation. Degenerative discs can present with extensive innervation, and nerve fibers can be reactive to substance P.[33] A loss of hydration of the disc itself and changes in type II collagen denaturation can result in decreased inherent stability of the disc.[32,34-36] Unlike a healthy disc, a degenerative disc is slow to resist creep and will deform at smaller loads, so its reparative process must be considered in appropriate rehabilitation.[37] Pain can come from the endplate, the outer annulus, or torn annular fissures that can change the inherent structure of the disc.[38] The intervertebral disc also contains nerve fibers with neuropeptides that have pain-transmitting effects.[39,40] Patients with degenerative disc disease demonstrate increased vascularity and calcitonin gene–related peptide and substance P sensory nerves in the endplate region; these signs can also be seen in various tendon pathologies.[40]

Chemical stimuli can play a role as well. Herniated disc material has a high glutamate concentration.[41] This neuroprotective response could affect receptors in the dorsal root ganglion and drive nociception.[40-42] Patients undergoing fusions and diagnosed with sciatica may have different levels of proinflammatory mediators (IL-6, IL-8, and prostaglandin E2).[43,44] Disc herniations may cause changes in nerve root structure and function through nerve injury as well as actual deformation to the disc or neighboring structures.[45] Changes in the extracellular matrix of the disc can also create inflammatory reactions. Mast cells can promote a chemotactic environment, secrete nerve growth factor, and promote angiogenesis; this process may lead to increases in inflammatory mediators such as substance P neurotransmitters, which may sensitize the intervertebral disc.[46]

Tumor necrosis factor alpha (TNF) is a proinflammatory cytokine that can be found in disc material of symptomatic patients.[47] This exposure to nuclear material and TNF may lead to apoptosis at the surface of the dorsal root ganglion and sensitize the sensory neurons.[48] In addition, high levels of phospholipase A2 can present in herniated and degenerative discs.[49] The nucleus pulposus from a herniated disc can create leukotaxis and increased vascular permeability.[50] An autoimmune response to the nucleus pulposus may also attract T and B cells and create a local immune reaction.[51] Thus, during rehabilitation the clinician must consider the biochemical and biomechanical status of the tissue and use research recommendations in clinical practice in the treatment of the spine (and all tissues).

Tendon

Anatomically, the tendon comprises tendon cells (tenocytes), an extracellular matrix (with ground substance), and parallel arrays of collagen fibers as the dominant fiber. Among fibers, collagen structurally has a triple helix region in its molecule that aids in its ability to withstand tensile load. The ground substance is made of proteoglycan and glycosaminoglycan chains. The tenocytes produce the collagen molecules that line up to produce collagen fibrils. Collagen fibrils produce the basic unit of a tendon, the collagen fiber, with elongated tenocytes packed between them. Tendon fascicles are connective tissue–bound collagen fibers, and the endotenon separates the tendon fascicles. Groups of fascicles are bounded by the epitendon, which is a fine connective tissue sheath comprising the tendon organ.[52,53]

In the presence of nociceptive:inflammatory and nociceptive:ischemia pain, tendon rehabilitation can be confusing, and semantics can interfere with rehabilitation. Consider the way clinicians discuss tendinopathy and tendonitis. True tendonitis can present like the nociceptive:inflammatory pain mechanism; however, chronic inflammation that is degenerative in process is technically a tendinosis and will not present like inflammatory pain because no inflammatory cells are present in the tissue. *Tendonitis* is an acute inflammatory condition in the tendon that can occur for a variety of reasons. *Tendinosis* is a histopathological degeneration in the tendon that causes a breakdown in connective tissues and a failed healing response.[52] Chronic tendonitis as a diagnosis can present with an ischemic mechanism that needs frequent movement and remodeling for appropriate rehabilitation.

Typically, tendon overload injuries occur with high training loads and overuse.[53] Tendons are slow-healing structures that show significant changes in pathology when they undergo trauma or stress. Pathological tendons have increases in ground substance and a greater proportion of large proteoglycans in their composition.[54] In chronic Achilles tendinopathies, specific degenerative changes can occur, with tendinosis changes involving "abnormal fiber structure, focal hypercellularity and vascular proliferation."[55(p151)] Pain typically signals paratenonitis, which can then lead to the ischemic lesion tendinosis.[54]

Chronic tendon injuries may reveal subjective and objective evaluation components similar to those of the nociceptive:inflammatory pain mechanism. At the cellular level, however, typically it is not inflammation that is present, but rather a chronic degenerative cellular process. This condition typically is treated like most ischemic pain mechanisms with a remodeling process that produces pain during the exercise or movement but gets no worse through the evening or next day. Repetitive icing of tendinosis will not move the patient toward tissue remodeling but rather will retard healing.

In addition, the subjective evaluation should include questions about the patient's activities because if the area feels better with increased stress, then telling the patient to cease activities could hinder the rehabilitation process; for example, a patient with chronic tendinopathy that worsens during the day as he or she sits at a desk at work but improves with running should interrupt the sitting rather than ease the running. Tendon biopsies in chronic tendinosis have shown an absence of inflammatory cell infiltration with no upregulation of proinflammatory cytokines. They also have shown higher glutamate levels, calcification, degenerative changes, and poor vascular supply, and higher lactate levels have been found in painful or ruptured tendons.[56,57] Most tendinopathies histologically do not have inflammatory cells in their composition; however, the tissue may still present with pain that results from the mechanical loading as opposed to true inflammation. It is important to reflect on tissue healing properties based on the stresses needed for appropriate rehabilitation.

Significant research supports the use of eccentric exercise with chronic healing tendons that have undergone degenerative changes. The use of eccentric strengthening has been supported with upper extremity as well as lower extremity tendon injuries.[52,58,59] Therapeutically, eccentric training has resulted in decreased tendon thickness and no remaining neovascularization in tendons of patients with midportion Achilles tendinosis.[56] The concept behind this finding is that the load that created the initial injury may have been an eccentric one, but this eccentric load could also restart and complete the healing process in chronic tendons. Vasculoneural ingrowth has been observed in chronic tendinosis tendons.[60] Interestingly, however, an 8-year study of patients with Achilles tendinosis found that 41% of patients eventually developed pain on exertion or with overuse in the uninvolved tendon, but the difference was not significant between the subchronic and acute pain patient groups.[61] In addition, researchers found no differences between surgically treated and nonoperative patients with acute to subchronic Achilles tendinopathy and noted that long-term prognosis is favorable.[60]

It has been speculated that many tendon injuries are based on excessive load; however, the specific mechanism of Achilles, patellar, and epicondylar tendinopathies is unclear. Some have speculated that malalignments, joint mobility, or training errors may play a role.[57] What is important to understand is how to rehabilitate acute and ischemic pain mechanism.[57] Conscious communication, boundaries on activity, and a well-implemented rehabilitation regimen are integral to the treatment of patients with chronic tendon pathology who experience repetitive inflammatory reactions because of a lack of understanding of the cycle of pain production (see **Appendix 4.C**).

When educating patients about appropriate tissue stresses, the clinician should counsel them to avoid activity that produces an increase in pain 2 hours later, 12 hours later, and 24 hours later, or they run the risk of creating an acute inflammatory process by doing too much too fast. Patients should be aware of their symptoms over this timeline because this information helps the clinician advise them on appropriate remodeling guidelines, whether for a new exercise following surgery or a return to running after a period of inactivity.

A significant amount of research has examined the use of eccentric exercise in chronic tendinitis in the Achilles and patellar tendons. A critical review of the literature on patellar tendinopathy supported the idea that use of a decline board should produce some level of discomfort in the tendon itself.[62] The patient is shown barefooted highlighting the final progression of exercise encouraging the greatest amount of eccentric end range load of the foot, ankle, and knee (**Figure 4.3**). Patients with painful eccentric and concentric patellar pain were compared, and only eccentric quadriceps training on a decline board reduced pain in jumper's knee with patellar tendinopathy.[63] It appears that the decline board supports greater improvement than a foot flat, eccentric squat alone.[58]

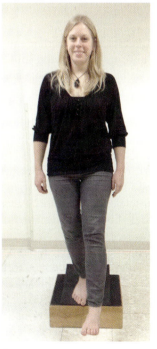 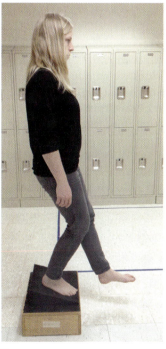

A B

FIGURE 4.3 Step down decline wedge. (**A**) Frontal plane mechanical view. (**B**) Sagittal plane mechanical view.

Stanish et al[64] discussed an eccentric training program based on increasing the length of the musculotendinous unit, increasing the load of the tendon, and increasing the force developed through speed of the contraction. Their initial program started with static stretching repeated several times and then eccentric exercise. This was progressed in 2/3/2-day increments from slow to moderate to fast progression over the week (day 1–2, slow; day 3–5, moderate; day 6–7, fast). The patient then ended with a stretch and icing program for 5 to 10 minutes.[64]

In addition to patellar tendinopathy, eccentric training has been shown to be effective with midportion Achilles tendinosis but less successful in insertional tendinopathy. Jonsson et al,[65] in a pilot study, showed promising results with insertional tendinopathy if the eccentric exercise was modified to eliminate loading in dorsiflexion.

There is no agreement on how much discomfort should occur or the frequency or duration of the exercise regimen. From a patient education perspective, Jonsson and Alfredson[63] recommended that the patient decide how much pain is acceptable, whereas Visnes and Bahr[62] recommended a pain level of 4 to 5 on a scale of 0 to 10 during training sessions and progressively increasing activity as pain decreases. Both forms of patient education are sound in logic; however, because of variations in patient anxiety, pain tolerance, and ability to self-manage, one strategy may make more sense than the other for an individualized rehabilitation program.

At best, all of these eccentric techniques are appropriate and need to be studied with more comparisons between rehabilitation programs. Eccentric exercises should be considered with nociceptive ischemic tendinopathy rehabilitation, but more research is needed with regard to specific frequency, intensity, duration, and type of tendinopathy or tissue.

Muscle

Skeletal muscle damage can occur through the same mechanisms that cause inflammation, including physical, chemical, thermal, infection, autoimmune insult, and degenerative disease processes. Contusions, lacerations, strains, ischemia, and complete ruptures to the muscle itself also occur. Ischemia can further skeletal tissue damage to the muscle through a lack of oxygen to necessary tissues.[66,67] Disruptions to the musculotendinous unit are more susceptible to injury than normal muscle tissue.[68] With tendon rehabilitation, muscle can take a prolonged period to achieve sufficient tensile strength. Return to sport or activity can increase the risk of injury if it occurs too quickly. In addition, if injections are used to diminish the pain and facilitate return to sport, the potential for complete rupture can increase.[68] Although muscle fiber after injury shows significant reparative qualities, microscopic damage to the contractile element of the muscle can occur with eccentric contraction of the muscle. Lengthening the contraction of muscle fibers or eccentric muscle contraction has also been shown to lead to skeletal muscle damage.[69]

Eccentric exercises have been linked to disturbance of calcium dynamics, Z-line disruption, and damaged sarcomeres.[67,69] Morgan and Allen[69] identified factors in mechanisms for reduced tension following eccentric exercises in muscle that included fatigue (weaker sarcomeres can be overstretched during eccentric contraction), electrical inexcitability or fiber death, shifts in the length-tension curve of muscle, and reductions in excitation-contraction coupling. Greater tension or force to the muscle results in greater muscle damage.[70] In a controlled situation in the muscle belly, tensile strength was not significantly different at any time period in an experimentally controlled nondisruptive muscle strain injury. Although strength trended toward lower values at 7 days, risk of rupture did not increase significantly.[71] This finding is consistent with the fact that the muscle was able to develop 90% of the tension produced by its contralateral control muscle in a week's time.

Typically, therefore, muscle returns to full function in a reasonably quick time frame, but rupture is a risk if the patient returns to a sport with increased eccentric movement too soon. Sufficient warm-ups help increase temperature in the muscle, and preconditioned muscles are able to stretch to a greater length from rest before failing than unconditioned muscles, although exact parameters in sport have not been sufficiently assessed.[72]

Nociceptive Pain Mechanism Evaluation

The subjective and objective pain evaluations reveal characteristics that help the clinician classify the dominant pain mechanism. Symptom characteristics specific to the nociceptive:inflammatory and nociceptive:ischemia pain mechanisms are described in the sections that follow. Table 4.3 summarizes typical features of evaluation findings with the nociceptive pain mechanisms.

TABLE 4.3 Subjective and Objective Features of the Nociceptive:Inflammatory and Nociceptive:Ischemia Pain Mechanisms

Feature	Nociceptive:Inflammatory	Nociceptive:Ischemia
Subjective Findings		
Location	Localized	Localized
Frequency	Constant or intermittent	Intermittent
Descriptors	Swollen, throbbing, aching	Fatigue, weakness, tightness
Onset	Within 3 weeks of injury or a recent flare-up of a chronic condition	Onset may be for no apparent reason; onset can be positional or cumulative or greater than 21 days after connective tissue injury in a remodeling phase
24-hour behavior	Increased pain in the morning; gets better throughout the day, then worsens at the end of the day and during the night	Typically better in the morning and worse in the afternoon or after maintaining an activity or position for 1-3 hours
Objective Findings		
Mechanical diagnosis for preferred direction (derangement, dysfunction, posture, other)	A close stimulus-response relationship is found. Pain responds to a mechanical diagnosis for preferred direction.	Dysfunction (contractile or articular) = pain produced at end range loading, loss of movement that is as a result no worse on repeated movements. Patient may have a painful arc of motion or region where contractile tissue is challenged in contractile dysfunction. Pain related to quality, function, activation, or positioning. Poor remodeling and healing are present.
Chemical	Every movement increases pain. Pain gets worse with static and repeated movement testing. Mechanical outcome is inconclusive.	

Subjective Evaluation

Pain Location, Description, and Frequency

Both inflammatory and ischemic pain present with localized pain complaints. The patient may be able to point to a specific joint or area of pain when these mechanisms dominate. Patients almost never complain of diffuse generalized pain throughout the body but rather report a local constant dull ache or throb at rest in one region.[73] The clinician should clear all other regions of the body to ensure the symptoms really are local. Many patients have symptoms that appear local because of intensity, but when asked they admit to having other locations of lower intensity, thereby requiring the clinician to investigate further.

Patients with nociceptive pain typically describe it with words such as *aching, dull,* or *throbbing.* Patients may describe an element of sharpness with certain movements and may complain of warmth or swelling as well.[74] Patients with inflammatory pain use words such as *swollen, stiffness, cracking, gnawing,* and *aching,* whereas those with ischemic pain typically describe it as *fatigue, weakness,* or *tightness.* Inflammatory and ischemic pain may be described using similar words, but ischemic pain tends to cause complaints that echo the need for movement.

Regarding frequency of pain, inflammatory pain may be either constant or intermittent because inflammation can be chemical, mechanical, or a combination of the two. Chemical inflammatory pain does not shut off; it is constant. There is not one moment when the pain is not present. Chemical pain may persist and may need time or chemicals (ie, medications) to diminish the inflammatory process and calm the tissues. Typically, as the chemical inflammation decreases, the patient is left with mechanical inflammation or pain that is affected by directions and positions. Directional preference indicates a direction-sensitive mechanical problem that can maintain inflammation if not addressed.

Ischemic pain presents with intermittent symptoms. By the nature of the mechanism, it never produces constant chemical pain. Deconditioned tissues that need blood and oxygen are able to shut off the pain or find a position of relief when the tissues are at rest and under no stress.

Onset or Mechanism of Injury

Inflammatory pain has a precipitating event, movement, or activity. It becomes evident to the patient quickly or, in a chronic condition, within 1 to 2 days of a flare-up after an increase in activity. Ischemic pain can come on for no apparent reason. It can be positional or cumulative and can occur more than 21 days after an injury as tissues progress to the proliferation and remodeling stages of healing.

24-Hour Behavior of Symptoms

Inflammatory pain presents with a diurnal pattern; the pain is worse in the morning and tends to get better as the day goes on. If the patient mechanically irritates the pain, it may worsen again by the evening. The pain is persistent through the night, and the same pattern occurs the next day. Patients with the ischemic pain mechanism report pain that is worse in the evening or after 1 to 3 hours of sustained activity or positioning. Pain typically is better in the morning because of rest and positions of minimal stress.

Thoughts, Beliefs, and Cultural Attitudes Toward Pain

Patients with inflammatory and ischemic pain typically do not present with fears, worries, concerns, beliefs, depression, anxiety, or personality disorders as contributing factors to the pain experience. These patients usually have a negative psychosocial screen.

Past and Current Treatments

Patients with inflammatory pain may respond to ice or simple nonsteroidal anti-inflammatory drugs.[73] Nociceptive:ischemia pain does not respond to medications directed at nociception.

Readiness for Treatment

Patients who are not ready for treatment typically do not perform as well in rehabilitation as patients who are ready to change their behavior. It is important for clinicians to determine how ready the patient is to change and accept potential treatment regardless of the dominating mechanism (see Chapter 3).

Objective Evaluation: Repeated Movement Examination

Repeated end range testing of the lumbar spine has been shown to aid clinicians in predicting the likelihood of successful response to conservative rehabilitative care, even in the presence of neurological deficits.[75] Improvement in pain location in response to end range spinal loading (ie, centralization) can occur when testing a direction of movement. Directions typically tested in the lumbar spine include flexion, extension, and right- and left-side glide and in the cervical spine, flexion, extension, side bending, and rotation. In the extremities, positions are tested according to the physiological motions of the joint. Differing amounts of load on the joint in a gravity-eliminated (unloaded) or gravity-assisted (loaded) condition can also be examined to determine the patient's functional mechanical pattern with progression of load. An example of a varied loading position in the lumbar spine is repeated forward bending in standing versus lying supine.

Repeated movements can be applied to a joint in a specific direction to determine whether symptoms improve or are aggravated in response. Centralization, or movement from distal to more proximal and diffuse to localized, is a positive response to repeated movement testing. A systematic progression of force allows the clinician to determine whether the patient will respond rapidly or more slowly to conservative care. Many patients can be treated successfully when they are given information about directional movement for symptom relief.

A comprehensive repeated movement examination involves enough repetition of the motion to determine a response (whether positive, negative, or no effect). Using an arbitrary number of repetitions (eg, 10) will not give the clinician a true grasp of the patient's ability to tolerate direction-specific load and therefore will not provide an accurate picture of the patient's mechanical syndrome and rehabilitation potential.

In patients with inflammatory pain from initial injuries and chemical pain processes, every movement tested tends to increase pain; as a result, pain worsens with static and repeated movement testing. At times, the mechanical outcome may be inconclusive with chemical inflammatory pain. When the patient has primarily mechanical inflammatory pain, there is a close stimulus-response relationship to movement, and the pain may respond to a preferred direction of movement. The patient may demonstrate an MDT classification diagnosis of derangement or other syndrome when chemical pain is present. Intermittent pain may occur in derangement, dysfunction, and posture syndromes, or other condition (see Chapter 2).

In patients with ischemic pain, repeated test movements often produce no symptoms, indicating that the ischemic pain is more related to sustained positions or cumulative functions. Certain patients with ischemic pain can have end range pain in the joint in question and a loss of movement in that direction. As a result of the repeated movement, there may be a production or increase in pain; however, the pain gets no worse. The movement may also have no effect on the symptoms. With ischemic pain, it is important to encourage patients that pain gets no worse. If movement is restricted, the clinician should encourage the patients to move into the pain and emphasize that this process is safe. Prior pain reactions may have taught the patients that "if it hurts, don't do it." With ischemic pain, the opposite is true: "If it hurts, move it. Move it often, and move it further than it's gone before, and you will get no worse." Conveying to the patients the no-worse concept as a measure of success for that treatment day may be all that is required; the clinician can explain that although pain may be produced with a movement, the pain ceases once the movement has ceased and the tissues are no worse as a result. Patients with this type of pain typically take between 8 and 24 weeks to resolve the joint and tissue remodeling process.

Patients who present with a chronic derangement that has underlying tissue dysfunction have a range of motion restriction that obstructs movement in one direction and reduces it in another. Over time these patients begin to respond more quickly when they are moved in their preferred direction (sometimes 4-8 weeks). For example, a patient who sustained an injury less than a week ago is in the inflammatory stage of healing. The pain mechanism is acute chemical inflammatory pain. Initially, the clinician should educate the patient on the importance of using pain as a guide, of not increasing or reproducing the pain, and of using ice. Gentle midrange movement should be performed with a sufficient number of repetitions to promote the appropriate healing response, depending on the tissue that was stressed. In contrast, an office worker whose pain gradually becomes worse over 6 months while using the computer may have suffered an initial injury, but the healing process should be completed after 6 months. If no trauma occurred, the pain may be associated with a lack of blood flow from repetitive typing movements or sustained posturing, indicating its ischemic nature.

Appendix 4.D describes a patient with ischemic pain in the proliferation phase of healing. Initially, the clinician should educate the patient that the pain is simply a message to the tissue that the tissue needs movement in order to receive nutrition. Tissue nutrition can be facilitated through heat or reciprocal movement to the tissue stresses.[18,74] **Appendix 4.E** describes a patient with ischemic pain and end range loading to his tissue structures without loss of motion. This patient requires education to correct his resting posture and avoid extremes of end range tissue loading. **Figure 4.4** is a patient education handout for ischemic pain, referred to as *overuse pain*.

FIGURE 4.4 Nociceptive:Ischemia (Overuse) Pain Mechanism Patient Education Handout

Overuse Pain

WHAT IS OVERUSE PAIN?

Overuse pain is one of the most common forms of musculoskeletal pain. Muscles and joints of the body do not receive proper blood flow or oxygen. The lack of oxygen allows acid and chemicals to build up in the muscles and joints, causing local tissue irritation and pain.

WHAT CAUSES OVERUSE PAIN?
- In the end stages of healing, blood supply is minimal, and regular movement to the end of your range of movement is necessary to encourage blood flow to the tissue. This blood flow is necessary to finalize the tissue's healing, repair, and recovery.
- Maintaining muscles or joints in the same position without change does not allow the tissues to get proper circulation and oxygen. Positions maintained for longer than an hour can cause overuse pain, especially if done on a regular basis.
- Moving muscles and joints repetitively in the same direction without taking a break prevents the tissues from getting proper circulation and oxygen. Moving tissues for longer than an hour in the same direction can cause overuse pain, especially if done on a regular basis. The tissues may not be strong and healthy enough for this continued stress.

WHAT DOES OVERUSE PAIN FEEL LIKE?
- The pain comes and goes and is usually located in one area of the body.
- The pain often starts for no apparent reason; you may be unable to remember a trauma or injury, or the injury may have occurred over a month ago.
- The pain usually worsens as the day or week goes on.
- You may describe the pain as *tightness, weakness,* or *fatigue*.

WHAT CAN YOU DO FOR OVERUSE PAIN?
1. Recognize and change the position or movement that causes the pain.
    - Take a break from positions sustained for more than 60 minutes; a break may consist simply of moving out of the posture for several repetitions and then readjusting the position to continue work.
    - Take a break from doing movements in the same direction for more than 60 minutes; a break may consist simply of moving in the opposite direction 10 times and then resuming the original movement.
    - For example, sustaining your wrists in certain positions while typing at the computer may not hurt for short periods, but sustaining those positions for longer periods may cause pain, and doing this day after day may have a cumulative effect that causes pain. Move your wrists out of sustained positions into the opposite direction or position.

(continues on next page)

FIGURE 4.4 Nociceptive:Ischemia (Overuse) Pain Mechanism Patient Education Handout

(continued from previous page)

2. Choose a "movement pill," or movement that alleviates stress on tissue that causes pain, and perform it 2 to 4 times a day.
   - Manage your pain with the movement pill. Your pill may be as simple as moving out of the sustained position several times into the opposite direction.
   - Seek the help of a health care provider to get specific instructions about proper body mechanics and energy-efficient positions and postures to complete daily tasks.
   - For example, if you feel back pain after working at the computer for 3 hours, you can use the movement pill of standing up and bending backward several times to increase the blood flow to that area. Take this pill (backward bending) every hour; it may even prevent the pain from occurring at all.

3. Consider using heat for relief when overuse pain occurs.
   - Use heat to promote blood flow and ice to decrease blood flow. Increased blood flow promotes healing.
   - Apply heat using a hot water bottle, heat wrap, or hot shower. The heat should always feel comfortable.
   - For example, if you work on an assembly line and perform the same movement for 8 hours a day, at the end of each shift your back will be tired. Use heat at home and motions not used during the day to reduce your pain and restore the tissue to a healthy balance.

SHOULD I TAKE A MEDICATION FOR OVERUSE PAIN?
Anti-inflammatory medications typically are not effective in treating overuse pain. Contact your physician if you cannot control your pain with a movement pill or heat. Your physician will be able to recommend the best medication for your condition.

Intervention for Nociceptive Pain Mechanisms

When treating patients with nociceptive:inflammatory or nociceptive:ischemia pain mechanisms, the clinician can use several strategies to ensure that the patients easily transition through the stages of connective tissue healing and restore function as comfortably as possible. Using the PMCS to gain an understanding of each pain mechanism guides the clinician to select an intervention that the patient can perform with confidence. Patient education is a valuable means of ensuring that patients quickly transition through inflammation, proliferation, and remodeling. The following sections provide guidelines to help patients and treating clinicians establish the activity baseline and manage flare-ups. Refer to **Table 4.4** for interventions of nociceptive pain mechanisms. **Appendices 4.F, 4.G,** and **4.H,** the peripheral nervous system characteristics summary charts, provide subjective, objective, and intervention guidelines to aid in the classification of peripheral nervous system mechanisms.

TABLE 4.4 Nociceptive:Inflammatory and Nociceptive:Ischemia Pain Mechanisms

Mechanism	Intervention
Mechanical inflammation	
Use pain as a guide: Identify directional or positional preference	
MICE	Mid-range OKC movement, ice, compression, and elevation for 30 min, three to four times daily
Kinetic chain	Extremity focus on indirect movements such that proximal segments help distal segments involved and vice versa
Spine	Unloaded neutral spine stabilization exercises; utilize activities of daily living, occupation tasks; incorporate directional preference into treatment
Neural	Unloaded mid-range sliders; propose using the joint one segment away from symptom area
Chemical inflammation	
Use pain as a guide	
MICE	Mid-range OKC movement, ice, compression, elevation for 30 min, three to four times daily
Medication	Oral nonsteroidal; progress to oral steroids or steroid injection; continue until movement exam reveals a preferred direction or restored function.
Modalities	Create a decreased blood flow response, decrease edema-electrical stimulation
Nociceptive:ischemia	
Motion	Progressed to end range and into pain; no worse as a result
Kinetic chain	Direct extremity focus; restore quality biomechanical principals of loading and unloading with triplanar motion. Pain response produced, and remains no worse.
Spine	Progress to weight bearing upright posture stabilization with emphasis on passing through neutral. Pain response produced, and remains no worse.
Graded exposure/pacing	Build low aerobic capacity 2 to 5 hours weekly, heart rate 55%–75% of maximum. Pain response produced, and remains no worse.
Strength training	1 to 3 times a week, total body movement patterns, weight lifting. Pain response produced, and remains no worse.
Manual therapy	Overpressure, mobilization, and manipulation applied as patient plateaus with active exercise associated with tissue dysfunction. Pain response produced, and remains no worse.
Modalities	Create an increased blood flow response by warming before and/or after exercise, ie, hot packs, ultrasound, heat wraps (active), massage.

Abbreviations: OKC = open kinetic chain.

Guidelines for Establishing the Activity Baseline

Inflammatory pain responds well to passive and active movements that help reduce discomfort and stiffness. When beginning to treat any patient with pain, it is important to establish his or her baseline level of activity for function. The patient's baseline is the level (eg, frequency, intensity, duration) of any specific desired functional activity that the patient is able to accomplish without increasing his or her pain rating on an 11-point visual analog scale

FIGURE 4.5 Baseline Activity Tolerance (BAT) Tool

Directions: For each hour of the day and night, list the specific activity and note how it made you feel compared with your everyday pain using the following codes: W = worse, S = same, B = better, NP = no pain. Then answer the questions at the bottom of the form.

Date:	Self-care (eg, bathing, dressing, grooming)	Work (eg, job, school, household, chores)	Recreation and leisure (eg, movies, reading, exercise)	Sleep and rest (eg, naps, evening)	Sample entry
7 AM					Showered—B
8 AM					Dressed—NP
9 AM					↓
10 AM					Did computer work—W
11 AM					
12 PM					↓
1 PM					Ate lunch—NP
2 PM					↓
3 PM					
4 PM					
5 PM					Drove—W
6 PM					↓
7 PM					Watched a movie—W
8 PM					
9 PM					↓
10 PM					Slept—B
11 PM					
12 AM					
1 AM					
2 AM					
3 AM					
4 AM					
5 AM					
6 AM					↓

When were you most tired or stressed?

When did you have the most pain?

by greater than 3 points (On a scale of 0 to 10, where 0 = *no pain* and 10 = *worst pain ever*, what level of pain are you experiencing?). The pain produced by the activity should abate within 15 to 20 minutes after the session and remain better after a night's rest. Movement that is too vigorous may increase pain, often not until hours after the treatment session, that night, or the next morning. The clinician should ensure that the patient understands that if an increase in pain occurs, he or she should curtail the activity level and identify the baseline level of activity that caused no increase in pain or worsening the next day.

The Baseline Activity Tolerance (BAT) tool (**Figure 4.5**) helps patients establish their baseline by recording their functional levels of activity and relative pain levels. The BAT allows the clinician to determine how the patients' pain responds to an activity (worse, better, or the same) in a diurnal pattern. After establishing activities and times of the day when the patients' pain is worse, the clinician can work with them to develop guidelines for restoring function and progressing functional activities. **Figure 4.6** is a patient education handout on use of the BAT tool.

Once the baseline activity level has been established, the clinician can create a program and educate the patient about the progression of rehabilitation using the 10% rule: The patient cannot increase the frequency, intensity, or duration of the task by greater than 10% each time he or she performs it. For instance, a patient who knows he is able to run for 10 minutes without increased pain should next try to run for 11 minutes (a 10% increase), not for 20 minutes (a 100% increase). This is a safe and reasonable expectation to guide patients in problem solving how to self-manage their progress. This generalized rule may be modified if 10% appears too aggressive based on each individual patient.

FIGURE 4.6 Baseline Activity Tolerance Tool Patient Education Handout

Once you have established your baseline activity level using the Baseline Activity Tolerance (BAT) tool, you can begin to focus on returning to the activities you enjoyed before you started having pain.

The body is designed for movement. Movement is essential to heal completely and restore prior activity levels. Consider your entries on the BAT in light of the following:

- Performing and increasing your activities should make your pain no worse. You may feel pain while doing activities, but if the pain is no worse that night and the next morning, your body was able to safely perform that level of activity. The pain simply indicates that you need to perform the activity to get better.
- If your pain is worse that night or the next day, a flare-up has occurred. The BAT can help you and your clinician to identify the activities that cause flare-ups and determine your baseline activity level so you can adjust your activities accordingly.

To progress from your baseline, add 1% to 10% more to each activity per day. This may mean doing one extra repetition of an exercise or adding 1 more minute to walking or sitting. Your progression has been successful when you are no worse as a result of the increase in activity that night and the next morning.

Flare-ups can happen, and you should not be afraid of them. It can be a balancing act to find just the right amount of activity. If you have a flare-up, reduce your activity but do not stop moving—find a new baseline. Refer to the flare-up management plan your clinician provided for strategies to avoid and address flare-ups.

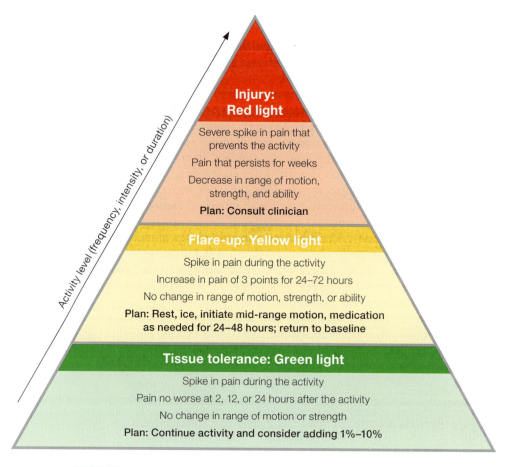

FIGURE 4.7 Activity Pyramid: Guidance for avoiding flare-up and reinjury.

The Activity Pyramid shown in **Figure 4.7** summarizes the effects of increased activity and describes how patients can tell whether they have increased their activity level too quickly. If patients cross the line between the green light and yellow light activity levels, they may produce a flare-up of discomfort or pain. If they manage the flare-up appropriately, within 2, 12, or 24 hours they will be no worse. As patients' function improves, it takes more stress on the tissues to create a flare-up or injury. Increasing their activity level adjusts the capacity of their tissues, or tissue tolerance, upward.

Guidelines for Management of Flare-Ups

Flare-ups are bound to happen regardless of the pain mechanism in operation. A *flare-up* is defined as an increased level of pain of at least 3 points that lasts more than a day. Flare-up pain during healing results from a variety of stressors such as poor positioning during daily activities, activity exceeding baseline tolerance, unnecessary tissue stresses, and awkward sustained postures. Flare-ups can be a normal part of the recovery process; they do not necessarily mean that damage has occurred, but they can delay the healing process. Early, effective management of flare-ups is critical to ongoing success in treating pain, restoring functional independence, and preventing chronic pain.

Patient education about flare-ups is a necessity in any type of pain mechanism intervention. The basis for a flare-up plan is to allow healing and repair of connective tissue. The patient must avoid overstressing the tissue with activity that, if continued, could create mild sprains and strains on connective tissue. This stress can sensitize the central nervous system toward chemical inflammatory production, creating lasting stress reactions and immune changes. The clinician must educate, mentor, test, and motivate the patients to take an active role in controlling flare-ups by

- Identifying the mechanical, social, or emotional causes of the flare-up in the patients' daily routine and confirming that the range of motion is no worse
- Teaching the patients how to manage flare-ups with the BAT tool (**Figure 4.5**)
- Teaching the patients to move in ranges that maintain the tissues in a no-worse state
- Teaching relaxation strategies that put the patients' bodies in a state of physical and emotional calmness

Clinicians can provide patients with the following strategies for managing flare-ups:

- Take action, and maintain a positive attitude. The sooner you take control of the pain, the sooner you can restart the healing process.
- Do not imagine the worst.
- Use relative rest for a maximum of 48 hours.
- Ice up to 72 hours after a flare-up to manage inflammatory pain.
- Use compression, elevation, or support garments to aid in swelling reduction if necessary.
- Check your range of motion. If it is no worse, do not worry; you have just challenged the tissues.
- Continue with your activities of daily living, household and job activities, and exercises for range of motion, but avoid new or more advanced activities.

If the patient has pain and significant loss of motion and pain is generally 3 or more points worse on an 11-point scale, he or she may have experienced a reinjury to the tissues. In this case, the clinician should provide education similar to that for a flare-up, but with the primary goals to decrease the pain, reassess tissue injury possibility, and restore range of motion to preinjury status. The clinician should also encourage the patient to avoid catastrophizing about the situation and remain calm, reassure the patient that he or she may be able to recover quickly despite the reinjury, and reeducate the patient to use the Activity Pyramid as a guide for preventing injury and flare-ups.

KEY MESSAGES

- Nociceptors are activated by thermal, chemical, and mechanical irritants.
- Chemical pain is a cascade that results when tissues are inflamed or irritated, whereas mechanical pain originates in deformation of tissues.
- Connective tissue goes through three stages of healing: inflammation, proliferation, and remodeling.
- Healing time varies depending on the type of tissue.
- Identifying inflammatory versus ischemic mechanisms is imperative throughout the rehabilitation process.
- Tendinosis is a degenerative process and not an inflammatory one. *Tendonitis* and *tendinosis* are often incorrectly used interchangeably. An understanding of the mechanical process in each is necessary for effective treatment.
- Use of a tool such as the Baseline Activity Tolerance tool to identify patients' baseline activity tolerance can help them avoid and manage flare-ups.
- Patients should be encouraged to progress from their baseline activity level using the 10% rule: Increase the frequency, intensity, or duration of the task by only 10%. If the pain is no worse at 2, 12, and 24 hours, tissue tolerance has adjusted upward, as illustrated by the Activity Pyramid.
- Clinicians must recognize and educate patients about flare-ups, which involve a chemical inflammatory process. The Activity Pyramid guides patients in avoiding and managing flare-ups.
- It is important for clinicians to reevaluate patients in each treatment session because the pain mechanism may change and treatment must change accordingly.

References

1. Treede RD, Meyer RA, Raja SN, Campbell JN. Peripheral and central mechanisms of cutaneous hyperalgesia. *Prog Neurobiol*. 1992;38:397-421.
2. Meyer RA, Campbell JN, Raja SN. Peripheral neural mechanisms of nociception. In: Wall PD, Melzachk R, eds. *Textbook of Pain*. 3rd ed. Edinburgh, Scotland: Churchill Livingstone; 1994.
3. Issberner U, Reeh PW, Steen KH. Pain due to tissue acidosis: A mechanism for inflammatory and ischemic myalgia? *Neurosci Lett*. 1996;208:191-194.
4. *Stedman's Medical Dictionary*. Baltimore, MD: Lippincott Williams & Wilkins; 2006.
5. Schaible HG, Schmidt RF. Time course of mechanosensitivity changes in articular afferents during a developing experimental arthritis. *J Neurophysiol*. 1988;60:2180-2195.
6. Brenn D, Richter F, Schaible HG. Sensitization of unmyelinated sensory fibers of the joint nerve to mechanical stimuli by interleukin-6 in the rat: An inflammatory mechanism of joint pain. *Arthritis Rheum*. 2007;56:351-359.
7. Kidd BL. Osteoarthritis and joint pain. *Pain*. 2006;123:6-9.
8. Bogduk N. *The Anatomy and Physiology of Nociception*. Oxford, England: Butterworth Heinemann; 1993.
9. Long A, Donelson R, Fung T. Does it matter which exercise? A randomized control trial of exercise for low back pain. *Spine*. 2004;29:2593-2602.
10. Bogduk N. On the definitions and physiology of back pain, referred pain, and radicular pain. *Pain*. 2009;147:17-19.
11. Culav EM, Clark CH, Merrilees MJ. Connective tissues: Matrix composition and its relevance to physical therapy. *Phys Ther*. 1999;79:308-319.
12. Evans P. The healing process at a cellular level: A review. *Physiotherapy*. 1980;66:256-259.
13. Serhan CN, Savill J. Resolution of inflammation: The beginning programs the end. *Nature Immunol*. 2005;6:1191-1197.
14. Linley JE, Rose K, Ooi L, Gamper N. Understanding inflammatory pain: Ion channels contributing to acute and chronic nociception. *Pflugers Arch*. 2010;459:657-669.
15. Best TM, Hunter KD. Muscle injury and repair. *Phys Med Rehabil Clin N Am*. 2000;11:251-266.
16. Ghivizzani SC, Oligino TJ, Robbins PD, Evans CH. Cartilage injury and repair. *Phys Med Rehabil Clin N Am*. 2000;11:289-307, vi.

17. McKenzie R, May S. *The Lumbar Spine: Mechanical Diagnosis & Therapy.* Waikanae, New Zealand: Spinal Publications; 2003.
18. Nadler SF, Steiner DJ, Erasala GN, Hengehold DA, Abeln SB, Weingand KW. Continuous low-level heatwrap therapy for treating acute nonspecific low back pain. *Arch Phys Med Rehabil.* 2003;84:329-334.
19. Nadler SF, Steiner DJ, Petty SR, Erasala GN, Hengehold DA, Weingand KW. Overnight use of continuous low-level heatwrap therapy for relief of low back pain. *Arch Phys Med Rehabil.* 2003;84:335-342.
20. Mayer JM, Ralph L, Look M, et al. Treating acute low back pain with continuous low-level heat wrap therapy and/or exercise: A randomized controlled trial. *Spine.* 2005;5:395-403.
21. Moseley L. *Pain* [DVD]. Aptos, CA: On Target Publications; 2013.
22. Peng B, Wu W, Hou S, Li P, Zhang C, Yang Y. The pathogenesis of discogenic low back pain. *J Bone Joint Surg Br.* 2005;87:62-67.
23. Buchanan CI, Marsh RL. Effects of exercise on the biomechanical, biochemical and structural properties of tendons. *Comp Biochem Physiol A Mol Integr Physiol.* 2002;133:1101-1107.
24. Turner CH. Three rules for bone adaptation to mechanical stimuli. *Bone.* 1998;23:399-407.
25. Turner CH. Bone strength: Current concepts. *Ann N Y Acad Sci.* 2006;1068:429-446.
26. Hagen KB, Dagfinrud H, Moe RH, et al. Exercise therapy for bone and muscle health: An overview of systematic reviews. *BMC Med.* 2012;10:167.
27. Novicoff WM, Manaswi A, Hogan MV, Brubaker SM, Mihalko WM, Saleh KJ. Critical analysis of the evidence for current technologies in bone-healing and repair. *J Bone Joint Surg Am.* 2008;90(suppl 1):85-91.
28. Borhanuddin B, Mohd Fozi NF, Naina Mohamed I. Vitamin E and the healing of bone fracture: The current state of evidence. *Evid Based Complement Alternat Med.* 2012;2012:684510.
29. Eschle D, Aeschlimann AG. Is supplementation of vitamin D beneficial for fracture healing? A short review of the literature. *Geriatr Orthop Surg Rehabil.* 2011;2:90-93.
30. Frank CB, Hart DA, Shrive NG. Molecular biology and biomechanics of normal and healing ligaments—A review. *Osteoarthritis Cartilage.* 1999;7:130-140.
31. Benani A, Pottie P, Fauchet M, et al. How a daily and moderate exercise improves ligament healing. *IRBM.* 2008;29:267-271.
32. Stokes IA, Iatridis JC. Mechanical conditions that accelerate intervertebral disc degeneration: Overload versus immobilization. *Spine.* 2004;29:2724-2732.
33. Coppes MH, Marani E, Thomeer RT, Groen GJ. Innervation of "painful" lumbar discs. *Spine.* 1997;22:2342-2349; discussion 2349-2350.
34. Buckwalter JA. Aging and degeneration of the human intervertebral disc. *Spine.* 1995;20:1307-1314.
35. Gruber HE, Hanley EN Jr. Ultrastructure of the human intervertebral disc during aging and degeneration: Comparison of surgical and control specimens. *Spine.* 2002;27:798-805.
36. Taylor J, Twomey L, Levander B. Contrasts between cervical and lumbar motion segments. *Crit Rev Phys Rehabil Med.* 2000;12:345-371.
37. Adams MA, McMillan DW, Green TP, Dolan P. Sustained loading generates stress concentrations in lumbar intervertebral discs. *Spine.* 1996;21:434-438.
38. DePalma MJ, Lee JE, Peterson L, Wolfer L, Ketchum JM, Derby R. Are outer annular fissures stimulated during diskography the source of diskogenic low-back pain? An analysis of analgesic diskography data. *Pain Med.* 2009;10:488-494.
39. Brown MF, Hukkanen MV, McCarthy ID, et al. Sensory and sympathetic innervation of the vertebral endplate in patients with degenerative disc disease. *J Bone Joint Surg Br.* 1997;79:147-153.
40. Gronblad M, Virri J, Tolonen J, et al. A controlled immunohistochemical study of inflammatory cells in disc herniation tissue. *Spine.* 1994;19:2744-2751.
41. Harrington JF, Messier AA, Bereiter D, Barnes B, Epstein MH. Herniated lumbar disc material as a source of free glutamate available to affect pain signals through the dorsal root ganglion. *Spine.* 2000;25:929-936.
42. Coderre TJ. The role of excitatory amino acid receptors and intracellular messengers in persistent nociception after tissue injury in rats. *Mol Neurobiol.* 1993;7:229-246.
43. Burke JG, Watson RW, McCormack D, Dowling FE, Walsh MG, Fitzpatrick JM. Spontaneous production of monocyte chemoattractant protein-1 and interleukin-8 by the human lumbar intervertebral disc. *Spine.* 2002;27:1402-1407.
44. Burke JG, Watson RW, McCormack D, Dowling FE, Walsh MG, Fitzpatrick JM. Intervertebral discs which cause low back pain secrete high levels of proinflammatory mediators. *J Bone Joint Surg Br.* 2002;84:196-201.
45. Olmarker K, Rydevik B, Nordborg C. Autologous nucleus pulposus induces neurophysiologic and histologic changes in porcine cauda equina nerve roots. *Spine.* 1993;18:1425-1432.
46. Freemont AJ, Jeziorska M, Hoyland JA, Rooney P, Kumar S. Mast cells in the pathogenesis of chronic back pain: A hypothesis. *J Pathol.* 2002;197:281-285.

47. Weiler C, Nerlich AG, Bachmeier BE, Boos N. Expression and distribution of tumor necrosis factor alpha in human lumbar intervertebral discs: A study in surgical specimen and autopsy controls. *Spine.* 2005;30:44-53; discussion 54.
48. Murata Y, Nannmark U, Rydevik B, Takahashi K, Olmarker K. Nucleus pulposus–induced apoptosis in dorsal root ganglion following experimental disc herniation in rats. *Spine.* 2006;31:382-390.
49. Saal JS. The role of inflammation in lumbar pain. *Spine.* 1995;20:1821-1827.
50. Olmarker K, Blomquist J, Stromberg J, Nannmark U, Thomsen P, Rydevik B. Inflammatogenic properties of nucleus pulposus. *Spine.* 1995;20:665-669.
51. Geiss A, Larsson K, Rydevik B, Takahashi I, Olmarker K. Autoimmune properties of nucleus pulposus: An experimental study in pigs. *Spine.* 2007;32:168-173.
52. Ashe MC, McCauley T, Khan KM. Tendinopathies in the upper extremity: A paradigm shift. *J Hand Ther.* 2004;17:329-334.
53. Cook JL, Khan KM, Purdam C. Achilles tendinopathy. *Man Ther.* 2002;7:121-130.
54. Benazzo F, Stennardo G, Valli M. Achilles and patellar tendinopathies in athletes: Pathogenesis and surgical treatment. *Bull Hosp Jt Dis.* 1996;54:236-240.
55. Astrom M, Rausing A. Chronic Achilles tendinopathy: A survey of surgical and histopathologic findings. *Clin Orthop Relat Res.* 1995;316:151-164.
56. Alfredson H. The chronic painful Achilles and patellar tendon: Research on basic biology and treatment. *Scand J Med Sci Sports.* 2005;15:252-259.
57. Jarvinen TA, Kannus P, Maffulli N, Khan KM. Achilles tendon disorders: Etiology and epidemiology. *Foot Ankle Clin.* 2005;10:255-266.
58. Purdam CR, Jonsson P, Alfredson H, Lorentzon R, Cook JL, Khan KM. A pilot study of the eccentric decline squat in the management of painful chronic patellar tendinopathy. *Br J Sports Med.* 2004;38:395-397.
59. Alfredson H, Pietila T, Jonsson P, Lorentzon R. Heavy-load eccentric calf muscle training for the treatment of chronic Achilles tendinosis. *Am J Sports Med.* 1998;26:360-366.
60. Ohberg L, Alfredson H. Sclerosing therapy in chronic Achilles tendon insertional pain—Results of a pilot study. *Knee Surg Sports Traumatol Arthrosc.* 2003;11:339-343.
61. Paavola M, Kannus P, Paakkala T, Pasanen M, Jarvinen M. Long-term prognosis of patients with Achilles tendinopathy: An observational 8-year follow-up study. *Am J Sports Med.* 2000;28:634-642.
62. Visnes H, Bahr R. The evolution of eccentric training as treatment for patellar tendinopathy (jumper's knee): A critical review of exercise programmes. *Br J Sports Med.* 2007;41:217-223.
63. Jonsson P, Alfredson H. Superior results with eccentric compared to concentric quadriceps training in patients with jumper's knee: A prospective randomised study. *Br J Sports Med.* 2005;39:847-850.
64. Stanish WD, Rubinovich RM, Curwin S. Eccentric exercise in chronic tendinitis. *Clin Orthop Relat Res.* 1986;208:65-68.
65. Jonsson P, Alfredson H, Sunding K, Fahlstrom M, Cook J. New regimen for eccentric calf-muscle training in patients with chronic insertional Achilles tendinopathy: Results of a pilot study. *Br J Sports Med.* 2008;42:746-749.
66. Tabebordbar M, Wang ET, Wagers AJ. Skeletal muscle degenerative diseases and strategies for therapeutic muscle repair. *Annu Rev Pathol.* 2013;8:441-475.
67. Garrett WE Jr. Muscle strain injuries. *Am J Sports Med.* 1996;24(6 suppl):S2-S8.
68. Taylor DC, Dalton JD Jr, Seaber AV, Garrett WE Jr. Experimental muscle strain injury: Early functional and structural deficits and the increased risk for reinjury. *Am J Sports Med.* 1993;21:190-194.
69. Morgan DL, Allen DG. Early events in stretch-induced muscle damage. *J Appl Physiol.* 1999;87:2007-2015.
70. McCully KK, Faulkner JA. Characteristics of lengthening contractions associated with injury to skeletal muscle fibers. *J Appl Physiol.* 1986;61:293-299.
71. Obremsky WT, Seaber AV, Ribbeck BM, Garrett WE Jr. Biomechanical and histologic assessment of a controlled muscle strain injury treated with piroxicam. *Am J Sports Med.* 1994;22:558-561.
72. Safran MR, Garrett WE Jr, Seaber AV, Glisson RR, Ribbeck BM. The role of warmup in muscular injury prevention. *Am J Sports Med.* 1988;16:123-129.
73. Smart KM, Blake C, Staines A, Doody C. Clinical indicators of "nociceptive," "peripheral neuropathic" and "central" mechanisms of musculoskeletal pain: A Delphi survey of expert clinicians. *Man Ther.* 2010;15:80-87.
74. Bloodworth D, Calvillo O, Smith K, et al. Chronic pain syndromes: Evaluation and treatment. In: Braddom RL, ed. *Physical Medicine and Rehabilitation.* 2nd ed. Philadelphia, PA: Saunders, 2001:913-933.
75. Wetzel FT, Donelson R. The role of repeated end-range/pain response assessment in the management of symptomatic lumbar discs. *Spine.* 2003;3:146-154.

APPENDIX 4.A Orthopedic Outpatient, 31-Year-Old Male

Physical Therapy/Occupational Therapy Initial Evaluation

SUBJECTIVE FINDINGS

Chief complaint:	R shoulder and chest pain
Descriptors:	Stiffness with occasional cracks, feels swollen, sharp pain with movement
Onset:	1 wk ago when stepping off a curb, he grabbed a sign pole to prevent falling
Frequency:	Intermittent
24-hr behavior:	Worse in AM, better as day progresses, worse in evening (diurnal pattern)
Subjective pain:	(Likert) / Faces scale: 3-8/10
Aggravating factors:	Lifting arm, holding objects
Relieving factors:	Disuse, gentle movements, ice, meds (Ibuprofen)

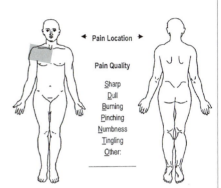

Pain Location

Pain Quality
 Sharp
 Dull
 Burning
 Pinching
 Numbness
 Tingling
 Other:

PATIENT EDUCATION CONSIDERATIONS

Readiness to learn:	(Ready and self-motivated) Extrinsically motivated Limitations (see below)
Limitations to learning:	Cognitive Physical Language Financial Cultural (Other:) None
Teaching method preferred:	(Handout) Verbal (Demonstration) (Practice) Other:
Explain:	

MEDICAL HISTORY

Past medical history:	Healthy other than arm pain
Family history:	Unremarkable
Surgery and invasive procedures:	Prior history of L knee anterior cruciate ligament reconstruction with a positive rehabilitation outcome
Medications:	Ibuprofen 2-3x/d for past week—reported helpful, no negative side effects Allergies: No known drug allergies
Previous treatments:	PT previously for L ACL injury
Diagnostic tests:	X-ray: Negative MRI: Inquisitive about an MRI CT scan: EMG: Other:

(continues on next page)

APPENDIX 4.A Orthopedic Outpatient, 31-Year-Old Male *(continued from previous page)*

PSYCHOSOCIAL FACTORS

Living situation:	Patient is a single male who lives alone. Family lives out of town, but he has good friends and a strong support system.
Behavior:	No maladaptive pain disorders
Occupation:	Schoolteacher, 5th and 6th grades
Recreation and leisure:	Active in sports; performs a regular fitness routine 3-4x/wk
Functional disability:	Workouts have been limited since injury a week ago because of fear of reinjury
Concerns:	Concerned about why he is not better yet and whether his X-rays show something significant

PROVISIONAL PAIN CLASSIFICATION

Nociceptive:inflammatory; *inflammatory* phase of healing

PAIN EDUCATION TOPICS

1. Connective tissue healing and repair; movement guidelines and pain
2. What the inflammatory pain mechanism involves
3. Soft tissue injuries and what may and may not show on X-ray; no need for further imaging
4. A flare-up plan should the patient begin to stress his healing tissues too quickly
5. Typical tissue healing rates and what he can expect
6. Refer to the Activity Pyramid to guide the appropriate stress of healing

Physical Therapy/Occupational Therapy Objective Evaluation

OBJECTIVE FINDINGS

Posture:	No abnormalities
Active range of motion:	Active elevation with pain during motion; no limitation to motion
Passive range of motion:	No pain during motion; no limitation to motion
MMT:	Pectoralis major (horizontal adduction) R 5/5 painful, everything else bilaterally WFL without complaints of pain
Repeated test movements:	Repeated horizontal adduction: produces pain, increases, worse as a result, each motion getting worse
	Repeated horizontal abduction: produces pain, increases, worse as a result, each motion getting worse
	Repeated shoulder flexion: produces pain, increases, worse as a result, each motion getting worse
	Repeated shoulder extension: produces pain, increases, worse as a result, each motion getting worse

PROVISIONAL MECHANICAL CLASSIFICATION

Other—trauma/healing state, pectoralis major, 7-day-old sprain

PROVISIONAL PAIN CLASSIFICATION

Nociceptive:inflammatory; *inflammatory* phase of healing of a mild sprain

TREATMENT

Treatment:
- Midrange active ROM 2-3x/d (patient is no worse as a result), progressing to full ROM
- Lower-extremity cardio, continue as before
- Pacing strategies for overhead work at school
- Icing at the end of the day after work and before bedtime
- Heat during the day if needed

Treatment summary: **3 visits over 4 wk,** 1x/wk

Goals:

	PSFS	
	Initial	Discharge
Return to fitness routine 3-4x/wk	0	10
Write on blackboard at work consistently	2	10
Pain limitation to function	5	10
Pain intensity rating	3	0

Abbreviations: ACL = anterior cruciate ligament; CT = computed tomography; EMG = electromyography; L = left; MMT = manual muscle testing; MRI = magnetic resonance imaging; PSFS = Patient-Specific Functional Scale; PT = physical therapy; R = right; ROM = range of motion; WFL = within functional limits.

APPENDIX 4.B Orthopedic Outpatient: 53-Year-Old Female

Physical Therapy/Occupational Therapy Initial Evaluation

SUBJECTIVE FINDINGS

Chief complaint:	Low back pain
Descriptors:	Tightness, dull ache, throbbing
Onset:	2-3 wk ago; acute onset when helping transfer a patient in the cardiac care unit
Frequency:	Intermittent
24-hr behavior:	Worse in AM, better as day progresses, worse in evening
Subjective pain:	(Likert) / Faces scale: 0-8/10
Aggravating factors:	Lifting patients, sitting, being still
Relieving factors:	Rest, lying down (unloading), ice at end of day, walking, movement

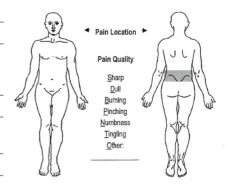

Pain Location

Pain Quality
- Sharp
- Dull
- Burning
- Pinching
- Numbness
- Tingling
- Other:

PATIENT EDUCATION CONSIDERATIONS

Readiness to learn:	(Ready and self-motivated) Extrinsically motivated Limitations (see below)
Limitations to learning:	Cognitive Physical Language Financial Cultural (Other:) None
Teaching method preferred:	(Handout) Verbal Demonstration Practice Other:
Explain:	

MEDICAL HISTORY

Past medical history:	Cardiac history of hypertension and mild obesity
Family history:	Unremarkable
Surgery and invasive procedures:	Hysterectomy 15 years ago
Medications:	Ibuprofen—no relief, no negative side effects Allergies: No known drug allergies
Previous treatments:	
Diagnostic tests:	X-ray: DDD: L4-5, L5-S1 MRI: Negative CT scan: EMG: Other:

PSYCHOSOCIAL FACTORS

Living situation:	Patient is a married female who lives with her husband and daughter.
Behavior:	Appropriate and calm
Occupation:	Nurse in the critical care unit
Recreation and leisure:	Currently inactive other than walking to and from the train (previously had done workouts at the gym 2-3x/wk)
Functional disability:	Workouts have been limited since the injury because of fear of reinjury
Concerns:	Concerned why the pain is persisting, what exercises she can do at the gym to avoid further weight gain

PROVISIONAL PAIN CLASSIFICATION

Nociceptive:inflammatory; *proliferation* phase of healing

PAIN EDUCATION TOPICS

1. Connective tissue healing and repair; movement guidelines and pain
2. What the inflammatory pain mechanism involves
3. Soft tissue injuries and what may and may not show on X-ray
4. A flare-up plan should the patient begin to stress her healing tissues too quickly
5. Typical tissue healing rates and what she can expect
6. How quickly she can expect to return to functional activities
7. What exercises she is able to resume

(continues on next page)

APPENDIX 4.B Orthopedic Outpatient: 53-Year-Old Female *(continued from previous page)*

Physical Therapy/Occupational Therapy Objective Evaluation

OBJECTIVE FINDINGS

Posture:	Decreased lumbar lordosis, forward head, and increased thoracic kyphosis
Active range of motion:	Minimally limited lumbar flexion with pain during movement and end range pain
	Moderately limited lumbar extension, pain during movement, end range pain
	Minimally limited R & L side glide equally, without complaints of pain
Neurological exam:	Positive lumbar slump test with pain on R & L lower extremity
	Normal reflexes and lower-extremity dermatomes on manual muscle testing
Repeated test movements:	**Baseline loaded exam:** no pain
	Standing lumbar flexion (10x): produces, increases, remains worse as a result
	Standing lumbar extension (10x): increases low back pain, no worse as a result
	Baseline unloaded exam: no pain
	Unloaded lumbar flexion (10x): produces, increases, remains worse as a result
	Unloaded lumbar extension: end range low back pain decreases, better mechanically
	Mechanically: slump better and all motions 25% better on reassessment after completion of unloaded exam

PROVISIONAL MECHANICAL CLASSIFICATION

Derangement—central, symmetrical lumbar, 17 days old

PROVISIONAL PAIN CLASSIFICATION

Nociceptive:inflammatory, mechanical; *proliferation* phase of healing and demonstration of preferred direction

TREATMENT

Treatment:	• Unloaded lumbar extension 5-8x/day for 10-15 reps • Pacing strategies for sitting and lifting at work (sit no longer than 20-30 min) • Icing at the end of the day if worse; use of continuous low-level heat during the day, if desired • Use of a lumbar roll, lordosis, and hip hinging with lifting, sitting, and transitions
Treatment summary:	**5 visits over 6 wk:** 1st wk 2x, then decrease to 1x/wk. She returns to sitting and lifting patients without pain and begins to commit herself to a walking program of 10,000 steps a day. By her discharge from therapy, she is happy to report that she has lost the weight she gained and is 10 pounds lighter just with healthier eating and her step walking program.

		PSFS	
		Initial	Discharge
Goals:	Return to sitting 60 min for computer documentation	2	9
	Lift patients consistently with aides throughout the workday	2	10
	Walking program 3x/wk	0	10
	Pain limitation to function	5	10
	Pain intensity rating	8	0

Abbreviations: CT = computed tomography; DDD = degenerative disc disease; EMG = electromyography; L = left; MRI = magnetic resonance imaging; PSFS = Patient-Specific Functional Scale; R = right; ROM = range of motion.

APPENDIX 4.C Orthopedic Outpatient: 37-Year-Old Male

Physical Therapy/Occupational Therapy Initial Evaluation

SUBJECTIVE FINDINGS

Chief complaint:	R Achilles pain
Descriptors:	Long distance running created an achy pain
Onset:	6 mo ago, twisted his ankle
Frequency:	Intermittent
24-hr behavior:	Worse in PM and on day of a long run
Subjective pain:	Likert / Faces scale: 0-3/10
Aggravating factors:	Running
Relieving factors:	Rest, ice, stretching occasionally

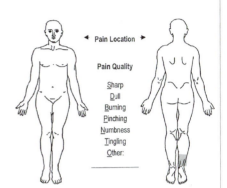

PATIENT EDUCATION CONSIDERATIONS

Readiness to learn:	Ready and self-motivated Extrinsically motivated Limitations (see below)
Limitations to learning:	Cognitive Physical Language Financial Cultural Other: None
Teaching method preferred:	Handout Verbal Demonstration Practice Other:
Explain:	

MEDICAL HISTORY

Past medical history:	Reported healthy other than psoriasis
Family history:	None
Surgery and invasive procedures:	None
Medications:	None Allergies: No known drug allergies
Previous treatments:	Physical therapy for 4 wk, consisting of ultrasound, soft tissue mobilization, and gastrocsoleus stretching
Diagnostic tests:	X-ray: Negative MRI: Negative CT scan: EMG: Other:

(continues on next page)

APPENDIX 4.C Orthopedic Outpatient: 37-Year-Old Male *(continued from previous page)*

PSYCHOSOCIAL FACTORS

Living situation:	Patient lives in a condo with his life partner.
Behavior:	Frustrated with the medical profession secondary to multiple opinions from physiatry, advice ranging from aggressive rehabilitation to orthopedic immobilization
Occupation:	Radiology technologist
Recreation and leisure:	Running intermittently 3-4 miles 2x/wk
Functional disability:	Unable to run distances >6 miles
Concerns:	Concerned why he was discharged from PT when pain and disability are still present

PROVISIONAL PAIN CLASSIFICATION

Nociceptive:ischemia; *remodeling* phase of healing

PAIN EDUCATION TOPICS

1. Connective tissue healing and repair; movement guidelines and pain
2. No-worse concept of healing; pain during exercises permitted and beneficial for continued healing
3. Proper return to running program; eccentric functional training exercises for success
4. Benefits of heat and ice
5. Expectation to return to marathon running

Protocol for Returning to Running After Prolonged Inactivity

Walk	Jog	Cycles per Running Trial	Total Time
30 min	—	—	30 min
9 min	1 min	x3	30 min
8 min	2 min	x3	30 min
7 min	3 min	x3	30 min
6 min	4 min	x3	30 min
5 min	5 min	x3	30 min
4 min	6 min	x3	30 min
3 min	7 min	x3	30 min
2 min	8 min	x3	30 min
1 min	9 min	x3	30 min
—	30 min	—	30 min
Once you can tolerate 30 min of running, you can increase distance and speed as tolerated. If needed, the patient can repeat each stage 6 times before progressing for a slow return to running progression.			

Unpublished chart used with permission from Ellen Casey, MD.

Physical Therapy/Occupational Therapy Objective Evaluation

OBJECTIVE FINDINGS

Active/passive range of motion:	End range pain with active and passive unloaded dorsiflexion of R ankle, minimal loss of motion
	Normal plantarflexion unloaded range of motion, pain on full heel raise R
Functional testing:	Mechanical functional test: Produces pain with active single-leg heel raise, no worse as a result
Repeated test movements:	Repeated R ankle dorsiflexion non-weightbearing: end range pain produced in ankle, pain on weight-bearing heel raise on R no different x20, no immediate change in ROM
	Repeated R ankle dorsiflexion weightbearing: end range pain produced in ankle, pain on weight-bearing heel raise on R no different x30, no immediate change in ROM
	R ankle plantarflexion non-weightbearing: no symptoms with AROM, pain on weight-bearing heel raise on R no different x20, no immediate change in ROM
	R ankle plantarflexion weightbearing: pain on weight-bearing heel raise on R no different x20, no immediate change in ROM, no worse as a result
	Patient sent home with repeated plantarflexion weightbearing 3-4x/d, returns no worse as a result in 48 h

PROVISIONAL MECHANICAL CLASSIFICATION

Dysfunction—contractile tissue, Achilles tendon

PROVISIONAL PAIN CLASSIFICATION

Nociceptive:ischemia; stuck in *remodeling* phase of healing

TREATMENT

Treatment:	Aggressive remodeling of end range dorsiflexion and active strengthening of plantarflexion progressing to end range plantarflexion off a step, eccentrically adding weights in backpack for increased load. Progressing to functional calf strength with medial reach slow descent to power up calf raise with speed. Patient continues with foot intrinsic strengthening with single-leg stance retraining progressing to power runner posterior reach single-limb squat.
Treatment summary:	**3 visits over 9 wk**, 1x every 2-3 wk. Patient returns to running up to 3 miles pain free at normal speeds by 8 wk and is able to perform active and passive dorsiflexion and plantarflexion comfortably. Patient has a home exercise program and is able to perform plyometrics without pain. Patient is discharged after 3 visits.

		PSFS	
		Initial	Discharge
Goals:	Return to running 6 miles, 2x/wk	0	9
	Pain limitation to function	5	10
	Pain intensity rating	3	0

Abbreviations: AROM = active range of motion; CT = computed tomography; EMG = electromyography; MRI = magnetic resonance imaging; PSFS = Patient-Specific Functional Scale; PT = physical therapy; R = right; ROM = range of motion.

APPENDIX 4.D Traumatic Brain Injury Inpatient: 37-Year-Old Female

Physical Therapy/Occupational Therapy Initial Evaluation

SUBJECTIVE FINDINGS

Chief complaint:	R anterior knee pain, R femur open reduction internal fixation
Descriptors:	Sharp, achy
Onset:	3 wk ago, patient was struck by auto. Pain initially increased 7 d ago when she was transferred to the inpatient rehabilitation hospital and increased her activity level. She has had an increase in mobility and pain since this time.
Frequency:	Intermittent
24-hr behavior:	Worse in AM, at end of day, with movement, and after therapy sessions
Subjective pain:	(Likert) / Faces scale: 0-6/10
Aggravating factors:	Too much movement, therapy, sit to stand, sitting longer than 20 min; unable to walk more than 100 ft weight-bearing as tolerated with a rolling walker and standby assistance for safety
Relieving factors:	Rest, ice, motion

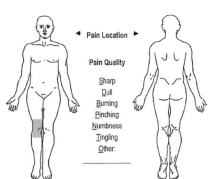

Pain Location

Pain Quality
Sharp
Dull
Burning
Pinching
Numbness
Tingling
Other:

PATIENT EDUCATION CONSIDERATIONS

Readiness to learn:	Ready and self-motivated (Extrinsically motivated) Limitations (see below)
Limitations to learning:	(Cognitive) Physical Language Financial Cultural Other: Difficulty communicating; decreased memory, speech, and comprehension of day-to-day tasks
Teaching method preferred:	(Handout) (Verbal) (Demonstration (frequent)) (Practice) Other: Visual handwritten directions and verbal reinforcement
Explain:	

MEDICAL HISTORY

Past medical history:	Reported healthy prior to the accident
Family history:	None
Surgery and invasive procedures:	2 prior C-sections and ORIF 21 d ago
Medications:	Anti-inflammatories (helpful in relieving pain) Allergies: No known drug allergies
Previous treatments:	Physical therapy for 3 wk at inpatient hospital
Diagnostic tests:	X-ray: Negative MRI: Negative CT scan: EMG: Other:

PSYCHOSOCIAL FACTORS

Living situation:	Patient is married with 2 children (3 and 5 years old) and a supportive family.
Behavior:	Anxious with all therapy disciplines (PT/OT/SLP); cognitive limitations to learning
Occupation:	Homemaker
Recreation and leisure:	Active runner prior to accident
Functional disability:	Unable to walk short distances
Concerns:	Family concerned about how she will take care of herself and her family and "how much she will heal"

PROVISIONAL PAIN CLASSIFICATION

Nociceptive:ischemia; *proliferation* phase of healing undergoing intermittent chemical inflammation from flare-ups

PAIN EDUCATION TOPICS

1. What the ischemia pain mechanism involves
2. No-worse concept of healing; exercises she is able to resume, gradual exposure
3. Connective tissue healing and repair; movement guidelines and pain using the Activity Pyramid to guide inflammation and ischemia understanding and action
4. Discussion with her caregivers and family members regarding her healing progression and how to help with her HEP
5. Flare-up plan; icing for inflammation if present
6. Explicit written directions and expectations regarding pain response during and after therapy; continuous reinforcement with the patient of appropriate healing guidelines

(continues on next page)

> **APPENDIX 4.D** Traumatic Brain Injury Inpatient: 37-Year-Old Female *(continued from previous page)*

Physical Therapy/Occupational Therapy Objective Evaluation

OBJECTIVE FINDINGS

Active/passive range of motion:	Pain during movement with knee flexion. Minimally limited with knee flexion and extension. Both movements painful at end ranges. Patient has a concordant sign of pain with knee flexion while stepping up and nonverbal pain responses with loading/stance phase of gait. Pain with active range of motion in flexion and extension of R knee.
Repeated test movements:	Repeated knee extension: produces pain in the knee that is no worse as a result
	Repeated knee flexion: produces pain in the knee that is no worse as a result

PROVISIONAL MECHANICAL CLASSIFICATION

Dysfunction—flexion and extension
Other: trauma—3 wk post injury

PROVISIONAL PAIN CLASSIFICATION

Nociceptive:ischemia[a]; *remodeling* phase of healing[b]

TREATMENT

Treatment:	Gentle ROM and restoration of function with a kinetic chain program focusing on R lower extremity strengthening and R knee ROM in a no-worse state.
	Over the next 4 wk, patient progresses to a straight cane with minimal assistance for safety and balance. Balance is more of an issue from a neurological perspective than lower extremity strength. After 4 weeks, patient transfers from IP to OP.
Treatment summary:	**16 total visits over 12 wk for OP care**, 2x/wk for the first 4 wk, decreasing to 1x/wk. From a strengthening and functional perspective, patient returns to sitting through a movie and ambulating community distances without knee pain and begins to tolerate going down stairs reciprocally and independently. Patient has a home exercise program, and her husband provides occasional assistance with higher level balance exercises.

		PSFS	
		Initial	Discharge
Goals:	Sit 1-2 h to allow her to ride in a car or sit through a movie	2	10
	Ambulate community distances with appropriate assistive device	1	10
	Pain limitation to function	5	10
	Pain intensity rating	6	0

Abbreviations: AROM = active range of motion; CT = computed tomography; EMG = electromyography; HEP = home exercise program; IP = inpatient; L = left; MRI = magnetic resonance imaging; OP = outpatient; ORIF = open reduction internal fixation; OT = occupational therapy; PSFS = Patient-Specific Functional Scale; PT = physical therapy; R = right; ROM = range of motion; SLP = speech-language pathology.

[a]This patient also demonstrates the nociceptive:inflammatory characteristics in her history; however, the dominating mechanism during her initial evaluation based on the objective evaluation is nociceptive:ischemia. The clinician, however, also needs to educate the patient on inflammation and the potential increase in pain with increases in her activity level that are too fast, too soon, or too sudden.

[b]For patients in the early remodeling phase of healing after trauma, regardless of mechanical diagnosis, the pain mechanism always drives the clinician to remodel the tissue under question in a no-worse state. In Appendix 4.C, the mechanical classification is dysfunction, and the patient is treated based on his contractile remodeling issues. The postsurgical patient in this appendix has a diagnosis of healing state after trauma and requires monitoring to ensure normal tissue remodeling; however, end range stress to the tissue will ensure healthy tissue stresses and restoration of normal ROM. Both patients have the same pain mechanism of nociceptive:ischemia, but the patient in Appendix 4.C is stuck in the remodeling phase of healing and needs significant education. The patient in Appendix 4.D is passing through remodeling to restoration of function; because of her head injury, education needs to be explicit and clear.

APPENDIX 4.E Orthopedic Outpatient, 17-Year-Old Male

Physical Therapy/Occupational Therapy
Initial Evaluation

SUBJECTIVE FINDINGS

Chief complaint:	Thoracic pain inferior to the scapulas
Descriptors:	Fatigue and achy, crampy feeling
Onset:	2 mo ago for no apparent reason
Frequency:	Intermittent
24-hr behavior:	Better in AM, worse as day progresses, worse in evening
Subjective pain:	Likert / Faces scale: 5/10
Aggravating factors:	Sitting through class, playing the guitar; unable to reproduce with movement
Relieving factors:	Stopping the activity, moving

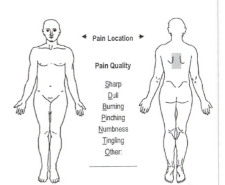

Pain Location

Pain Quality
Sharp
Dull
Burning
Pinching
Numbness
Tingling
Other:

PATIENT EDUCATION CONSIDERATIONS

Readiness to learn:	Ready and self-motivated Extrinsically motivated Limitations (see below)
Limitations to learning:	Cognitive Physical Language Financial Cultural Other: None
Teaching method preferred:	Handout Verbal Demonstration Practice Other:
Explain:	No limitations; however, patient appears distracted and frustrated to be in therapy

MEDICAL HISTORY

Past medical history:	Seasonal allergies, irritable bowel syndrome
Family history:	Unremarkable
Surgery and invasive procedures:	None
Medications:	None Allergies: No known drug allergies
Previous treatments:	None reported
Diagnostic tests:	X-ray: Negative MRI: CT scan: EMG: Other:

(continues on next page)

APPENDIX 4.E Orthopedic Outpatient, 17-Year-Old Male *(continued from previous page)*

PSYCHOSOCIAL FACTORS

Living situation:	Patient lives with his parents and is a junior in high school.
Behavior:	Distracted and frustrated
Occupation:	Student
Recreation and leisure:	Active in playing the guitar
Functional disability:	He has had problems sitting extended periods of time and playing the guitar longer than 1 hr
Concerns:	Concerned about why he is not better yet

PROVISIONAL PAIN CLASSIFICATION

Nociceptive:ischemia

PAIN EDUCATION TOPICS

1. What the ischemic pain mechanism involves with respect to pain production and Activity Pyramid
2. Correction of posture correlated with elimination of pain
3. Conditioning of posture with graded exposure to functional activity as opposed to merely strengthening

Physical Therapy/Occupational Therapy
Objective Evaluation

OBJECTIVE FINDINGS

Active/passive range of motion:	No ROM limitations in any directions in cervical or thoracic spine
Repeated test movements:	No effect of repeated movement testing. Patient is able to produce his pain only with >20 min of sustained sitting posture in thoracic flexion; reversal of posture abolishes all symptoms.

PROVISIONAL MECHANICAL CLASSIFICATION
Posture syndrome

PROVISIONAL PAIN CLASSIFICATION
Nociceptive:ischemia

TREATMENT

Treatment:	Postural correction and slouch overcorrect exercise; graded exposure to erect posture with guitar playing and sitting during classes at school unsupported, increasing 1-5 min each day or guitar session		
Treatment summary:	**2 visits over 3 wk.** Patient is aware that postural correction is important and is all that is necessary to eliminate his thoracic pain.		

		PSFS	
		Initial	Discharge
Goals:	Sitting 1-2 hr to allow him to play the guitar	3	9
	Pain limitation to function	5	9
	Pain intensity rating	6	0

Abbreviations: CT = computed tomography; EMG = electromyography; MRI = magnetic resonance imaging; PSFS = Patient-Specific Functional Scale; ROM = range of motion.

APPENDIX 4.F Clinical Reasoning for Subjective PNS Pain Characteristics

Peripheral Nervous System Pain Mechanisms: Subjective Characteristics		
Nociceptive:Inflammatory Mechanical vs. Chemical	**Nociceptive:Ischemia**	**Peripheral Neurogenic**

Location: Localized
Frequency:
  Chemical: Constant dull ache or throb at rest
  Mechanical: Intermittent and sharp with movement
Descriptors: Swollen, throbbing, aching
Onset: Recent trauma within 3 weeks or recent flare-up of chronic pathological condition
24-hour behavior: Increased pain in the morning; gets better throughout day, then worsens at end of day and during night
Course: Improving rapidly according to expected tissue healing/pathology recovery times
Alleviating factors: Ice, responds to simple NSAIDs / analgesia medications, certain directions or positions
Aggravating factors: Heat; clearly related to certain directions or positions
Psychosocial screen: Negative
	Location: Localized
	Frequency: Intermittent
	Descriptors: Fatigue, weakness, tightness, sharp with movement
	Onset: Onset may be for no apparent reason; onset can be positional or cumulative or >21 days after connective tissue injury in a remodeling phase
	24-hour behavior: Typically better in the morning and worse in the afternoon or after maintaining an activity or position for 1-3 hours
	Course: Unchanged, plateau
	Alleviating: Heat, change position, gentle stretching/exercise, limited movement
	Aggravating: Related to prolonged movements, positions, activities
	Psychosocial screen: Negative
		Location: Localized to dermatome or cutaneous nerve field
		Intensity: High, irritable
		Frequency: Constant, intermittent, spontaneous, or paroxysmal pain
		Descriptors: Sharp, deep ache, cramp = muscle; superficial burning, parasthesia, pins and needles, shooting, electric shock like, crawling = skin; numbness, heavy, tingle, weakness = root
		Onset: History of nerve injury, pathology, or mechanical compromise
		Alleviating: Heat; antiepileptic (gabapentin, pregabalin), antidepression (amitriptyline) medications; activities or postures associated with no movement, less tension, pressure of neural tissues
		Aggravating: Mechanical pattern involving activities and postures associated with movement; loading or compression of neural tissue; stress, mood can alter pain
		24-hour behavior: Worse at night, disturbed sleep

APPENDIX 4.G Clinical Reasoning for Objective PNS Pain Characteristics

Peripheral Nervous System
Pain Mechanisms: Objective Characteristics

Nociceptive:Inflammatory Mechanical vs. Chemical	Nociceptive:Ischemia	Peripheral Neurogenic
Objective findings: **Mechanical** • Close movement/pain relationship with active, passive, resisted repeated motion testing • Classification of mechanical diagnosis for derangement; identified preferred direction • Sprain/strain identified with pain, weakness, pain laxity, palpation • Absence of neurological signs, allodynia/hyperalgesia **Chemical** • All static/repeated movement tests increase pain; remains worse • Unable to identify position or motion to abolish symptoms • Ice temporarily eases pain with midrange position of affected area • Evidence of warmth, swelling • Antalgic posture movement pattern	**Objective findings:** Classification of mechanical diagnosis for dysfunction, posture, other • Contractile or articular tissue dysfunction: Symptoms present *during* for contractile and at *end range* for articular on repeated movement assessment; no worse as a result *after* repeated movement assessment • Patient may have a painful arc of motion or region where contractile tissue is challenged in contractile dysfunction. • **Posture syndrome:** Reproduction of symptoms is often difficult on movement exam and no loss of motion is present. Symptoms are produced with static end range posture and are abolished when stress is removed. • **Other condition:** Often this kinetic chain impairment and/or pathology affects the quality of movement or muscle activation during movement; produces symptoms and remains no worse as a result.	**Objective findings:** **Posture:** Antalgic of affected body part **Palpation:** Provoke symptoms with palpation of involved nerve **Neurological findings:** Positive for altered reflexes, sensation, muscle power, hyperalgesia/allodynia/hyperpathia in a dermatome, myotomal, cutaneous path **Repeated movement tests:** Identify preferred direction and signs of centralization with mechanical inflammation present **Repeated neurodynamic tests:** Identify nerve irritation as nerve or container dependent. **Nerve dependent:** Restriction in ROM; can produce or increase symptoms with additional movements that increase force to the neural tissues. Repeated neural tension movements *during* may increase or decrease; as a result, *after* symptoms will be no better or worse and no change in ROM will occur. **Container dependent:** May be restriction in ROM but not always; unexpected response of symptoms with additional neural tension. Latency symptom response after testing: Pain at release, decreased pain with loading. Repeated neural movements *during* increase and worsen symptoms. Symptoms change when manual muscle test or joint play test is performed in a neural tension position, which can isolate the nerve container tissue source.

APPENDIX 4.H Clinical Reasoning for PNS Pain Intervention

Peripheral Nervous System Pain Mechanism Intervention		
Nociceptive:Inflammatory Mechanical vs. Chemical	**Nociceptive:Ischemia**	**Peripheral Neurogenic**
Mechanical **Patient education:** Use pain as a guide **MICE:** Mobility, Ice, Compression, Elevation *Mobility:* Midrange motion of the involved tissue; identify directional or postural preference; use every 1–2 hours as a guideline for exercise; modify ADLs and occupational tasks. *Ice:* 30 min, 3-4x/day; light covering on skin *Compression:* Use compression garments on involved tissue during activity. *Elevation:* Typically use at end of day; may need to support involved tissue above heart. **Chemical** Patient education: Use pain as a guide **RICE:** Rest, Ice, Compression, Elevation *Rest:* Use corset or brace on involved tissue during activity; modify ADLs and occupational tasks. *Ice:* 30 min, 3-4x/day; light covering on skin *Compression:* Use compression garments on involved tissue during rest. *Elevation:* At end of day, elevate involved tissue above heart when appropriate. **Medication:** Use oral nonsteroidal medication every 4–6 hours; progress to steroid oral or injection if no effect is seen after 72 hours. **Modalities:** Use electrical stimulation to decrease edema.	**Patient education:** Repair/remodeling phase of tissue healing. Pain is no longer a guide. No worse after 20 minutes of activity is a guide. **ROM:** Progressed to end range and into pain of involved tissue in all directions; no worse as a result. **Extremity function:** Restore quality biometrics and progress from isometric to concentric to eccentric function; progress the return of ADLs, occupational tasks, and sports function. **Spine function:** Begin in antigravity position; restore neutral spine; progress through weightbearing activities with posture, body mechanics, ADLs, occupational tasks, and sports function. **Cardiovascular exercise:** Build on the patient's low aerobic capacity 2–5 hours weekly, HR at 55%–75% of max; progress to high-intensity interval training 2-3x/wk, HR at 75%–90% of max for exertion intervals (10 seconds to 1 min) followed by recovery intervals (30 seconds to 2 min) for 3–9 sets for a total of 10–30 min. **Strength training:** Weightlifting for 1-3x/wk; total body functional movement patterns **Manual therapy:** Massage, overpressure, mobilization, and manipulation applied as patient plateaus with active exercise associated with tissue dysfunction **Modalities:** Increase blood flow response before or after exercise, using hot packs, ultrasound, heat wraps (active), or electrical stimulation.	**Patient education:** Based on inflammatory or ischemic pain properties, follow previous guidelines. **Neural-dependent guidelines** *Neurodynamic movement:* Slider neural movement pre and/or post low aerobic (LA) exercise. Start movement at extremity joint away from symptom area. Progress neural movement to tension on the nerve pre and/or post LA exercise toward location of symptoms. *Manual therapy:* Neural rubbing at abnormal impulse generating site (AIGS); work away from the nerve, then move directly onto palpation of the tender region of the nerve. *Graded exposure/pacing cardiovascular exercise:* Build low aerobic capacity 2–5 hours weekly, HR at 55%–75% of max; add 1–5 min every 24–72 hours. Progress to high-intensity interval training 2-3x/wk, HR at 75%–90% of max for exertion intervals (10 seconds to 1 min) followed by recovery intervals (30 seconds to 2 min) for 3–9 sets for a total of 10–30 min. **Container-dependent guidelines** Treat container first. *Muscle:* Soft tissue massage; stretch and strengthen muscle or apply eccentric strength if tendon. *Joint:* Overpressure, mobilization, manipulation; restore ROM in 3 planes. *Neurodynamic movement:* Neural slider movement after container treatments; progress to neural tension movement if necessary.

CHAPTER 5

Peripheral Neurogenic Pain Mechanism

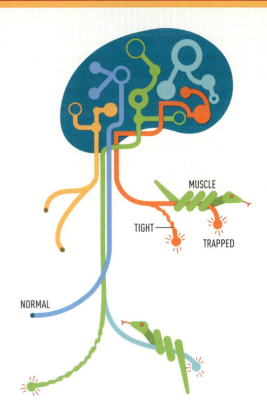

To be effective, treatment must somehow reach and reverse the painful process at its source in a lasting fashion. If one is not successful reversing the pain-generating disorder, it will persist, allowing pre-existing psychosocial factors to become operative, flourish, and even dominate.

—James Cyriax, MD
Father of Orthopedic Medicine

POINTS TO DISCUSS

- Characteristics of neurogenic pain
- Role of neurodynamics in classifying mechanical problems related to the peripheral neurogenic pain mechanism (PNPM)
- Peripheral nerve clinical anatomy, including peripheral nerve mobility, peripheral nerve dynamics, spinal cord dynamics, axoplasm, and peripheral nerve conduction
- Peripheral nerve injury and impairment, including nerve conduction impairment and abnormal impulse generating sites
- PNPM connection to central sensitization
- Nerve pain subjective evaluation
- Nerve pain objective evaluation, including nerve conduction and neurodynamic examination
- Classification of PNPM mechanical dysfunction as container dependent or neural dependent
- PNPM management and intervention

Pain is necessary for survival, no matter how unpleasant a stimulus may be perceived. With injury to the body, nerve cells detect the injury and send an electrical message via the spinal cord to the brain. The brain perceives that the body tissues are in danger and generates a response to protect or prevent further damage. Most pain is short lived; however, for some individuals it persists for weeks, months, years, or throughout life. Sometimes chronic pain results from damage to the peripheral nervous system (PNS) itself, and other times pain is present with no damage or pathology. Experts have referred to peripheral nerve pathology as *peripheral neurogenic pain* (eg, radicular low back pain, sciatica). In this chapter we explore the peripheral neurogenic pain mechanism (PNPM), including neurodynamics and recovery, and explain the connections with and differences from chronic central neurogenic pain. This chapter also highlights subjective history characteristics and objective sensory, motor, and neurodynamic testing that allow the clinician to classify the mechanical elements of PNPM and screen for central nervous system (CNS) pain mechanisms.

Characteristics of Peripheral Neurogenic Pain

The scientific literature uses many terms to describe peripheral neurogenic pain, including neuropathic, neurogenic, neural-dependent, container-dependent, intraneural, and extraneural pain; neuralgia; double crush syndrome; radiculopathy; entrapment; and perineural fibrosis. Regardless of the terminology used, this musculoskeletal pain mechanism results from alterations in nerve structure, nerve dynamics, or the interface with other tissues in the anatomical path of the peripheral nerve. The PNPM applies to situations in which nerve roots and associated nerve trunks have been injured or irritated by mechanical and/or chemical stimuli that exceed the physical capabilities of the nervous system. This mechanism may be associated with trauma, disease, postural strain, positional effects of certain links in the kinetic chain, and unhealthy tissues adjacent to the peripheral nerve causing a nociceptive process of inflammation and/or ischemia.[1]

The PNPM is a unique category because inflammatory and ischemic characteristics simultaneously occur. The target connective tissue with this pain mechanism is the peripheral nerve originating outside the dorsal horn and continuing to terminal cutaneous branches. An understanding of the nervous system as both a peripheral and a central system is essential to enable clinicians to effectively address the neurobiological pain mechanisms described in this chapter and in Chapter 6.

The quantitative evaluation procedures of sensory testing, nerve conduction studies, evoked potentials, functional imaging, skin biopsies, and genetic screening provide valuable information about neurobiology. These investigations are labor intensive and expensive and require a level of technical expertise usually available only at highly specialized centers. These tests, however, may not be necessary for routine evaluation of a patient's nerve-related pain. The PNPM is recognizable by specific subjective characteristics of pain-related symptoms. Objective clinical characteristics of conduction and neurodynamic testing can then provide sufficient information to allow the clinician to forgo more elaborate testing and initiate a treatment plan of patient education and active care.

Patients with neurogenic pain are typically classified based on disease diagnosis. The only correlation study of neurogenic pain–related symptoms and disease addressed one pain subtype associated with a subgroup of patients with diabetic polyneuropathy.[2] Disease itself does not predict the occurrence or natural course of neurogenic pain; the etiological factors and pathological changes that define a neurological disease do not necessarily correlate with mechanisms responsible for the manifestation of spontaneous pain. Hyperalgesia, an exaggerated response, or allodynia, a painful response to a stimulus that does not typically evoke pain, are both common features of neurogenic pain.[3,4]

Different pain mechanisms can operate in patients with the same disease, the same pain mechanisms can be present in patients with different diagnoses, and the relative contribution of particular mechanisms to the pain in individual patients may change over time.[5] Changes in the nervous system can become autonomous and persist long after the primary disease has disappeared (eg, postherpetic neuralgia).

Role of Neurodynamics in Classifying Mechanical Problems Related to PNPM

The interdependence between the mechanics and physiology of the nervous system was termed *neurodynamics* by Shacklock[6] in 1995. An understanding of neurodynamic concepts sets the foundation for discussion of the mechanical problems of container-dependent and neural-dependent dysfunctions associated with the development of peripheral neurogenic pain.

The relatively new concept of neurodynamics is just beginning to be applied in medicine and physical and occupational therapy despite the universal attention it has received throughout the past 25 years.[7-12] The study of neurodynamics investigates how the mechanics and physiology of the nervous system relate to each other and to patients' symptoms.[6] A neurodynamic test assesses the mechanics and physiology of a part of the nervous system (eg, root, axon, cutaneous branch).

Neural tension is tightness within a part of the nervous system; some forms of neural tension are normal end range responses to stretch and should not be assumed to be pathological when found on neurodynamic testing. Neurodynamic testing is not just an assessment of the length capabilities of the neural structures; it also includes how the neural tissue interfaces with adjacent structures and tissues. For example, the straight leg raise (SLR) test is an assessment of sciatic nerve length, the production of symptoms, and the interface with structures including but not limited to lumbar discs, lateral foramina, sciatic notch, posterior hip capsule musculature, and posterior thigh, knee, and lower leg tissues. The SLR test evaluates the sciatic nerve throughout its path as it continues to terminal branches of the tibial and common peroneal nerve.

The PNPM is the only mechanism directly affiliated with an anatomical tissue. Hence, reference to neurodynamics of the peripheral nerve allows clinicians to understand the function of the nervous tissues and the need for therapeutic exercises directed at the peripheral nerve when rehabilitation needs are present. Appreciating the mechanical continuity of the nervous system may also assist clinicians and their patients in understanding why different areas of the body may be used to mobilize involved neural tissues. The impact that movement has on the nervous system is not only mechanical, as in amount of load, but is also related to fluid dynamics, connective tissue interfaces, and ability to dissipate pressures. The next section includes physiological explanations of how intraneural circulation, axoplasmic flow, and nociceptors in neural connective tissues can be affected by mechanical loading.[6] This knowledge can help clinicians direct patient education and exercise prescriptions depending on the type of PNPM mechanical problem.

Peripheral Nerve Clinical Anatomy

This section summarizes peripheral nerve clinical anatomy. For a more complete description, refer to Butler's *The Sensitive Nervous System*.[12]

The peripheral nerves, formally referred to as the *peripheral nervous system*, originate as part of the CNS from the brain. Peripheral nerves connect via the brainstem to the spinal cord. They continue through the tracts of the spinal cord and evolve into the dorsal root ganglion. The peripheral nerve axon exits as a spinal nerve root, changing into a nerve trunk and reaching its final destination as terminal cutaneous branches throughout the upper and lower limbs. This tissue anatomically is one of the longest in the body, hence the complexity of patient education and exercise prescription.

Peripheral nerve is made up of connective tissue that is continuous with the strong dura mater and epidural tissues in the spinal cord canal. These strong connective tissues protect neural tissue from excessive compression, allow movement distribution though their tensile load properties, and maintain the environment for adequate nutrition to neural structures. As with other connective tissues, the nerve fibers, axons, and fascicles are designed for movement. They do not run in straight lines. They unfold and fold during activities based on the way they are stressed. The neurodynamic properties that dissipate loads and accommodate positions exist at the axon cylinder and myelin levels as well. This movement design allows for efficiency in force distribution for tensile and compression loads and anchoring to surrounding somatic tissues for added stability in the path. Anchor points can contribute to some of the somatic symptoms present in patients with PNPM. Because the nervous system is one system, access is essential to communication among the endocrine, immune, and autonomic nervous systems. Education of patients about nerve pain should include a review of how long and strong neural tissues are and their need for blood, space, and movement.

The three major connective tissues comprised by the peripheral nerve are the epineurium, perineurium, and endoneurium. Surrounding all these connective tissues is a sheath called the mesoneurium[13] or paraneurium.[14] The sheath allows the nerve to glide alongside adjacent tissues, and it folds or contracts.[13] With injury, the sheath commonly becomes fibrotic and shrinks like a tight stocking.[14] Neurogenic massage and neural sliding and neural tension stretching exercises may be helpful to remodel fibrotic connective tissues after injury.

Peripheral Nerve Mobility

Function dictates the mobility requirements of each patient. Typical anatomic tissue mechanics also drive function in each patient; this is especially true with the peripheral nerve. The electrochemical processes involved in neural conduction occur through a variety of movements that develop the nervous system's strength, mobility, and nutritional scheme. The tissues that interface with peripheral nerves can affect normal mobility, conduction, and nutrition. Consider the physical forces placed on the neural structures when ballet dancers, athletes, or contortionists perform their respective activities. Each discipline requires a different set of technical movements to complete these activities. If the nerve cannot move, glide, undulate, and stretch to enable these people to function, then the nerve's primary function of conduction will be altered. Just as function dictates motion, so does motion dictate function.

Inman and Saunders[12,15] and Louis[12,16] noted that from spinal extension to flexion, a spinal canal may elongate up to 7 to 9 cm and longer. Breig[12,17] showed that during cervical flexion, the brain stem elongates a full centimeter or more. These studies indicate the ability of nerves not only to elongate, but also to adapt to surrounding tissues. When the clinician performs an SLR test, the patient's sciatic nerve must adapt in length to the surrounding tissues by at least 12% of its normal length.[12,18] Consider what tight hamstrings and myofascial tissues mean to this adaptability: The nerve needs to elongate in excess of 12% to account for the interfacing tissue mobility loss. When a person raises an arm above the head, the median nerve must increase in length by 20%; it accomplishes this by sliding, bending, and stretching through all the adjacent tissues and structures.[12,19] In a patient with forward shoulder posture, the tight pectoralis minor will greatly affect that 20% adaptability. Wright et al[12,20] noted that in any location along the peripheral nerve, the nerve needs the ability to slide around the surrounding body tissue interfaces by 2 cm to prevent ongoing injury and allow normal excursion.

The elongation aspect of nerve dynamics is critical, but the ability to absorb pressure from the forces of compressing tissues is just as important. It has been shown that the pressure within the nerve doubles or even quadruples during elongation.[21] Compression occurs

TABLE 5.1 Clinical Findings Differentiating Tight Muscle from Tight Nerve

Tight Muscle	Tight Nerve
Straight leg raise (SLR) test is positive.	SLR test is positive.
Repeated SLR test results in an increase of symptoms from baseline and more apprehension in SLR test. When in SLR tension position, the SLR test is altered with isometric hamstring manual muscle test.	Repeated SLR test produces an increased symptom response but afterward has no immediate effect on symptoms or SLR test apprehension.
Palpation of the muscle identifies tender muscle–nerve interface points. Repeated hamstring muscle stretching alters SLR test with improved range of motion and less apprehension, which indicates that interface tissue is the issue.	Repeated neurodynamic stretching indicates that nervous tissue tightness is the issue.

as the ulnar nerve flattens around the bend in the elbow or as the spinal cord shortens or folds to go from flexion to extension. These neurodynamic abilities to lengthen, slide, and dissipate compression are crucial and need to be restored when PNPM dominates.

As a general rule, the amount of neural movement is proportional to the movement of the surrounding tissue. Patients with tight muscles or scars attaching the nerve to surrounding tissues may place additional demands on the system with which the nerve interfaces. When patients stretch their hamstrings, for example, sometimes the SLR test for sciatic nerve improves in length and tension, indicating the interfacing tissue's effect on neural function. The opposite is true as well if hamstring length is normal but the patient's SLR test is positive and limited and produces the painful symptom; in this case, the neural tissue is more dysfunctional. If the SLR test is positive, a neurodynamic exercise is required to lengthen the dysfunctional nerve or the tight hamstring. The decision of whether to treat the nerve with neurodynamic exercise or to treat the entrapping interfacing tissue is an important clinical reasoning step in prescribing exercise in PNPM patients, and the source must be differentiated. **Table 5.1** summarizes the clinical findings that differentiate tight muscle from tight nerve.

Routinely, patients are injured while moving, and initially movement may need to cease or decrease to jump-start recovery. Recovery requires progressive movement of the injured tissue; this is no different with a peripheral nerve. The peripheral nerve could sustain an injury by being overstretched or pinched, resulting in edema causing an abnormal impulse-generating site (AIGS). Patients may become fearful of movement or reinjury, immobilizing themselves in their own minds. All of these situations have a different movement-symptom relationship on neurodynamic testing, but all of these situations will improve through organized movement approaches.

Neurodynamics and mobilization of nerves are not new. Athletic stretching, running, Tai Chi, yoga, martial arts, and wrestling have been putting the nervous system through an array of body movements for centuries. What is new is the inclusion of movement of neural tissues when pain and symptoms are involved and the accompanying education about those movements and symptoms that is given to the patients with dominating PNPM.

Peripheral Nerve Dynamics

The nerve root and plexus are designed for movement transmission. The peripheral nerve axons take a circuitous route through the extremity. Because of this spiraling and interfascicular sliding, the nerve can assist in tension transmission, as demonstrated when the elongating force of one nerve is transmitted to several cervical nerve root complexes.[10,22] These micro motions allow the nerve root to dissipate mechanical forces and receive nutrition.[23] For example, with immobilization from disc pathology, surgery, or stenosis, the resultant fibrosis and tissue irritation affect not only motility but also nutrition and oxygenation of the peripheral nerve and contribute to its ischemic-like pain mechanism. Neurodynamic movement retrains micro motions and provides nutrition.

Spinal Cord Dynamics

The spinal cord elongates and contracts with spinal movements in both the sagittal and frontal planes.[3,24] To handle these forces, the neurons are arranged in folds and spirals that straighten with elongation and refold as the cord contracts. These folding-unfolding and spiral arrangements of neurons protect the spinal cord. The cervical spinal cord is most mobile in the direction of flexion to extension. The cervical cord is approximately 20% longer[10,12] and the sagittal canal diameter is about 30% narrower,[12,25] creating neural pressure. This pressure throughout the cord aids in its stability and strength. The ability to transmit tension throughout the cord is a necessity, as demonstrated by reported elongations of 5 to 9 cm.[8-10,12] Because of the spinal cord's ability to elongate, its continuity in cervical spine flexion mechanically challenges tension of the neural tissue cord, roots, and axons in the lumbar spine.[2,9] In general, cervical flexion increases neural tension, and cervical extension decreases neural tension.

Axoplasm

Cytoplasm is present in all cells. In the peripheral nerve, it is called *axoplasm*. Different dynamics of flow occur to maintain health in peripheral nerves. The fast flow carries ion channels and neurotransmitters, and the slow flow carries cytoskeletal proteins and neurofilaments distally from the cell body of a peripheral nerve. In the PNPM, this essential flow can stop or slow down with mechanical nerve dysfunction or entrapment.[12,26,27] Axoplasm is a viscous substance that is five times the density of water, and consequently it flows better with movement.[12,28,29]

Educating patients about the nerve axoplasm's need for movement using an analogy such as "nerve lubricant" can help them understand the remodeling process for restoring nerve dynamics. For example, with diabetes and its abundance of nerve entrapments, the fast axoplasmic flow becomes sluggish when under excessive compression from entrapment peripheral nerve dysfunctions.[12,30,31] As the flow slows or stops, so do blood supply and tissue oxygenation. The peripheral nerve is blood thirsty at the cellular level. The brain and spinal cord are about 2% of body mass; however, they consume 20% of available oxygen circulating in the blood.[12,32] The blood system for the peripheral nerve was designed for movement, with a well-developed microvascular system through multiple feeder vessels.[12,33] Fascicles have arteries with slack built in to allow for intrafascicular sliding that is essential for nerves to glide through tissues.[10,12,32,33] Regular movement directed at the peripheral nerve can have profound effects on the axoplasm and thus on the symptoms of PNPM patients. In these patients, cardiovascular exercise helps meet the need for blood flow to these tissues. A patient with comorbidities will have more difficulty meeting this blood flow need.

Peripheral Nerve Conduction

Genetics provides a predetermined blueprint of neural connections and the activity associated with those connections. Many of these connections can run unconsciously. Throughout development, responses to various triggers, such as accidents, positions, chemicals, emotions, motivations, and the words we use, dictate the genetic movement presentations. One neuron can represent how the entire system behaves because it receives many inputs at different places and times. The response of the neurons can be excitation or inhibition. The brain of an adult contains about 100 billion neurons, and these are interconnected with multiple other synapses.[12,34] Each neuron has numerous spines that can create more synapses. Most of the synapses are feedback synapses; repeatability of the nervous system is explained by the continued checks and balances of its actions. It is a system that allows for many micromanagers.

The potential for connections and synapses also demonstrates the plasticity that is needed in the PNS and CNS for recovery. Plasticity is the coding behind each connection and combination of connections that typically dictates a pattern of activity. These patterns of activity can be replayed if needed or quickly adapted based on responses and additional triggers. The behaviors clinicians witness in their patients are the result of this genetic and environmental coding. The responses and triggers of a patient include joyful and painful experiences, past and present, and ultimately will guide the context in which the neurodynamic exercise needs to be understood and performed to aid full recovery.

Various chemical substances called *neurotransmitters* and *neuromodulators* of the PNS are needed for these synapses, and activation requires receptors and ion channels. The most important substances are the inhibitory and excitatory amino acids, neuropeptides, acetylcholine, serotonin, and noradrenalin. Clinically speaking, symptoms can be triggered by words, thoughts, memories of injury, and feelings, which can drive the production of inhibitory or excitatory amino acids and therefore compromise the neurodynamics and conduction of the peripheral nerve. In the most simplistic form, conduction is dependent on open ion channels. Movement-based therapy is focused on reversing closed ion channels to open by facilitating new patterns and behaviors and by changing the patient's context, environment, thoughts, words, and feelings. The channel's receptors have proteins associated with a chemical stimulus neurotransmitter; agonistic protein receptors open and antagonistic receptors close the ion channel. The mechanosensitive channels that respond to stretch, pressure, or temperature exist mainly in the PNS.[12,35]

The number, kind, and activity of ion channels vary with each individual. The plasticity of the CNS and PNS is based on ion channel expression. When injury happens, ion channel expression and numbers increase dramatically in the amygdala, hippocampus, and dorsal root ganglia.[12] With demyelination, after injury the demyelinated segment of the peripheral nerve has a high density of channels because the myelin sheath resists channel insertion.[12,36] This process is the basis of the AIGS commonly observed in peripheral neurons related to the PNPM.[12,37] Clinically, understanding the AIGS is critical to understanding peripheral neurogenic pain that has CNS pain mechanism characteristics. In contrast, this chronic neural mechanosensitivity at the spinal cord and ultimately brain level is referred to as *central neurogenic pain* and (a less traditional example) *fibromyalgia*.

Peripheral Nerve Injury and Impairment

This section summarizes peripheral nerve injury and impairment. For a more complete understanding, refer to Butler's *The Sensitive Nervous System*.[12]

Peripheral nerves can generate pain in several ways. The most common ways are dysesthetic pain and nerve trunk pain.[12,38] The epineurium, perineurium, and endoneurium that provide mechanical support can be injured by overstretch or pinch or can be caught within adjacent interfacing tissues. Chemicals are released that result in chemical inflammatory pain from the reaction to the damaged nerve. As healing progresses, immobilization sets in and scarring occurs. Inflammation gradually decreases, and ischemia may occur as neural adaptations continue.

As discussed in Chapter 4, neurons within connective tissues may be irritated by temperature, chemical, and mechanical stimuli; this is true in neural tissue as well. Mechanical forces such as repeated tensile load, compression, vibration, and friction can cause mechanical irritation. This irritation occurs near anatomically narrow tissue interfaces where the nerve needs significant room to pass through.[10,12,39] Neural irritation can be complicated by a chemical inflammatory process when the connective tissues adjacent to the nerve release inflammatory substances.[40-42] Nerve injury challenges the vascular, connective tissue, and impulse conduction aspects of the peripheral nerve both chemically and mechanically.

Initially after nerve injury, a decrease in intraneural circulation and axoplasmic flow occurs, creating venous congestion from mechanical and chemical stimuli that exceed the physical capabilities of that peripheral nerve.[12,43,44] The low axoplasmic flow maintains the neurogenic inflammation and increases fluid pressure; both are caused by the anoxia and microvascular permeability alterations that occur during the inflammatory response in nerve trunks and dorsal root ganglia.[12,43,45] Inflamed neural connective tissues become sensitive to additional mechanical and chemical stimuli, causing the enhanced mechanosensitivity seen with PNPM patients.[46,47] The edema is slow to leave because the diffusion barrier resists the escape of inflammatory exudates.[48,49] Typically, this edema leads to intraneural fibrosis that can reduce the elasticity of the peripheral nerve and interfere with functional movement.[43,50]

In mechanosensitive tissue, additional mechanical force from intraneural fibrosis provides greater mechanical stimulation to the peripheral nerve. This additional load may come from simple activities of daily living, physical examination movements, or demanding sport activities.[21,47] The decreased capacity of the peripheral nerve to move and conduct and the decreased capacity of surrounding connective tissues to move add to the PNPM. This example of PNPM with mechanical contributions from both container (interface) and intraneural fibrosis inputs is discussed in greater depth later in this chapter (see sections on container-dependent and neural-dependent mechanical dysfunctions).

Nerve Conduction Impairment

In addition to the dynamic changes that occur with intraneural fibrosis, the extent of endoneurial edema has been correlated with the amount of degradation in myelin content and axon structure.[12,43] It has been suggested that these myelin changes and disruption of axoplasmic flow alter the cell body.[50] Varying degrees of pathology have been found to be present in adjacent fascicles within the affected nerve segments.[51] With the degree of pathology so visible, many patients report significant peripheral neurogenic pain, but the clinical examination of motor function and electrodiagnostic testing may be normal.[52] Electrodiagnostic testing cannot be specific to one nerve fascicle; therefore, normal electrodiagnostic tests are associated with normal nerve fascicles. The abnormal adjacent inflamed nerve fascicle, however, could be responsible for the symptoms,[51,52] which may be why PNPM patients who complain of positive symptoms of pain, paresthesia, dysesthesia, and spasm may have no clinical signs of hypoesthesia or anesthesia (numbness) and weakness.[12,51,53] These patients display the primary presentation of mechanosensitivity in the neurodynamic exam.

Pain does not always relate to injury; this is a feature of nerve injuries as well. In a study of cadavers (asymptomatic in life), connective tissue injuries such as nerve entrapments in the upper extremity were demonstrated with nerve fiber changes.[12,54] Imaging reveals abnormally compressed nerves in many adults whose clinical exams do not reveal symptoms. The process of turning pathology into pain in the human being is a complex biopsychosocial phenomenon of which the PNPM is only a small part.[12] In a nervous system that has lost its normal ability to strain and glide, forces can no longer be normally dispersed and mechanical forces on peripheral nerves may increase. In addition, chemicals can no longer be dispersed and irritate the surrounding peripheral nerve and target tissues.

Research indicates that mechanosensitive nerve roots often are associated with the presence of scar.[12,55] Kuslich et al[12,55] attempted to define the origin of low back pain and sciatica in patients receiving local anesthesia for surgery of herniated discs or stenosis. They concluded that scar tissue and perineural fibrosis keep the nerve in one position and can compound nerve pain. More complex pain experiences can be explained by the long conducting fibers and the development of an AIGS. In an AIGS, a segment of the nerve develops the ability to repeatedly generate its own impulses. Increasing sensitivity occurs at the peripheral nerve level and may explain the sensitivity and irritability of symptoms that persist longer than normal healing. This spontaneity of impulse generation combined with the mechanosensitivity of the nerve is the main feature of an AIGS. Neurodynamic tests in all three nerve impairment situations evoke symptoms and assist in clinical reasoning regarding the dominant mechanical dysfunction of the PNPM.

Abnormal Impulse-Generating Sites

Any injured segment of the peripheral nerve and/or its associated dorsal root ganglion can develop into an AIGS. AIGSs can repeatedly generate their own impulse in areas of a neuron that normally do not initiate impulses and create a source of ectopic discharge.[12,37] AIGSs are able to form more frequently in the bare spots of demyelinated neurons. These bare spots allow ion channel insertion, increasing the membrane potential needed for activation.[12] A small amount of inflow into mechanosensitive channels causes a spike in the membrane potential, which is called an AIGS. An impulse is fired independently of a stimulus.[12] The areas that are most susceptible to the development of AIGSs are demyelinated patches of peripheral nerves, neuromas, regenerating axon sprouts, cells in the dorsal root ganglia and spinal cord, as well as near the cross-excitation that occurs with adjacent bare neurons.[12]

An AIGS in a dorsal root ganglion or midportion afferent axon can fire an impulse from proximal to distal toward the periphery (ie, antidromic impulse) and from distal to proximal toward the spinal cord (ie, orthodromic impulse).[12,56,57] Afferent depolarization in the dorsal horn of the spinal cord leads to dorsal root reflexes. It is proposed that these reflexes contribute to inflammation. Antidromic impulses arise from injury along the nerve, nerve terminals, or dorsal root ganglion or spinal cord (known as *dorsal root reflexes*), causing the release of proinflammatory chemicals into the interfaces of target tissues.[12,58,59] An injured segment of a peripheral nerve can have an impact on the physical health of the tissue it innervates.[12,60] Inflammation in target tissue can perpetuate the chronicity of syndromes such as stubborn lateral epicondylosis or Achilles tendinosis. Generally, the longer nerve pain persists, the more likely it is that an AIGS will develop and continually sensitize the nervous system.

Ion channel type and number dictate the stimuli that cause symptoms in PNPM. Many stimuli can activate an AIGS. Mechanical stimuli such as lengthening movements, pinching, friction forces, palpation of nerves, or neurodynamic tests can open mechanosensitive channels. Repetitive movements from activities such as running or sustained positioning from cycling can activate symptoms from an AIGS. Emotional stress can exacerbate symptoms of nerve injury by increasing neurotransmitters such as adrenaline or noradrenaline, thereby stimulating an AIGS as well.[12,61]

Temperature affects different nerve fibers differently. Thermal sensitivities exist in injured nerves such that cooling a tissue excites C fibers and heating excites A-δ fibers.[12,62] This quality is a function of alterations in the injured axon as opposed to any potential thermal mechanisms. Clinically, it may explain why some patients do not tolerate cold weather and why phantom limb pain may be aggravated by cold intolerance.[12,62]

Metabolic changes, anoxia, blood gas, and certain chemicals arising from ischemia can excite the damaged and altered membrane of an AIGS.[12,37] Cytokines and catecholamines have been linked to demyelination associated with an AIGS.[12,63,64] Neuromas contain large numbers of mast cells, which contain serotonin, a proinflammatory chemical stimulus shown to activate an AIGS.[12,65]

Because there are so many triggers, it is easy to see how AIGSs can manifest in patients with persistent nerve pain and symptoms. Spontaneous activity is a main characteristic of an AIGS, especially when the dorsal root ganglion is involved. Clinically, patients may express that they are unable to identify aggravating activities or that symptoms occur without any stimulus.[61] This lack of relation to a stimulus may be the result of the spontaneous firing that is common with AIGSs. The A-δ and C fibers that innervate deep structures appear to develop spontaneous discharge related to neural inflammation secondary to the mechanosensitivity.[66] This feature has been hypothesized as a reason why patients with PNPM complain of deep painful symptoms and why dermatome pain charts may be inaccurate, and thus a thorough patient symptom history is critical.[67]

The term *double crush syndrome* has been used to refer to a secondary nerve problem created from an initial nerve injury. A study found that male gender and increased age were independent risk factors for double crush syndrome.[68] Research is needed to better understand the process that occurs with nerve injury. It is crucial that clinicians consider all proximal areas and conduct an electrophysiological screen for patients with symptoms consistent with double crush syndrome.

Cross-excitation occurs when a peripheral nerve is injured and excites adjacent neurons, sometimes very quickly.[12] The anatomical connection occurs between the demyelinated segments of both neurons. A patient with pain that keeps returning and lasting longer with each recurring episode may be experiencing cross-excitations that cause chain reactions that recruit more neurons with each episode and sensitize the nervous system over time. Pain that spreads after a nerve injury has been shown to be due to central mechanisms; however, some have suggested that maintenance of CNS sensitization is attributable to the uninjured afferents and AIGSs.[12,68-70] Clinicians must understand the clinical importance of identifying all operant pain mechanisms and then the mechanism that dominates; treatment is always focused on the dominating mechanism. With AIGS development and maintenance, a patient's PNPM may progress to pain dominated by central sensitization.

PNPM Connection to Central Sensitization

It is not uncommon for patients with the PNPM to have central sensitization characteristics in the background of their pain experience. (Chapter 6 discusses the central sensitization pain mechanism.) Central sensitization develops because alterations in afferent input result from changes in the chemicals transported from the periphery, causing sprouting of low-threshold afferent fibers into superficial layers of the dorsal horn involved in nociception, immune activation, and finally alterations in central descending control mechanisms.[71,72] Alterations in descending control mechanisms indicate that the brain is not a passive recipient of pain[73]; the brain actively modulates the input it receives and directs the motor response via the descending control mechanisms.[74]

Pain is produced by the brain when it perceives that body tissues are in danger and a response is required.[75] During a pain experience, areas of the brain responsible for sensory perception, emotion, attention, cognition, and motor planning are all activated; this activation of neural activity has been referred to as the *pain neurosignature*.[12,73,75,76] Multiple areas are involved, which explains why psychosocial factors, such as confidence in the ability to recover, satisfaction with life and work, distress, false beliefs about the nature of pain, and fear avoidance behaviors related to activity and reinjury, can increase pain and slow recovery.[12,74,75,77] Recognition of when a patient with PNPM is presenting with dominating yellow flags is imperative, because the clinician needs to address the patient's pain behaviors and distress before addressing the nociceptive aspect of the PNPM.[12,74,75]

Peripheral nerve symptoms can simultaneously be inflammatory (related to too much activity) and ischemic (related to not enough activity). Positive symptoms from sensory axons consistent with an AIGS are described as painful sensations of burning or feelings of coldness, crawling, tightness, and prickling.[12,78] Negative symptoms are related to a decrease in conduction, with complaints described as sensory loss and weakness.[78] Using this information to guide questions helps clinicians diagnose the PNPM. The subjective pain evaluation identifies characteristics consistent with PNPM patterns, aiding clinicians in distinguishing mechanically dominated nerve pain from centrally sensitized nerve pain. The subjective history provides clinicians with the best indication of how many pain mechanisms are involved and which one is dominating in the treatment session.

Nerve Pain Subjective Evaluation

Location

Pain associated with peripheral nerve mechanical dysfunction can be variable even though the anatomical pathways of peripheral nerves, dermatomes, and cutaneous fields coursed by nerves can be similar.[12,67,79] Variability in location of symptoms is related to the nervous system's continuous nature. Dermatomes can vary because sensory and motor fibers contain intradural connections between spinal cord segments next to each other.[12,80] Nerve pain location can manifest as mere spots along a nerve path to severe debilitating nerve root disorders along the entire path. Often the pain associated with a nerve trunk may be represented in patient drawings as a line or a path. Most authors recommend using dermatome maps, cutaneous nerve fields, or myotomal or sclerotomal charts in the diagnostic process to allow for a comparison with the patient's drawings of his or her relative symptoms during a painful episode.[12,67,79] Location characteristics of pain or symptoms referred to in a dermatome or cutaneous distribution were correlated with PNPM in a study supporting pain mechanism classification.[81]

Description

Manifestations of peripheral neurogenic pain include positive symptoms of pain, dysesthesia, and spasm, reflecting abnormal levels of excitability, and negative symptoms of hypoesthesia or anesthesia (numbness) and weakness, indicating a reduced level of impulse conduction.[12,37,71,82] Dysesthetic pain and nerve trunk pain are also associated with peripheral nerve injury.[12,38] Dysesthetic pain has been characterized as an unfamiliar or abnormal sensation associated with AIGS development; common descriptors include *burning, tingling, electric shocklike, searing, drawing,* and *crawling*.[12,37,38,71,81] It is typically cutaneous, and there is little that makes it better mechanically. It is thought to arise from damaged or abnormal excitable nerve fibers. Nerve trunk pain is described as *deep, aching,* and *throbbing* sensations that have been linked to the neural connective tissue's mechanosensitive and chemosensitive nociceptors.[12,38,82] It can improve with positioning, stretch, or palpation and massage. The nerve trunk generates pain via stimulation of endings of nociceptive afferents that innervate the nerve sheath.[12,38] Symptom descriptions may indicate motor involvement with weakness of certain muscles; a burning sensation, especially with cutaneous nerves; deep diffuse cramping sensations, especially with deeper nerves to muscles; paresthesia in a neural zone; spots along a nerve path; and symptom presentation at night.[12]

In patients with neurological injury (eg, spinal cord injury, traumatic brain injury, stroke), it is not uncommon for spasticity to be described as a symptom of PNPM. In a compromised neurological system in which spasticity is a familiar response, peripheral nerve irritation may be expressed as changes in spasticity patterns, intensity, and behaviors.

Frequency

As discussed in Chapter 4 with respect to the pain mechanisms of nociceptive:inflammatory and nociceptive:ischemia, peripheral nerves can have the presence of both simultaneously. Chemical inflammatory pain may be constant pain that does not appear to change in intensity. Nerve pain may present with mechanical inflammatory characteristics, meaning patients can report that symptoms are constant but the intensity can change to intermittent based on the position or movements performed. Ischemia, if dominating, is always intermittent because it is related to mechanical loading of impaired tissue or the decrease in vascularity that occurs with prolonged posturing and cumulative repetitive movements. In addition, nerve pain presents with high severity and irritability. It is easily provoked and takes longer to settle than nociceptive pain from other connective tissues.[81]

Onset or Mechanism of Injury

It is important that clinicians understand the nature of peripheral neurogenic symptoms. Questions such as when the patient's symptoms started, how often they occur, and how many episodes of each particular symptom the patient has had in his or her lifetime may help the clinician understand the acute or gradual onset of symptoms. Many tissue entrapments related to peripheral neurogenic dysfunctions are gradual-onset episodes after an initial injury of another tissue. The interfacing tissue entrapping the peripheral nerve may be the original culprit, but the nerve is the recurring victim as a result of immobilization. With these types of recurring problems, identifying the last time the patient was symptom free can aid the clinician in diagnosis and prognosis. If the patient reports that symptom-free time frames occur, then the possibility that symptoms will resolve is greater. If a symptom-free time frame has not occurred in years, then the possibility of resolving symptoms is lower. In this case, management of symptoms and restoration of function may become a more primary management focus than identification of tissue impairment.

An important characteristic of the PNPM is a history of nerve injury, pathology, or mechanical compromise.[5,81] It is important to note the date of the injury to identify the stage of healing of the peripheral nerve involved. Healing of the peripheral nerve is similar to that of ligamentous tissue; in healthy patients, 95% of the mechanical tensile properties are recovered after 16 weeks of healing, and roughly 48% of normal strength is recovered in the first week. Injured nerves can acquire tensile strength stability in 1 week[83] and can maintain this relative tensile strength stability within 6 weeks, but continued remodeling can occur over a longer period.[84] The time frame from injury and repeated neurodynamic movement assessment assist the clinician in identifying the movements and forces needed for a restoration of function exercise prescription.

When a patient reports that symptoms started for no apparent reason, the clinician should consider the possibility of prolonged postural positions and/or cumulative repetitive movement situations that mechanically could have caused irritation over time. If the patient has no mechanical explanation, then understanding the stress the patient was undergoing at the onset of symptoms may help the clinician identify a trigger for the symptoms.

24-Hour Behavior of Symptoms

Knowledge of how the patient's symptoms behave over a 24-hour period helps the clinician understand whether nociceptive:inflammatory and/or nociceptive:ischemia mechanisms are dominating in a particular session. If the patient has a diurnal pain pattern, that is, the pain or symptoms are worse in the morning, improve as the day progresses, but are worse again at night, through the night, and into the next morning, then a chemical inflammatory mechanism may be dominating. Worse means that the symptoms have significantly increased above baseline intensity by at least three points on an 11-point pain scale. Alternatively, the symptoms may spike but are no worse. It is important for the clinician to confirm the meaning of "worse" with the patients, because it helps him or her establish the best education for activity analysis and progression.

In contrast, a pattern of 24-hour symptom behavior that is good in the morning, worse as the day progresses (especially related to certain activities), worse at the end of day, but back to baseline through the night and next day supports an ischemic dominating mechanism. Patients' dominant pain mechanisms can change based on the day of the week and amount of activity they undertake. The clinician should reassess the patients' 24-hour behavior at each visit to identify acute chemical inflammatory mechanisms for quick symptomatic resolution.

Aggravating and Alleviating Factors

Education on the three dimensions of pain—mechanical, emotional, and social—helps patients understand the scope of involvement that triggers their symptoms. By asking direct questions regarding aggravating and alleviating factors in these dimensions, the clinician can differentiate dominating pain mechanisms. Nerve trunk pain commonly has a direct mechanical aggravating stimulus,[12,38,53] whereas central pain mechanisms can have a wide range of clinical behaviors.[12,37,79] It is not uncommon for patients to admit to experiencing a burst of pain with a direct motion but subsiding pain as the motion is repeated. For example, a tennis player with peripheral neurogenic shoulder and arm symptoms might report that, during a forehand shot, the symptoms turn on when the shoulder initiates the forehand movement but subside by the end of the movement. Movement-related symptoms may be provoked after the movement has been removed. Dysesthetic pain may be related to the cumulative effects of many movements. For example, the tennis player might have an increase in symptoms after hitting multiple forehand shots in a rally as the shoulder goes through repeated forehand movements.

Many PNPM patients experience spontaneous pain that may have no direct mechanical connection, and they may relate the worsening of their symptoms to times when life pressures were too great to manage. These situations can be related to an over-excitable nervous system with increased afferent discharge related to an AIGS.[5,12,37,46]

Often patients with peripheral neurogenic pain use accommodating postures in an attempt to alleviate the neurogenic symptoms. For example, in lower cervical nerve root irritation, elevation of the shoulder girdle might lessen stretch or pressure on the nerve. Sometimes patients attempt to physiologically adjust their posture by favoring or leaning toward one side to offload the weight impinging on neural structures through the lumbar spine. Lumbar shifts typically are an attempt to decrease tensile forces to lumbar nerve roots. These shifts could be ipsilateral or contralateral to the lesion or pain. Most importantly, many of these patients do not present with fixed deformities. They may be able to move out of the shift freely. Altering weightbearing or spinal position may be the only way patients can decrease, centralize, or abolish their symptoms. Prone may be a position of relief for certain neurogenic leg symptoms, revealing centralization and a possible preferred direction

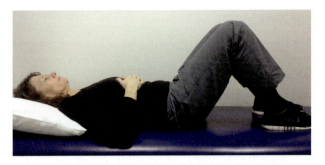

FIGURE 5.1 Unloaded neural position in which minimal or no tension is placed on the upper and lower peripheral nerves.

and confirming a mechanical interface irritation with lumbar spinal disc and nerve root. For upper and lower extremity complaints, the unloaded neural position, with the patient supine and resting the hands on the chest and both knees bent with the heels as close to the buttocks as possible, may be a position that can decrease or abolish symptoms (see **Figure 5.1**).

The PNPM may be related to recurring movement and automatic or unconscious postural habits. For example, a person may always tilt his or her head to the right while talking or reading or always cross one leg over the other. These unconscious activities are difficult for patients to identify and report. For an effective subjective evaluation, the clinician needs to listen carefully and also needs to observe the patients' postures and facial expressions when they describe situations.

A strong characteristic in the classification of PNPM regards the alleviating effects of medications. Pain experts have found that nerve pain is less responsive to simple analgesics or nonsteroidal anti-inflammatory drugs and/or more responsive to antiepileptic (eg, gabapentin, pregabalin) or antidepressive (eg, amitriptyline) medications.[81]

Thoughts, Beliefs, and Cultural Responses

Patients with the PNPM may, for the most part, present with mechanical mechanisms, meaning that their symptoms are directly affected by movements, positions, or activities. As discussed in Chapter 3, the following screening questions may help the clinician confirm that the patients' thoughts, concerns, fears, and worries are not contributing to their pain experience:

- What do you think is happening to the tissues when pain occurs?
- Do you believe that your pain has to abolish before you start returning to your functions and activities?
- What do you believe will help this pain?
- Do you believe something harmful is happening as a result of your symptoms?
- Do you have confidence in your ability to improve your symptoms?

Negative words, descriptions, and beliefs regarding symptoms and avoidance of certain activities indicate a dominating CNS mechanism. Chapters 6 and 7 describe the management of patients with dominating cognitive, emotional, psychological, and social dimensions.

Past and Current Treatments

The identification of how patients have successfully managed their symptoms, whether through exercises, body mechanics, or even manual procedures and modalities, can provide insight into whether the current pain episode is related to past episodes or is something new. For patients with reoccurring peripheral neurogenic pain, the results of previous treatments can indicate how the clinician can begin current treatment. For example, for a patient who reports that massage and different types of manipulation provided temporary relief of upper and lower leg peripheral neurogenic symptoms, the clinician can begin by evaluating active postures, positions, and movements that mimic the position in which the patient underwent those procedures to determine whether an effect occurs and to progress forces to manual medicine if indicated by the repeated movement exam.

The ability to identify and explain to the patient the connection between symptoms and the position in which treatment was provided can be an important avenue of patient education for continued symptom relief. For example, a patient whose hamstring symptoms were completely relieved by massage in a prone position may have benefited from the positioning rather than the tissue massage. Rather than devaluing procedures that patients have found beneficial, the clinician can educate patients to use the positions more readily during the day to gain more control of their symptoms. Likewise, for a patient who has been using the press up, or extension in lying, procedure to centralize lower leg neurogenic symptoms several times a day but cannot remain better between sessions, a clinician's understanding of the positive effect of extension may lead him or her to investigate progression of force in that direction with overpressure and mobilization techniques to progress the reduction process further and continue centralization effects. In all circumstances, the focus on treatment should be on showing the patients what they can do for their symptoms.

Nerve Pain Objective Evaluation

When the subjective evaluation suggests that the patient's symptoms are related to a mechanical PNPM, the goal of the objective exam is to investigate whether the mechanical pain is related to the nerve and/or the tissue that interfaces with the peripheral nerve. The objective evaluation described in this section focuses on the clinical reasoning to further classify mechanical PNPM as neural versus tissue interface mechanical dysfunction.

The objective evaluation for musculoskeletal pain is well established in neurological and orthopedic texts and may include gross observation; active, passive, repeated, and accessory motion analysis; resisted movement tests; special tissue tests; palpation; neurological examination; and diagnostic tests. Not all of these methods are necessary with every patient; the most difficult decision for a clinician is when to choose what test. For example, to mechanically assess the peripheral nerve for its capabilities of load acceptance, conduction, and elasticity, there is no need for electrodiagnostic testing and scanning.[12] If, however, the physical exam of conduction reveals significant impairment, electrodiagnostic testing at that point can help identify specifically what nerves are impaired and benchmark the impairment, allowing the clinician to monitor progression or regression with future electrodiagnostic testing.

Neurodynamic examination of the peripheral nerve is necessary when the classification is PNPM. The mechanical examination of the peripheral nerve has two parts: (1) the nerve conduction examination and (2) the neurodynamic examination.

Nerve Conduction Examination

The nerve conduction examination involves sensory and motor testing of the CNS and PNS. This evaluation can be therapeutic for patients because it provides an opportunity for the clinician to comment directly to patients "how strong the nerve conducts" or "how well those nerves are firing." Patients can learn about and identify some good things about their body. The clinician should not focus on the "bad" or abnormal evaluative findings; this style of communication can negatively affect patients and contribute to the development of dominating central pain mechanisms. Even when a test indicates impairment, the clinician can identify the connections to the patients' complaints and focus on how they can improve the test result rather than on how bad the result or impairment is. By comparing test results at each visit to patients' initial baseline, the clinician can help the patients become invested in changing their impairment and related functions, ultimately desensitizing their symptoms. Even noting small, subtle changes in the presentation and interpretation of their symptoms helps patients believe in themselves and gives them the confidence to alter their state of affairs.

It is essential for the clinician to perform nerve conduction testing in the same manner to maintain good intrarater reliability. One recommendation is for the clinician to perform the exam after the subjective interview so that he or she can be consistent in establishing mechanical baselines and reassessing outcome measures prior to any intervention. This helps the clinician to easily interpret patterns and will aid him or her in guiding the session, especially if central syndromes become apparent in the subjective interview. The nerve conduction examination consists of sensory and motor examinations. The next two sections summarize these examinations. For greater detail, refer to Butler's *The Sensitive Nervous System*.[12]

Sensory Examination

Two methods of sensory testing are available for patients: bedside sensory evaluation and quantitative sensory testing (QST).[12] QST generates specific physical vibratory or thermal stimuli or delivers electrical impulses at specific frequencies.[85] QST should be performed when red flags are present; QST requires specialized equipment, trained staff, and time to analyze data. For information regarding QST, refer to Bovie et al [12,86] and Omer and Bell-Krotoski.[12,87] This section covers bedside sensory testing, which can be performed with the patient in bed or on an ambulatory outpatient table.

Sensory examination terminology for clinical practice was developed by the International Association for the Study of Pain to define sensations related to the skin (excluding special senses).[88] Adopting the following terms when recording responses with nerve conduction and neurodynamic examination aids the clinician in multidisciplinary communication[12,88]:

- *Allodynia* is pain due to a stimulus that does not normally evoke pain. For example, a pain response to light touch is referred to as *tactile allodynia*.
- *Hyperalgesia* is an exaggerated pain response to a stimulus that is normally painful; for example, a pinprick may be more painful in one limb than another.
- *Analgesia* is the absence of pain in response to a stimulus that is normally painful. A patient may call this *numbness*, but that term does not validate the skin's absence of sensation with light touch. A clinician should test this description and report analgesic areas.
- *Hyperpathia* is a painful syndrome that involves allodynia and hyperalgesia and is discovered during repetitive testing or stimuli. An upper limb neurodynamic test that becomes increasingly painful with each repetition indicates a hyperpathic response to movement.
- *Hypoalgesia* is diminished pain in response to stimulation that would normally be painful; for example, the patient may describe the pinprick test as sharpness on one side and as pressure on other side, indicating a hypoalgesic response. Making a comparison between sides allows the clinician to identify an asymmetry. The clinician must be careful not to interpret the absence of pain as normal; the inability to detect a pinprick is a positive sensory loss.

- *Hypoesthesia* is diminished sensitivity to stimulation (excluding special senses). The clinician should specify the stimulus and site. Hypoesthesia differs from hypoalgesia in that responses to many types of stimulus (eg, light touch, pinprick, sharp vs dull), not just those considered painful, are lost.
- *Hyperesthesia* is an increased sensitivity to stimulation. The clinician should specify the stimulus and site. Hyperesthesia may overlap with allodynia and hyperalgesia because all tests elicit increased sensitivity, not just one test.
- *Dysesthesia* is an unpleasant but not painful sensation, such as tingling. Patients with dysesthesia may have normal findings on sensory testing.

In performing an examination of hyperalgesia, the clinician looks for increased sensitivity. Primary hyperalgesia is directly related to the peripheral nerve, and secondary hyperalgesia is related to central sensitization and secondary symptoms that occur as pain spreads, such as touch-evoked pain.

Dermatome and myotomal maps are widely used in bedside sensory testing; sclerotomal maps are available but are rarely used because stimulus to deeper structures is difficult in bedside testing.[12] A *dermatome* is an area of skin, a *myotome* is an area of muscle, and a *sclerotome* is an area of bone innervated by a single dorsal nerve root.[12] Other valuable maps include cutaneous nerve innervation fields, which are areas of skin innervated by post plexus peripheral nerves. Maps of these fields can be valuable to a clinician when clinical reasoning indicates that there is a tissue interface mechanical problem with the peripheral nerve; they may help identify where to search for the interface or entrapment site of neural mechanosensitivity. **Appendix 5.A** provides maps of the dermatome and cutaneous nerves.

The clinician needs to exercise some caution when using maps, because there are differences in the maps reproduced in texts.[12] Anatomical variations in nerve distribution are common, and symptoms of nerve injury are often represented in only part of the innervation field.[12,89] Many patients have nerve pain symptoms that do not resemble any of the patterns in these maps.

Appendix 5.B describes the sensory tests and summarizes the guidelines for their use.

Motor Examination

Two methods of motor testing can be performed at the bedside: reflex and manual muscle testing. In reflex testing, the tester interprets the results to identify a problem. Reflex testing can provide a mechanical baseline measure before and after repeated movement testing procedures or before guided interventions as an effective way of monitoring changes in patients' reflexes and the effects of certain movements. Manual muscle testing involves tactile and proprioceptive stimuli to the muscle and provides insight into the patient's PNS ability. Both motor examination methods provide information regarding the presence of motor loss.

Motor examination terminology is universal and more consistent than that of sensory testing. Adopting the following terms when recording responses with nerve conduction and neurodynamic examination aids the clinician in multidisciplinary communication:

- *Muscle wasting* is an objective change in measured muscle girth that allows for objective treatment goals. Often patients are unaware of wasting, especially in the posterior groups of gastrocnemius, hamstring, gluteus maximus, triceps, and scapular muscles. Muscle wasting could be the result of previous muscular or neurological injuries, and classification can be difficult. Muscle wasting also can predict certain diagnoses, such as sciatica. Kerr et al[12,90] showed in 136 patients with sciatica that calf muscle wasting had low sensitivity (.29) but very high specificity (.94) for diagnosis of lumbar disc disease.

- *Tremor* is an involuntary contraction of muscles producing sensations of trembling or quivering.[12] *Fasciculation* is a spontaneous, sometimes visible or palpable contraction of muscle fibers associated with a single motor unit.[12,91] Tremors in chronic pain patients are often triggered by emotional stress or fatigue.[12] Most fasciculations are benign, but some can result from peripheral nerve root disorders, poliomyelitis, and spinal cord disease or injury.[12,89] Many patients worry that fasciculations are harmful or indicate a neurological disease and do not understand that most are benign.[12] This is an important aspect of patient education.
- *Manual muscle testing* is an examination of muscle power and can be performed to localize sources of damaged or strained muscles, tendons, nerve roots, or peripheral nerves. Sometimes a functional movement reveals possible functional weakness better than a simple manual muscle test; for example, a single leg calf raise or standing mini squat can be used to screen for asymmetries or weakness. The following grading system is universal, according to the Medical Research Council[12,92,93]: 0 = no palpable contraction, 1 = flicker or trace contraction, 2 = full active movement with gravity eliminated, 3 = full active movement against gravity, 4 = full active movement against gravity with moderate resistance, and 5 = full active movement against gravity with maximum resistance.

Most authors recommend testing a motion rather than a specific tissue to clinically assess innervating motor roots or the peripheral nerve and major muscles involved. **Appendix 5.C** provides guidelines for manual muscle testing and summarizes common movement tests.[12,93]

Two types of reflexes in the upper and lower extremity can be tested: skin and muscle stretch reflexes. Muscle stretch reflexes are of interest to clinicians treating PNPM. They are monosynaptic between primary afferent fibers from muscle spindles and spinal cord motor neurons that innervate that muscle.[12,94,95] All reflexes are motor behaviors activated by a sensory input or a descending input from the brain. Reflex activity is affected by body position, gravity, and loads on a muscle and is dependent on CNS inhibitory and excitatory triggers. For these reasons, considerable interrater disagreement occurs in testing.[95]

Reflexes can be used to assess the integrity of both afferent and motor connections and the general sensitivity of the CNS. Common muscle stretch reflexes include biceps reflex (C5-6), triceps reflex (C7-8), quadriceps reflex (L2-3), Achilles reflex (S1-2), and CNS reflexes (clonus or Babinski) when CNS disease or injury is suspected. The following guidelines can help clinicians improve accuracy and repeatability in these tests:

- Place the patient in a relaxed pain-free position.
- Provide an explanation of the test and findings to the patient. A response such as a flicker of reflex muscle activity can be a sign of pathological changes or a positive sign of recovery, depending on the patient.
- Put the muscle tested on slight stretch. Check the reflex in different positions of stretch or with thumb pressure on the tendon if difficulty arises.
- Test the reflex for five or six repetitions to understand whether the reflex progressively stops.
- Describe the reflex using terms such as *absent, decreased, normal,* or *increased*. Comment on symmetry with the uninvolved side.[12]

Neurodynamic Examination

The neurodynamic examination involves mechanical movements that challenge the compression, tensile load acceptance, and transference properties of the CNS and PNS. Neurodynamic tests, which cover large tracts of neural tissues and their surrounding connective tissue interfaces,[10] are the mechanical tests for the peripheral nerve. Just as the Lachman test investigates the ability of the anterior cruciate ligament to accept shear load between the tibia and femur while transferring load to the lower extremity, the upper limb median nerve test investigates the ability of the median nerve to lengthen, accept, and transfer load through each link it passes through in the upper extremity. These tests are simple to use and require minimal components to ensure clinical test-retest reliability.

The neurodynamic examination is an opportunity for patients to understand how reactive the nerve is with tensile load. It can help patients understand how agile the nerve is in bending and twisting to complete its path to the hand and foot, how the nerve influences their symptoms and function, and most importantly how they should interpret their symptoms as a result of those movements. When patients relate their symptoms to certain movements, the clinician can use neurodynamic testing to help them understand the nerve's functional limitation and determine the safety of these movements.

During a neurodynamic repeated movement test, the clinician designates symptoms as "green lights" or "red lights" depending on the response they produce (similar to **Figure 4.7**). A *green light* refers to a symptom that indicates it is safe to proceed further with these movements, whereas a *red light* is a symptom that indicates that it is not safe to proceed further, prompting the patient and clinician to stop and consider next steps. Designating a symptom as a green light allows patients to interpret this message from their body as less threatening and to begin the desensitization process. Neurodynamic tests provide the clinician with mechanical baselines against which to compare the patients' progress at reassessment after spinal and extremity repeated movement tests and to identify improvement visit to visit with PNPM range of motion and reactivity. The clinician can work with patients to identify what tests are best based on the patients' functional limitations and symptom location. As symptoms improve, test results and function should improve; this is a hallmark of mechanical nociceptive mechanisms involved in PNPM.

Butler recommended neurodynamic tests in *Mobilization of the Nervous System*[10] and *The Sensitive Nervous System*[12]; see also *The Neurodynamic Techniques: A Definitive Guide From the Noigroup Team*.[96] **Appendix 5.D** reviews and summarizes the following tests: passive neck flexion, slump test, SLR test, side-lying slump test, median nerve test, radial nerve test, and ulnar nerve test.

The neurodynamic tests have a bias toward a particular nerve trunk, root, or section of the meninges. They cannot be specific because movement changes loads on all connective tissues simultaneously, and the neural and nonneural tissue relationships need to constantly change and adapt. Neurodynamic tests challenge the physical capabilities of the nervous system by using multijoint movements of the limbs and/or trunk to alter the length dimensions of the nerve bed surrounding the corresponding neural structures.[82]

Neurodynamic tests assist in clinical reasoning regarding the presence and type of neural tissue mechanosensitivity. Type of mechanosensitivity is related either to the nerve that mechanically lost its ability to accept load, transfer load, and become elastic or to the connective tissues interfacing with the nerve somewhere along the path that have become unhealthy and a neural irritant. It is important to understand these two situations because pain and symptoms typically are located in the same distribution. Patients with both types of mechanosensitivity use the same terms to describe their symptoms, which often can be made worse and better with the same mechanical activities but respond quite differently on repeated neurodynamic movement testing. For example, during the SLR and slump tests, the lumbar nerve root and disc interface alter, allowing the clinician to understand whether disc pathology is interfacing poorly, causing lumbar nerve root mechanosensitivity symptoms, or whether poor repair and remodeling healing stages in the lumbar nerve root are causing disorganized scarring and are responsible for the symptoms. In the latter case, the lumbar nerve root has lost the mechanical properties of load acceptance, transference, and elasticity, causing neural tissue mechanosensitivity symptoms. Lumbar nerve root and disc interface can cause the same symptoms but require completely different treatment strategies and exercises. In this chapter, the interfacing tissue mechanical problem is called *container dependent*, and the peripheral nerve's loss of mechanical properties to load is called *neural dependent*.

Container-dependent peripheral neurogenic pain refers to a mechanical problem in which the connective tissue surrounding a part of the neural tissue is in a state of ill health. Because of its proximity to the nerve, the unhealthy tissue indirectly affects the nerve's function. Examples of the many diagnoses that accompany container-dependent mechanical problems include stenosis, disc pathology, carpal tunnel syndrome, and muscular and fascia entrapments. Often these diagnoses are chronic, and neural-dependent mechanical problems can coexist. The clinician should use caution in assuming that a diagnosis has a mechanical problem.

Neural-dependent peripheral neurogenic pain refers to a mechanical problem in which the neural tissue (root, axon, terminal branch, meninges) has lost mechanical properties of tensile load, transference, and elasticity and the ability to glide and fold within the neural container. The interface involves a two-way relationship between the neural container tissues and the nerve itself. The interface tissue has to slide around the nerve, and the nerve has to slide around the neural container. Examples of the many diagnoses that accompany neural-dependent mechanical problems include adherent nerve root, neural fibrosis, cervical spine strain, immobilization-contracted neural tissue, neural tethering, and de Quervain's disease. The clinician uses the neurodynamic repeated movement assessment and symptom response to differentiate these types of mechanical problems, aiding in the treatment, prognosis, and outcome of PNPM patients.

Butler[12] described five patient considerations that can aid in neurodynamic testing: (1) joint axes; (2) movement and strain; (3) movement sequencing; (4) elongation, compression, and neural blood supply; and (5) unloaded neural position. These considerations guide the clinician in customizing the appropriate neurodynamic tests for each patient and identifying the best way to perform the testa based on the patient's situation.

Joint Axes

Listening carefully to the patient's history, especially involving aggravating and alleviating symptoms and mechanism of injury, can aid the clinician in identifying the relationships between the neural tissues and joint positions. Maneuvering joint position or axis can have profound effects on symptoms. For example, Rempel et al[12,97] discovered with the median nerve test that extension of fingers challenged the median nerve. Rempel et al[12,98] added wrist extension and forearm supination to the median nerve test and discovered more of a challenge. Kleinrensink et al[12,99] concluded that elbow extension, shoulder abduction, and cervical lateral flexion away from the test side presented the greatest challenge to the median nerve throughout its entire path.

Movement and Strain

Neural movement is a mixture of elongation and loading as well as gliding and undulating. The neurodynamic examination tests both elongation and gliding, depending on location and type of movement. Zoech et al[12,19] concluded that 22% of adaptation results from elastic elongation within the nerve and 78% from the nerve's ability to glide and undulate around tissues. Both elongation and gliding are important considerations in nerve exercise prescription and selection of the type and location of manual therapy procedures.

Movement Sequencing

Many clinicians and patients have noted that the order of movements appears to have an effect on nerve responses. Maitland[9,12] stated that in the slump test, neck flexion should precede spinal flexion components. Butler[12] advised that when testing the median nerve in carpal tunnel–related syndromes, the clinician's test sequencing should start at the wrist and add forearm, elbow, and shoulder movements as indicated in upper limb tension test 2. Neural structures are subjected to different mechanical loads depending on the order of joint movement during neurodynamic testing, and the testing sequence has been shown to alter the mobility and/or symptom response during the SLR, slump, and median nerve tests.[82] This movement sequencing concept stems from Breig's[7,12] described idea of the *tissue borrowing phenomenon*; the first movement tested "borrows" the neural tissue, allowing a better examination of it with each movement added. If the nervous system is on slack, then the first component of movement tested will be the local part of the nerve and its relationships with local surrounding structures. For patients who are highly sensitive or have CNS pain mechanisms, the clinician may want to start as far away as possible from the site of symptoms in the unloaded neural position to mechanically ensure the least chance of aggravating symptoms and the best chance of easing anxiety related to movement.

Regardless of the condition, neurodynamic testing that is performed in a certain order may not allow the clinician to fully understand the neural mechanical problem. Although reliability in testing is important among the same patients, it is also imperative to investigate how different movement sequencing affects the neural mechanical interface sensitivity. This assessment can help in clinical reasoning regarding the order of the exercise prescription. Movement sequencing should always start at the site of symptoms and then work proximally or distally, depending on the start point.

Elongation, Compression, and Neural Blood Supply

As discussed in Chapter 4 with the nociceptive:ischemia pain mechanism, the peripheral nerve is vulnerable to a lack of essential blood flow and nutrients. There is a clear relationship between the strain placed on a nerve and the amount of blood available to the strained neurons. With as little as 6% to 8% strain, blood flow to the peripheral nerve slows down.[12,100] If the strain is held for an hour, nerve conduction is affected.[12,101] Complete arrest of blood flow occurs at 15% elongation.[12,100] Compression forces, such as stretching forces, interfere with intraneural blood supply, impair axoplasmic flow, and ultimately alter nerve function.[12,102] The function of a nerve appears to alter at about 30 mm Hg of pressure.[12,103] The effects of pressure can last a long time; as little as 30 mm Hg pressure for 2 hours causes a sustained rapid increase in endoneurial fluid pressure for as long as 24 hours after compression is removed.[12,104] With high pressures held for long periods, long-term changes of endoneurial edema, fibrin deposits, demyelination, axonal sprouting (at 1 week), and endoneurial invasion of mast cells have all been noted.[12,105]

The response to nerve compression does not always need a mechanical stimulus; van Meeteren et al[12,106] showed that healing in sciatic nerve crush injury in rats was slower when the subjects were subjected to chronic lifestyle stressors (noise, nutrition irregularity, sleep deprivation). To handle the compression, the nervous system slides, glides, and elongates to keep the pressure at a minimum. If a nerve is entrapped within the neural container or a scar on a nerve is disorganized, the nerve cannot dissipate forces to allow necessary function and elongation and pressure capacity is reached sooner, which over time could result in neurogenic symptoms. Because of the effect of movement on neural blood supply, sustained stretching exercise should be avoided and on/off nonballistic repetitive movements may be more beneficial. Clinically, these characteristics explain typically aggravating symptoms that patients experience with sustained postures.

Unloaded Neural Position

Unloaded neural position (see **Figure 5.1**) is patient specific and depends greatly on the area of symptoms, injury, adjacent joints, and surrounding neural containers of the injured nerve. An MRI study of healthy volunteers showed that the most favorable position for the spinal canal in the cervical spine is the head elevated about 2 cm in a supine position.[12,107] When considering the upper extremity, carpal tunnel pressure is least with a few degrees of wrist extension with ulnar deviation.[12,108] This information guides the clinician to ensure proper wrist placement and allow elbow flexion at midrange and shoulder elevation to unload the median, ulnar, and radial nerves. This placement is especially beneficial when examination points to inflammation, heightened sensitivity, or positions needed to control tension situations. In the lower body, unloaded neural position is supine with neutral spine halfway between kyphosis and lordosis, hips at 60°, knees bent, and feet relaxed. This position is also beneficial to initiate patient education, breathing, relaxation, and early attempts to move the neurological system.

Neurodynamic Testing with Sensitive Patients

The clinician can use the following guidelines in neurodynamic testing with sensitive patients:

- Always perform an active screen. Patients are less likely to hurt themselves and the clinician can observe their behaviors, facial expression, and affect that indicate apprehension about movement.
- Consider the dominant mechanism behind the sensitivity to movement. Is it nociceptive (tissue-based) sensitivity, or are secondary (central) influences at play? This consideration can help the clinician decide whether passive testing for the neural structures is necessary.
- During passive neurodynamic tests, return to the start position to assess symptom latency after each movement sequence. The longer the latency effect after loading the neural tissues, the greater the likelihood of AIGS development and/or a possible central sensitization pain mechanism dominating the patient's pain state. This would indicate that passive testing is too much, too soon.
- Start the movement test away from the location of symptoms. An indirect method would be to evaluate how close to the location of symptoms can movements be introduced. This will help the clinician understand how far the sensitivity has spread from the original or most sensitive location.

Neurodynamic Examination Contraindications

The following patient characteristics are contraindications for neurodynamic testing[12,82]:

- Cervical and lumbar disc herniations with peripheralization present
- Severely irritable nerve root
- Progressive neurological deficits present
- General health problems such as circulatory disturbances, presence of Guillain-Barré syndrome, or localized abscess, either inflammatory or infective
- CNS signs such as dizziness or known spinal cord injury
- Severe unrelenting pain

Absolute contraindications to using neuromobilization as a form of treatment include the following[12,82]:

- Worsening neurological and peripheralization signs
- Cauda equina lesions
- Spinal cord direct injury
- Tethered cord (spinal cord adhered to meninges and canal)
- Spinal instability and osteoporosis
- History of transient quadriplegia
- Fracture

Neurodynamic Testing Procedures

This section summarizes procedures for neurodynamic testing described in Butler's *The Sensitive Nervous System*[12] and applies the principles of repeated movement testing from *The Lumbar Spine: Mechanical Diagnosis and Therapy*.[109] Structural differentiation of neural tissue mechanosensitivity can be further classified as container-dependent or neural-dependent mechanical problems.

One mechanical problem in neurodynamic testing involves the dynamic properties of the peripheral nerve itself (neural dependent), and the other affects the interfacing tissues surrounding the peripheral nerve (container dependent). These mechanical problems can exist individually or simultaneously. Terms also used to describe neural-dependent problems include neural tissue dysfunction and intraneural mechanical problems. Terms used to describe container-dependent problems include neural tissue interface irritation, entrapment, compression site, and extraneural mechanical problems. The following seven-step neurodynamic test aids the clinical reasoning process for mechanosensitivity to subclassify the PNPM mechanical problem as either container dependent or neural dependent:

1. Perform an active screen.
2. Examine the uninvolved side first.
3. Begin neurodynamic testing at the site of symptoms.
4. Maintain end range with each movement while sequencing additional movements.
5. Assess the need for repeated movement testing.
6. Perform repeated movement testing to formulate a provisional PNPM subclassification.
7. If the provisional classification is container dependent, identify the interface connective tissue irritant. If the provisional classification is neural dependent, identify the appropriate nerve stretch to produce a symptom and remain no worse.

Perform Active Screen

A full passive neurodynamic test is not needed to understand whether mechanical neurogenic symptoms are present. The active screen, if positive, indicates the need for further passive testing and further subclassification. An understanding of structural differentiation principles (ie, the effect different movements have on symptoms) is important in the active screening process. Structural differentiation guides clinical reasoning regarding neurogenic versus local tissue symptoms. For example, if a patient with an ankle injury has pain with ankle and foot plantarflexion and inversion, this pain could be related to the local tissue of the ankle and foot or to a number of other diagnoses. If that patient maintains ankle and foot plantarflexion and inversion, however, and adding an SLR evokes an increase in symptoms or reproduces actual symptoms at the ankle, a neurogenic pain mechanism is confirmed. Progressing to the SLR test and performing repeated movement testing can confirm whether neural mechanosensitivity is container dependent versus neural dependent.

A common example often seen in spine clinics is a patient with lower leg and lower back symptoms who, when asked to extend the knee in seated position, reports an increase in leg and back symptoms. When then asked to look up and extend the neck, the patient reports a decrease in both symptom areas. This active screen is positive as a relieving posture and indicative of the need for further passive neurodynamic testing, slump test, and repeated movement testing to further classify the mechanical PNPM as either container dependent or neural dependent. Another common example involving the upper extremity is a patient who reaches above the head and produces elbow, wrist, and hand symptoms. Bending the wrist into extension as far as possible increases symptoms, but laterally flexing the neck to the side of symptoms decreases all symptoms. The use of structural differentiation in this median nerve active screen indicates the need for a median nerve test with repeated movement testing to further classify the PNPM as either neural dependent or container dependent.

Examine the Uninvolved Side First

Examining the uninvolved side first helps the clinician and patients establish their normal end range response to their peripheral nerve stretch. Range of motion and end range spring of certain joints can be used as baselines for comparison between sides. It is important for the clinician to communicate appropriately regarding nerve movement when assessing sensitive patients with dominating CNS pain mechanisms. Proper explanations about mobility and side-to-side comparisons allow patients to experience what their normal is and what may be aberrant. Patients should be coached to comment on the normal location, description, and intensity of the response; how far they can stretch; and how springy the nerve presents at the end range of the motion. This information aids the clinician's clinical reasoning when evaluating the patient's involved side.

Begin Neurodynamic Testing at the Site of Symptoms

According to Shacklock,[6] the greatest mechanical challenge for a segment of neural tissue occurs when the joint adjacent to the nerve is loaded first during the testing sequence. The development of strain, excursion, and stress spreads to other portions of the neural tissue tract as more joint complexes participate in the movements.[6] Clinically, it is valuable to begin at the site of symptoms when they are related to small neuropathies below the elbow and knee. Meyer et al[110] showed that the sequence of dorsiflexion and eversion prior to the SLR may be more effective for detecting a peripheral neurogenic component to heel pain. The clinician should take up the slack in the range of movement in the area of symptoms first, maintain end range by repeating the movement three to four times, and assess pain and other symptom response. Does the movement produce, increase, or decrease symptoms? How does the response compare with that of the uninvolved side?

Maintain End Range of Each Movement While Sequencing Additional Movements

Neurodynamic movement sequencing has been shown to help clinicians determine whether the site of the peripheral neurogenic mechanical problem is more distal or proximal. Wainner et al[111] concluded that applying the median nerve test loading components in a proximal to distal sequence has clinical value in ruling out cervical radiculopathy, even when electrodiagnostically confirmed. A later study by Wainner,[112] however, showed that this same proximal to distal sequencing did not help in identifying electrodiagnostically confirmed carpal tunnel syndrome. The latter finding is different because of the movement sequencing mentioned earlier. Proximal to distal movement sequencing loads the proximal nervous tissue first, exposing the cervical radiculopathy. When applied to carpal tunnel patients, a distal to proximal sequencing exposes the neurogenic component in this neural entrapment. There is no one standard approach to sequencing movements to determine the presence of mechanical problems along the neural pathway, which is why these guidelines are helpful. To assist in subclassification of a PNPM mechanical dysfunction as container dependent or neural dependent, the clinician should add at least three additional sequencing movements or loads to the neural tissue and assess pain and symptom response at end range of each sequencing movement. Then the clinician can compare range of movement and spring with those of the uninvolved side and progress to repeated movement testing.

Assess Need for Repeated Movement Testing
After sequential loading to neural tissue, the clinician should assess the latency of pain and symptom response and decide whether the repeated movement test should occur. A green light for further repeated movement testing would be no latency of symptoms and symptoms that are no worse than when testing started, typically within 5 minutes. A red light for further repeated movement would be latency of symptoms and symptoms are worse than when testing started; typically, worse means persisting at a level indicated by a change in visual analog scale rating of at least 3 for longer than 5 to 10 minutes.

If a green light is present, the next step is to decide what link to use for the repeated movement test. This decision is based on the history and provisional dominant pain mechanism diagnosis. The longer the pain and symptoms persist with no chemical inflammatory signs or central pain mechanisms, the greater the clarity provided by using the link adjacent to the symptoms in terms of the container-dependent versus neural-dependent clinical question. For example, for a patient who has intermittent buttock and posterior thigh pain rated 5/10 over 6 months, is pain free in the morning but worse at the end of the day after sitting and walking, works full time, and has a negative yellow and red flag screen, the use of repeated hip movements with the SLR or slump test may elicit the best results because of the location of symptoms and the ischemic nature of the pain mechanism. This does not imply that repeated movement tests to clear the spine would not also be done. The presence of the ischemic pain mechanism allows for a more aggressive examination and ability to change the neural tissue. For a similar patient who has intermittent posterior buttock and thigh pain rated 5/10 over 1 year, whose symptoms in the morning depend on the previous day's activity level but are worse at the end of the day, who works full time, whose yellow and red flag screen is negative, and for whom latency is longer than 10 minutes after the SLR test, the use of repeated ankle dorsiflexion with the SLR or slump test may elicit the best results in neural repeated movement testing because of how easily the symptoms are irritated. The presence of latent, worsening symptoms warrants a cautionary modified examination with repeated movement tests; the clinician should select a link that elicits few or no symptoms. Repeating neural input at a location or link where symptoms are not aggravated with repeated movements allows further clinical reasoning regarding container-dependent versus neural-dependent mechanical problems and prevents the examination from irritating symptoms.

Perform Repeated Movement Testing and Formulate Provisional PNPM Subclassification
The clinician begins the neural repeated movement test using the previous sequencing that produced or increased the symptoms, ensuring that end range is maintained, and uses the link decided on in a pressure on/pressure off stretching manner for at least 10 repetitions before completely releasing all components. The clinician notes the effects of each repetition on symptoms and range of movement (ie, producing, increasing, or decreasing symptoms or

having no effect). After a minimum 5-minute break, the clinician records the overall effect on symptoms as better, worse, no better, no worse, no effect, and/or abolish. On reassessment, the clinician records the neurodynamic test baseline range of movement as increased, decreased, or no effect.

Provisional Container-Dependent Classification: Identify Interface Tissue Irritant
Adding palpation, muscle contraction, or joint play assessment in the pain-producing neurodynamic tension position can aid in localizing tissue interface sources.[12] The clinician returns the patient's limb to the position in which symptoms were at the highest intensity and palpates related neural structures or pathways, identifying mechanosensitive locations using deep pressure on the spot or indirectly over and around the area. If palpation either increases or decreases symptoms, the irritating interface or snag in the neural system can be identified.

If symptoms are located along a muscle, the clinician should use isolated muscle contractions. From the symptom-producing test position, the clinician resists isometrically various local muscles in an attempt to alter the symptom (increase or decrease) to identify the neural container that is indirectly affecting neural function. For example, hip external rotation in the SLR test may alter symptoms in the buttocks, indicating hip external rotator interface as the source of irritation for the sciatic nerve.

Joint play assessment techniques are used when symptoms are on the joint line or deep within the joint. From the symptom-producing test position, the clinician performs joint play assessment, gliding in different directions in an attempt to alter the symptoms (increase or decrease) and identify the articular neural container that is indirectly affecting neural function.

Provisional Neural-Dependent Classification: Remodel the Nerve
If the provisional classification is neural dependent, then the goal becomes remodeling of the nerve. The clinician should have the patient produce a stretch, or familiar painful symptom, but upon release the patient should feel no worse. Roughly 10 to 15 repetitions over 2 to 5 times a day should help to remodel this structure over 8 to 16 weeks. Assessment may determine which level of joint stress, tissue borrowing, or sequencing of movements is enough to stimulate a painful response, but not enough to be too aggressive and create a lasting inflammatory painful response.

Clinical Reasoning in Neurodynamic Testing
Clinical reasoning involves identifying factors that indicate the neurodynamic test is positive or relevant. A cluster of clinical findings indicates a positive neurodynamic test; the more clinical findings in a patient, the more confident the clinician can be in designating positive mechanosensitivity in neural tissues. The cluster of positive neurodynamic test findings includes the following[12,82,113]:

- The clinician reproduces the patient's symptoms or various sensations in the areas of symptoms through structural differentiation and sequencing of movements.
- The clinician notes differences between the involved and uninvolved sides in range of movement and symptom responses with similar movement sequencing. Differences can include asymmetry in sensory responses (eg, pulling, aching, tingling, burning) and resistance perceived by the clinician and altered with structural differentiation.[113]

For a patient with bilateral symptoms or amputation, known normal responses can be used for comparison. For a patient who experienced a motor vehicle accident more than 4 months previously and exhibits hyperalgesic responses in the neck and upper extremity with neurodynamic testing, a central sensitization pain mechanism is likely present.[114]

- The clinician perceives differences in resistance at end range spring testing, considered one of the most important signs of increased neural tissue mechanosensitivity.[115] The resistance perceived is not always tightness in the viscoelastic properties of peripheral nerve or the neural container but may be subconscious protective motor activity. The upper trapezius, brachialis, and biceps often contribute to resistance perceived with median nerve testing.[116] The hamstrings may have similar activity and perceived resistance in the SLR test. When performing upper limb neurodynamic tests, the clinician notes resistance while maintaining shoulder depression during increased load sequencing. In the lower extremity, the resistance is commonly felt when knee extension is maintained in both the slump and SLR tests.
- The clinician relies on other data already collected (ie, history, description, location, motor sensory testing, imaging, electrodiagnostic studies), if available. Certain symptoms or features may help identify a source. Symptoms that travel a dermatome may indicate more nerve root involvement, and a cutaneous neural zone may indicate more nerve trunk involvement.[12] Motor and reflex loss indicates nerve root or nerve trunk involvement. These features confirm mechanical changes in the nerve and can aid in concluding a positive neurodynamic test. History and palpation may lead to the container site of neural mechanosensitivity, indicating a neural entrapment or development of an AIGS.[12]

A positive test is not necessarily a relevant finding, and the clinician should further decide whether the positive test is relevant. The following questions aid the clinician in determining the relevance of a positive test[12,82,113]:

- Does the patient have dominant CNS pain mechanisms? If so, the patient's words, thoughts, worries, and concerns can cloud the brain's interpretation of the symptom message, affecting the patient's answers on testing and the clinician's ability to differentiate mechanical dysfunctions. In addition, the patient may display global sensitivities and alterations in sensory findings in other areas of the body. Many patients know that an SLR is painful, and some respond with answers that indicate a worsening response but after analysis are found to be no worse; in this case, the positive test is not relevant.
- Is the movement being tested meaningful and needed for the patient to function better and improve his or her quality of life? Patient-rated outcome measures can be used to ensure that movements are related to meaningful functions; measures can help the clinician provide an overview for the patient of the real-life implications of his or her symptoms.
- Is this test the best for ongoing reassessment? When mechanical pain dominates, mechanical function tests should be used to evaluate and support changes over each visit.

PNPM Mechanical Dysfunction

A positive relevant neurodynamic test, according to many researchers, does not identify the mechanical peripheral nerve tissue injury; rather, the tissue and its neural tract are demonstrating neural mechanosensitivity.[6,12,117] It is not until a clinician challenges the peripheral nerve using end range repeated test movements, palpation, resisted movement, and/or accessory glide in neural stretch positions that he or she can identify the dominating dysfunction causing neural mechanosensitivity as container dependent or neural dependent.

Container-Dependent Dysfunction

Nerve trunk palpation and isometric contractions are physical examination maneuvers used to identify enhanced neural mechanosensitivity related to a certain muscle.[12,53,118] The culprit for the neurogenic symptoms is the unhealthy neural container. Identifying neural mechanical dysfunction helps the clinician focus treatment on the unhealthy neural container tissue sources first. Patients are not treated with neurodynamic exercise first; rather, initial treatment addresses the container itself. For instance, a patient with a lumbar bulging disc who had symptoms that centralized with repeated lumbar extension procedures presented on the initial examination with a positive SLR test, and neurodynamic repeated test movements revealed a container-dependent neural mechanosensitivity involving the lumbar spine. As the examination changed focus toward the lumbar spine and a repeated lumbar spine movement assessment was performed, a reduction of the disc derangement occurred. The patient presented with signs of centralization with lumbar extension in standing. Reassessment of the SLR test indicated a change in the mechanosensitivity, confirming that the lumbar spine was the culprit and interfacing tissue the irritant. In this situation, the patient did not need neurodynamic exercise or mobilization to improve neural symptom baseline tests. **Appendixes 5.E** and **5.F** summarize subjective and objective evaluation findings for two patients with PNPM and container-dependent dysfunction.

Neural-Dependent Dysfunction

Neural-dependent dysfunction indicates that a change has occurred with the nerve's dynamics. The culprit for the neurogenic symptoms is the unhealthy neural tissue. The purpose of identifying these neural mechanical problems is to focus treatment on the unhealthy neural tissue along its entire path and to restore the nerve's mechanical properties. Patients presenting with neural-dependent problems need a neurodynamic exercise, either a slider or tensioner, tweaked and progressed based on the functional demands of the individual nervous system. These patients require neurodynamic movement exercise of the nerve because the nerve itself is the problem. **Appendixes 5.G** and **5.H** summarize the subjective and objective evaluation findings for two patients with PNPN and neural-dependent dysfunction.

Clinical Reasoning in Differentiating Container-Dependent and Neural-Dependent Dysfunction

Unexpected Responses: Container-Dependent Problems

Container-dependent problems often are indicated by unexpected responses on neurodynamic tests when the mechanical nerve pain is dominated by container-related interfacing tissues and/or central sensitization. Many researchers agree that these provocative tests alter the symptoms by increasing afferent discharges from the AIGS and sensitized nerve.[12,37,53] Documented unexpected responses on neurodynamic tests include the following[12,61,79,82]:

- Pain and symptoms increase at the release of a movement.
- Symptoms are produced or increase during and after movement and remain persistent.
- Symptoms increase with each cumulative repetition. The patient reports worsening, and the clinician perceives resistance or noticeable movement apprehension.
- Baseline reassessment of pain intensity indicates a change from initial measurement, and the patient reports worsening of greater than three visual analog scale levels.
- Manual muscle test or accessory joint motion tests performed in symptom-producing positions alter symptoms, identifying the interfacing tissue connected to symptoms.

Documentation of a neurodynamic evaluation should include the movement sequencing order the clinician used, along with the pain response location and range of motion comparison with the uninvolved side. The repeated test movement should indicate the joint, direction, number of repetitions, and pain and mechanical responses. Responses may be objective (eg, range of motion changes, motor responses from various muscles) and/or subjective (eg, when symptoms occur, change in intensity). Subjective findings may change before objective mechanical or symptomatic findings. For example, a patient classified as having a dominating PNPM with neural-dependent mechanical dysfunction involving the sciatic nerve and a few characteristics of central sensitization referred to his pain as a "raging wildfire down my leg." The clinician provided education and explanation about "tight nerves" and their need for space, blood, and movement. After a few weeks of stretching to remodel tensile properties, the patient referred to his pain as a "well-controlled brush fire down my leg." This statement, in addition to the gains the clinician observed in range of motion on the SLR test and improvements in function indicated by the outcome measure, reflects desensitization of the central mechanisms, and a mechanical approach continued to be the treatment focus.

Expected Responses: Neural-Dependent Problems

The responses of neural-dependent mechanical problems to movement sequences and repeated test movements are consistent, almost expected. Expected responses on neurodynamic tests indicating neural-dependent mechanical problems include the following[12,61,79,82,109]:

- Pain and symptoms are produced and increased from baseline with each additional neural load sequence.
- Neural range of motion of the involved side is restricted compared with the uninvolved side, correlating with function loss. Final neural stretch position is restricted on the involved side.
- Repeated movement test responses produce or increase pain symptoms near and/or at end range with each repetition, and no appreciable change in range of motion is sustained. Within 15 minutes of the end of testing, pain and symptoms are no worse, are no better, or show no effect from baseline intensity and range of neural movement.
- Resisted or accessory glide tests have no effect on pain and symptoms if maintained at end range.

Table 5.2 summarizes key subjective and objective characteristics of peripheral neurogenic pain as a reference for clinicians to guide clinical reasoning.

TABLE 5.2 Subjective and Objective Characteristics of Peripheral Neurogenic Pain

Characteristic	Findings for Peripheral Neurogenic Pain
Subjective	
Location	Localized to dermatome or cutaneous nerve field
Intensity	High, irritable
Frequency	Constant, intermittent, spontaneous, or paroxysmal
Descriptors	Muscle: sharpness, deep ache, cramping
	Skin: superficial burning, paresthesia, pins and needles, shooting, electric shock sensation, crawling sensation
	Nerve root: numbness, heaviness, tingling, weakness
Onset	History of nerve injury, pathology, or mechanical compromise
Alleviating factors	Heat and medications: antiepileptics (eg, gabapentin, pregabalin), antidepressives (eg, amitriptyline); low responsiveness to nonsteroidal anti-inflammatory drugs
	Activities or postures: no movement, low tension and pressure on neural tissues
Aggravating factors	Mechanical pattern involving activities and postures associated with movement that loads or compresses neural tissue, stress, and negative mood
24-hour behavior	Worse at night, causing sleep disturbance
Objective	
Posture	Antalgic of affected body part
Palpation	Symptoms provoked
Neurological findings	Positive for altered reflexes, sensation, and/or muscle power
	Hyperalgesia, allodynia, and/or hyperpathia in a dermatome, myotome, and/or cutaneous path
Repeated movement tests	Identify preferred direction, signs of centralization
Neurodynamic tests	Identify source as nerve or container of nerve
Nerve-dependent findings	Restriction in range of motion, production of and increase in pain with additional neural load movements
	Increased or decreased symptoms with repeated movements, leaving patient no better or worse and resulting in no change in range of motion
Container-dependent findings	Restriction in range or motion or none
	Unexpected response with additional neural loading: pain at release, decreased pain with loading, latency response; repeated movements as a result worse
	Manual muscle test or joint play test in tension position identifies container source through symptom change

PNPM Management and Intervention

PNPM management has two main goals: reduce the mechanosensitivity and restore the normal movement ability of the nervous system. Proper management entails acknowledging all the relevant cognitive, emotional, sympathetic, and immune triggers, which are sometimes more involved than the mechanical triggers. Sympathetic and immune inputs are managed by explaining the disorder to the patient, creating goals related to activity, decreasing the patient's fear, and returning patients to low- and high-intensity aerobic exercise. To alter sympathetic inputs, the clinician encourages increased circulation through simple vigorous cardiovascular exercises, lessening of mechanical adaptive postures, and alteration of hot and cold extremes in the workplace. Interventions should be targeted at the trigger or culprit. Treatments should address both the anatomical structures and the physiological mechanisms with the goal of dampening the sensitivity of the nervous system. Because maladaptive behaviors can negatively influence the CNS, making the overall pain state worse, the clinician needs to incorporate interventions for CNS pain mechanisms if features of these mechanisms are dominant.

Restoring normal function of the peripheral nerve includes treatment directed at conduction, dynamic properties, and connective tissue interfaces. Evidence-based medicine has produced no consensus concerning the optimal therapeutic strategy for neurogenic pain and its comorbidities. More recently, it has been suggested that clinicians should concentrate on the mechanisms underlying the symptoms of neurogenic pain (inflammation, ischemia, CNS contributions, chronic pain) and use this as a basis for treatment.[2,12,81,82,119] Research on the use of neurodynamic analysis in clinical reasoning regarding problems with neural and nonneural components indicates that intervention strategies should be selected based on the broad goals of reducing mechanosensitivity and restoring functional movement.[12,53,82,113,120]

Intervention Strategies

Patient Education

Educating patients with respect to the neurobiological mechanisms involved in the clinical presentation of their symptoms can have profound effects on their interpretation of the symptoms and may alter any unhelpful beliefs they have about the problem.[76,121] A study showed that patients with low back pain who were provided information about neurobiological pain mechanisms showed immediate changes in SLR mobility that correlated directly with reductions in unhelpful beliefs and attitudes about pain.[121] Neurobiology education in conjunction with clinician- or patient-generated therapeutic movement has been shown to be effective.[12,76,82,113,121]

Patients should understand the nervous system's strength, length, and interfacing tissue relationships. Five frequently asked questions can assist clinicians in starting the education session:

- What is nerve pain?
- How does a nerve heal?
- How does nerve pain behave?
- What does nerve pain feel like?
- What are the common treatments for nerve pain?

The key messages patients should hear with respect to neurobiology are as follows:

- The nervous system needs blood, space, and movement, like any other dynamic tissue.
- Intraneural circulation, axoplasmic flow, and nociceptors in neural connective tissue can be positively affected by mechanical loading or movement. Loading and movement help provide nerves with blood flow and restore dynamics and conduction.
- The nervous system was designed for movement involved in daily activities. Movement helps provide nerves with more space, even when pathology exists..
- Movements away from the site of symptoms can have an effect on symptoms and are typically prescribed as a treatment strategy to move neural tissue. Movement of nerves involves multiple links.

Figure 5.2 is a patient education handout that highlights key messages regarding the PNPM and nerve pain.

FIGURE 5.2 Nerve Pain Patient Education Handout

Nerve Pain

WHAT IS NERVE PAIN?
Your peripheral nerves connect your brain and spinal cord to your tissues. Your peripheral nerves typically follow a pattern that is easily traceable down your arm or leg. These nerves tell your brain when there is activity or potential danger in your body. A segment of the nerve can become the source of pain.

HOW DOES A NERVE HEAL?
A nerve heals just like any other tissue. Finding ways to encourage movement and blood flow promotes the best healing that is possible. Sometimes you need to glide the nerves, and sometimes you need to stretch them. Sometimes you need to do both to complete the healing process and restore the functions of the nerve.

HOW DOES NERVE PAIN BEHAVE?
Nerves can change with age and at sites of the body where there is wear and tear. This pain can increase with stress, pressure, lack of blood flow to the nerve, and many other factors. In addition, a nerve can be injured and not show symptoms until days, weeks, or months later.

Sometimes the symptoms you feel are influenced by the tissue that the nerve supplies or that interacts with the nerve. If the tissue near the nerve is unhealthy, the tissue may take longer to heal. You may need to work directly on this tissue before you affect the nerve itself.

Nerve pain can have a mind of its own; there may be days when your nerve pain does not have a physical cause. Nerve pain can be made worse in certain emotional states and social situations. So to help you understand the reason for an increase in pain, your clinician will work with you to identify the physical activities, emotional states, locations of the pain in your body, and your surroundings (eg, work, home, traveling) when the pain occurred.

WHAT DOES NERVE PAIN FEEL LIKE?
- You may have sensations such as shooting, burning, shocking, or stinging.
- You may feel numbness, weakness, a deep ache, cramping, and sensations of warmth and cold.
- You may prefer to use other words to describe your pain; descriptions of nerve pain are unique to each person. Describing your symptoms as precisely as possible will help your clinician target treatment to your specific needs.
- With time and treatment, your symptoms may change; this indicates that your nerve is healing.

WHAT ARE THE COMMON TREATMENTS FOR NERVE PAIN?
- Treatment for nerve pain is intended to turn off the firing nerve or change the factors that aggravate the pain, including emotions and system-wide body problems (such as immune and stress responses). The clinician will ask questions to determine what aggravates and relieves your nerve pain to assist in identifying treatments that may help.
- Movement is crucial in treating nerve pain. You may need to glide the nerve first to get it to move comfortably before you stretch the nerve and put tension on it. Don't push your nerves past a point of comfort, making you feel worse as a result. If you move your nerves and feel *no worse* after the action, this is a good thing. Your clinician will help determine the appropriate movement for you.
- Engaging in relaxation or visualization and changing the emotional context of your pain can help give your brain a less stressful state. When you are emotional about your pain, practice deep breathing and positive thinking.
- Remember, nerves are sensitive! Just as your body can react to changes in temperature, so can your nerves. It is important to take action if you are unable to tolerate cold and warm temperatures. For example, if you are sitting under the cold air vent at work and your neck or shoulder pain is aggravated, change your position at your desk or wear a warm sweater.
- Cardiovascular exercise is a good way to increase blood flow to your painful nerve. A brisk 5-minute walk increases blood flow throughout the body and helps relieve nerve pain that is related to sustained postures.

WHAT ELSE CAN HELP?
Your doctor may prescribe a number of medications for your peripheral nerve pain. Consult with your doctor regarding what type of medication will work best.

Active Movement

Restoring functional mobility of the nervous system includes restoring patient activities. Active movement is used to lessen disability and symptoms associated with nerve pain.

Much research is still needed to identify which activity is best for which patient and at which time. In the meantime, the clinician must rely on his or her biopsychosocial-based judgment with respect to what is meaningful to each patient. *Meaningful movement* is defined as movement that is important and positively received by that person's brain. Meaningful movement is different in different patients, and sometimes the only barrier to treatment success is not prescribing activities that involve fun or meaningful movement. There are two main considerations in the activity prescription: (1) healing tissue stage and nociceptive mechanisms and (2) pain system sensitivity and maladaptive CNS behaviors.

Healing tissues, especially those with large amounts of connective tissue, need appropriate movement to assist healing and best restore mechanical abilities. In this regard, the nervous system is no different from any other connective tissue; the healing stages of the peripheral nerve are very similar to the healing stages covered in Chapter 4. The presence of chemical or mechanical inflammation and ischemia influences active movement prescription. Therefore, activity needs to be prescribed that is based on tissue health and stage of healing (ie, inflammation, repair, and/or remodeling), which dictates the healing tissue's strength to handle increased mechanical loading. The dominant stage and mechanism can change weekly, sometimes daily, thereby altering the active movement prescription. The clinician should stress education regarding nociceptive pain mechanism behavior to enable the patient to change and redirect his or her own care as a step toward independence and confidence.

Pain system sensitivity is dictated by the presence of CNS mechanisms, so the activity prescription should include a strategy for managing maladaptive CNS behaviors. The general rule is to start with function and progress to focused mechanical movement exercises when managing peripheral neurogenic pain with CNS characteristics. Meaningful function for each patient drives all decisions regarding exercise. Putting the emphasis on fun and pleasure and changing the context or environment of the movement using distraction are good ways to dampen CNS mechanisms. Pleasure is a great pain liberator!

The following guidelines can aid the clinician in designing active movement prescriptions for nerve pain[12]:

- Break down the desired function into small, attainable movements. Meaningful functions divided into their component movements can be used to improve tissue health and retrain movements to reduce CNS pain and fear of movement. For example, a patient whose goal is to restore cervical rotation when driving may start by performing cervical rotation in an unloaded position (lying down), progressing to sitting cervical rotation, and finally moving to cervical rotation behind the wheel of the car. Likewise, restoration of standing forward bending can start with lumbar flexion in sitting or supine positions. The clinician begins by identifying movements that the patient is confident in initiating, using the no-worse principle to validate success, and establishing green lights for safe movement.
- Consider the order of the movement. The order in which the movement is directed at the nervous system affects the movement and strain perceived. It is best to take up slack and load the neural system at the joint adjacent to the symptoms and then add components in a way that produces less output activation. For example, median nerve pain involving the wrist and hand would be addressed by applying load to the carpal tunnel with the wrist in extension and moving the nerve via the shoulder first. Using the shoulder, an area that does not have symptoms, to initiate the movement of the

nerve at the wrist is a form of distraction. The median nerve is moving but is not using the wrist. This is a way to introduce movement to the median nerve without directly involving the site of symptoms. As the patient improves, the clinician can encourage him or her to move the nerve at the location of symptoms and progress from sliding to tensioning movements.

- Consider the use of trick movements. Trick movements involve directing a desired motion by moving an adjacent area or by using distraction to affect motion. For example, cervical rotation can be achieved by having the patient do a lateral gaze, rotate the neck by reaching across the body with the arms while maintaining a fixed gaze on an object or lying supine in a hook-lying position, and rotating the legs side to side. This noninvasive technique encourages movement when fear may be preventing movement and CNS pain mechanisms are dominating. The technique is most successful when the clinician follows up with education about how the patient was actually moving the painful area and how distraction aided acceptance by the brain.
- Understand the patient's capacity for movement. The clinician operates at the patient's pace by prescribing activity, techniques, and exposure to stimuli at a rate the patient accepts and that is beneficial to his or her health. On the basis of judgments regarding sensitivity related to the health of tissues and the mechanism of pain, the clinician encourages the patient to work into or gain control of the pain by knowingly stopping an activity before the pain occurs or willingly investigating ranges with painful responses. The clinician can teach the patient to pace by trialing different increments using the no-worse concept. Involving the patient is the best way to discover the optimum pacing interval. Pacing helps the patient avoid and acknowledge flare-ups. Some patients create better movement exercises than the clinician could ever think of simply by understanding the concepts and components of neural loading.

Peripheral nerve active movement exercises include sliders or gliding movements and tension movements. Sliders allow movement with less challenge using tension at one end of the system and slack at the other end. A slider provides a large excursion of neural movement and allows for slack in the tissue as opposed to a tensioning force. These movements produce a sliding movement between nerve and adjacent tissues, commonly executed in a nonpainful range and manner.[12,113] Sliders and gliding movements increase blood flow at the neural tissue and allow for better interface with surrounding adjacent tissue or neural containers. They are good techniques to start with for anxious and apprehensive patients.

Isolated research on sliding techniques in the form of cervical mobilization lateral glide has shown immediate reductions in pain and signs of neural mechanosensitivity in patients with lateral epicondylalgia or neurogenic neck-arm pain.[8,122,123] The research shows how treating the neural container in one area can affect symptoms and outcome at another site. This finding supports the importance of identifying the neural container causing the neural mechanosensitivity. Sliders are an effective active exercise, especially when dealing with container-dependent mechanical dysfunction.

A *tensioner* is an aggressive end range technique that places tensile load on the neural system at both ends. Tension movement concepts were developed by Shacklock, Slater, and Butler. A tensioner induces symptoms and protective muscle responses and is needed to stretch scar tissue formation, whether directly within the nerve or when adhered to other tissue interfaces because of immobilization. Typically it is necessary to produce symptoms to achieve remodeling levels of tension to create elasticity in peripheral nervous scar tissue. The patient should not feel worse 20 minutes later, that night, or the next day after remodeling-directed therapy. Remodeling connective tissue dysfunction requires 10 to 15 repetitions every 2 to 5 hours; in chronic conditions, change will occur over 2 to 6 months.[109]

The purpose of neurodynamic tension movements is to restore the mechanical capabilities to tolerate movements that lengthen the corresponding nerve bed. Tensile loading is not static stretching; movements are performed in an oscillatory fashion to gently engage resistance to the movement that is causing protective responses. These techniques are not indicated in patients with clinical evidence of impairments in impulse conduction such as motor loss in acute radiculopathy.[12,113] Tensile loading movements are more aggressive than neurodynamic sliders. Tension movements are indicated in neural-dependent mechanical dysfunction to assist with remodeling of the peripheral nerve and surrounding scar tissue.

A clinical trial on Australian soccer players with grade 1 hamstring strains found faster return to competition when players were prescribed a neurodynamic tensile loading movement, especially those who had positive findings on the slump test.[124] In a randomized controlled study to understand the most effective hamstring stretch, a qualitative perceived level of tightness measurement improved the most with a neurodynamic tension–type hamstring stretch.[125] Both studies suggest that the sciatic peripheral nerve, to a greater extent than the suspected local hamstring tissue, was the tissue in need of exercises to progress healing, return to function, and change patient perception of hamstring tightness. In addition, tensile loading techniques have been used successfully in case studies and single-subject design studies describing patients with signs of neural tissue mechanosensitivity associated with peripheral nerves in the heel,[110] lateral epicondylalgia, and cubital tunnel syndrome,[126] again suggesting that the peripheral nerve was the direct movement focus that had an effect.

Management of Container-Dependent Dysfunction

Many researchers agree that nonneural tissues that cause neural mechanosensitivity need to be addressed first during management of patients with the PNPM.[12,53,113,120] The health status of interfacing tissues can reduce the mechanical forces these structures place on sensitive neural tissue,[12,53] which in turn theoretically reduces nociceptive input from nervi nervorum and the AIGS.[12]

An understanding of the dynamics of the nervous system leads the clinician to examine the neural pathway, especially areas with local symptoms of increased mechanosensitivity.[12] For example, restoring joint play of the proximal tibiofibular joint is important in fully abolishing pain from a peroneal nerve that became mechanosensitive after an inversion ankle injury.

An understanding of the neural tract allows the clinician to identify contributing sites to pain states. Contributions may be seen in the form of physical forces on neural structures, but additional sites of inputs to the CNS from old injuries may also be present. An understanding of the neural tract also aids the clinician in realizing how general physical fitness is important for isolated lesions. When a patient presents with a significant container component, the clinician can try addressing the container first and then reassess the patient's response to neurodynamic tests. Many times, once the neural container mechanical problem is addressed, the neural mechanosensitivity with neurodynamic testing is abolished. Because this result is so common, it is recommended that the clinician treat the neural container first before progressing to direct neural tissue movement and mobilization techniques. Treating the neural container tissue first may involve one or more of the following direct interventions:

- With spinal containers, the clinician focuses on identifying preferred directions that cause centralization in the spine and localization in the extremity, which confirms the classification of derangement. Neural mechanosensitivity on neurodynamic tests often changes with signs of centralization and localization.
- With articular containers, the clinician focuses on restoring joint play and motion in all directions by achieving end range overpressure and end feel spring. Mobilization

and manipulation may be necessary with the classification of articular dysfunction. In most cases, neural mechanosensitivity changes as dysfunction is remodeled.
- With contractile containers, the clinician focuses on restoring length and strength of the muscle or tendon complex, progressing to restoration of kinetic chain tissue neuromuscular control and quality. The clinician can use soft tissue techniques at entrapment sites to focus on the tissue around the nerve, progressing if needed to direct neural tissue massage. Isolated stretching and eccentric strengthening exercises with progression to functional exercises to restore neuromuscular control may be necessary with the classification of contractile dysfunction. In most cases, neural mechanosensitivity changes as dysfunction is remodeled.

A clinician may find that addressing nonneural tissue impairments and mechanical diagnoses can be a starting point for the management of PNPM, especially if the clinician is less familiar with neural tissue exercise and mobilization. However, findings of neural tissue mechanosensitivity should be monitored closely, as the lack of adequate improvement in response to neural container management indicates the need to progress toward direct neural-dependent management interventions.

Management of Neural-Dependent Dysfunction

Direct neural tissue movement and mobilization techniques are passive or active movements that focus on restoring nervous system capacity to handle normal compressive, friction, and tensile forces associated with daily, occupation, and sport activities.[12] Some researchers have concluded that these neural tissue movements can have a positive impact on symptoms by improving intraneural circulation, axoplasmic flow, and neural connective tissue viscoelasticity and reducing the sensitivity of the AIGS.[12,113] Neurodynamic exercise may also reduce patients' fear of movement; they should be provided with appropriate neurobiology education about reducing the reactivity of the pain neuromatrix.[12,75,76,121] Methods of restoring active and passive properties of movement are determined on an individual basis because no two patients have the same complaints, limitations, interpretations, behaviors, or experience of nerve pain. Potential peripheral nerve restoration movements are best tailored, trialed, and progressed on the basis of the patient's stage of tissue healing and the dominant nociceptive mechanism.

Active Treatment Guidelines for Neural-Dependent Dysfunction

The following guidelines are recommended for active treatment in the inflammatory and repair stages of healing[10,12,82]:

- Initiate beginning to midrange range of motion at the site of symptoms with no neural loading. For example, with wrist pain, start with wrist extension directed at the median nerve, keeping attention directed at the elbow, shoulder, and neck position to ensure no neural load. For symptoms located at the peroneal nerve in the ankle, use plantarflexion, keeping the patient's knee bent and trunk erect while sitting to decrease neural load.
- Perform slider exercises. Take motion up at the site of symptoms, then move the neural system with a joint not associated with the symptoms through midrange. For the wrist example, the wrist is kept in midrange extension and the shoulder is used to move neural tissue. For the ankle example, the ankle is maintained in plantarflexion and inversion in midrange and the knee is extended to tension while the hip remains flexed using neck extension to release tension.

- Use pain as a guide, as the chemical inflammatory mechanism dominates. Do not produce or increase symptoms. The patient should perform exercises one to three times daily if the pain baselines indicate no worsening immediately after. Evaluate each patient's baseline or capacity for movement using the no-worse concept or traffic light guide for safe interpretation.
- Use clinical reasoning to determine whether it is advantageous to turn on the patient's symptoms with each repetition. If the response is increased and no worse, the tensile load is a green light and safe. If the response is increased and worse, the tensile load is a red light, and the symptom should not be turned on.

The following guidelines are recommended in active treatment in the repair and remodeling stages of healing[10,12,82]:

- Progress range of motion to midrange and then to end range at the site of symptoms with no neural loading. For the wrist example, progress to end range with wrist extension using a weightbearing position to assist in achievement of end range. Keep the elbow bent and shoulder elevated with neutral cervical posture to decrease the neural load. For the ankle example, progress ankle and foot range of movement to end range plantarflexion and inversion, managing knee flexion and an erect trunk to decrease neural load.
- Perform the tensioner exercise, taking motion up at the site of symptoms. Move the neural system from a joint away from the site of symptoms toward end range. For the wrist example, the wrist and elbow are maintained at end range extension and supination, shoulder is in abduction, and the neck is moved into lateral flexion for tension. For the ankle example, the towel maintains ankle plantar flexion and inversion using knee extension in the long sit slump position to create and minimize tension.
- Progress to a tensioner exercise using the site of symptoms as the moving component toward end range. For the wrist example, use wrist extension as the mobilizing force to the neural system. For the ankle example, maintain the trunk position and use ankle plantarflexion and inversion as the mobilization link and direction.
- Produce and increase symptoms with each repetition; further progression with each repetition is the goal in remodeling exercises at this stage. Use the no-worse concept or traffic light guide to identify successful loading amount, duration, and frequency. In some cases, the patient should perform the exercise every 2 to 5 hours for effective remodeling. Every patient should have a remodeling program dosage dictated by the number of repetitions it takes for them to perceive a change in tissue stiffness and frequency decided by the number of hours it takes to return to baseline stiffness. Most importantly, the clinician should identify the capacity of the ischemic mechanism without triggering the inflammatory mechanism.
- Finish the job! Progress movements to activities achieving tension positions in weightbearing or fine tune to involve direct function. Remodel the load capabilities of nervous tissue at end range; apply overpressure principles and eccentric loading principles. Incorporate the kinetic chain for function restoration. For the wrist example, use wrist extension in weightbearing postures such as physioball pushups. For the ankle example, progress the exercise to standing in the forward bend position or mimicking the follow-through of a soccer kick, exaggerating the foot and ankle finish.

Nerve tissue is elastic and has excellent load capabilities. The clinician should ensure that the home exercise program given to the patient at discharge maximizes these characteristics and, more importantly, the patient's functional abilities.

Passive Treatment Interventions for Neural-Dependent Dysfunction

When restoration of function programs plateau and the need to desensitize pain mechanisms persists, treatment should increase the load to nerve tissue. Passive neural mobilization is most effective. In sensitive nerve patients, active care should include passive neural unloading and gentle oscillations at certain entry points to inhibit neural system firing, along with effective patient education. The following guidelines should be followed for neurodynamic mobilization[10,12]:

- For a sensitive patient, start movements away from symptom location or pathology. For example, mobilize the brachial plexus from the wrist and hand when pathology or symptoms present proximally around the shoulder. Sometimes introducing movements from the less painful or uninvolved side can be beneficial, especially with a patient who has dominant CNS pain mechanisms.
- For a sensitive patient, start movement in an unloaded neural position. In acute cases, gently mobilizing tissues at painful areas with the hands is the best way to calm the patient's brain using the skin of affected areas. Because the skin is the largest organ with the most afferent input to the brain, using the skin is an effective way to start retraining movements in the nerve with gentle passive movements and light stroking or holding of affected areas.
- Use clinical reasoning to decide whether a slider or tension, or both, would be best for the functional goal. Sliders help warm up an area that is symptomatic, allowing progression to a tensioner as the area becomes more comfortable. Large movements are better for sliding nerve through tunnels, providing a gentle "milking" of venous congestion or "inflammatory soup" in the epineurium and mesoneurium, and decreasing fear of movement and motor responses. Small range of movement with progressive tension is better for challenging stiffness in neural tissues and organizing scar and longstanding intraneural edema.
- Use clinical reasoning to decide the order of movement sequencing based on stage of healing, repeated movement test findings, and functional goal. Movement taken up first at the site of symptoms allows for a better challenge of the neural tissue at that site and can assist in progressing and sequencing movement; this guideline is important for evaluation, treatment, exercise, and mobilization.
- Progress the mobilization technique. Progression may include increasing endurance by increasing repetitions and frequency, adding more load by increasing range of motion, or increasing neural container tension by using joint mobilization techniques at the joint that affects symptoms while positioned in neural tension position. For example, a posterior hip capsule mobilization in the SLR test position can help restore the capabilities of the peripheral nerve and its neural container, meeting the function desired by the patient of driving for prolonged periods.
- If neuromobilization techniques are used, it is essential that the clinician integrates active movements as soon as possible. No mobilization technique should be performed without the patient understanding and using an activity or specific movement pattern to reinforce the changes that occur with manual passive treatment.

Neurogenic Massage

Because the peripheral nerve is a connective tissue and local ischemic pain is a biological mechanism, neurogenic massage can be considered as a treatment option. Any segment of the nerve or tissues next to the nerve may be massaged. Biological indications for direct massage to the peripheral nerve include swelling around the nerve, venous stasis, organizing scar, and the need to restore the peripheral nerve's local tissue interface play of 2 cm in all directions within the neural container.[12] The clinician can consider neurogenic massage if there are swelling pockets around a nerve (eg, sural nerve lateral to the Achilles), in tunnels (eg, carpal tunnel, posterior tibial tunnel), and especially where nerves pass through potentially tight fascia (eg, cutaneous branches of the thoracic spinal nerves in the interscapular region, areas of trauma or surgery).[12]

Neurogenic massage would not be appropriate with elevated CNS sensitization in disorders such as fibromyalgia or acute or active AIGSs. In these situations, it is best to have patients self-massage because they are less likely to irritate themselves; this option also supports their self-efficacy and active coping strategies. This is especially useful at night and when dominating CNS mechanisms are present.

Neurogenic massage begins with rubbing along the longitudinal axis of the nerve for about 2 to 5 minutes to produce a change in blood flow. Initially symptoms increase, but after several minutes the patient experiences relief or a decrease in sensitivity. The best place to start is next to the nerve or neural container that is sensitive, progressing to the nerve if necessary.

Interventions to address the PNPM should first seek to reduce mechanosensitivity through patient education and then to restore movement through active cardiovascular exercise. **Table 5.3** summarizes interventions appropriate for the PNPM.

Refer to PNS characteristics summary charts for subjective, objective, and intervention guidelines for clinical use to aid in the classification of PNS mechanisms (**Appendices 5.I, 5.J,** and **5.K**).

TABLE 5.3 Peripheral Neurogenic Pain Mechanism Intervention Summary

Mechanism	Intervention
Neural-dependent dysfunction	
Movement	Prescribe slider neural movement before and/or after low aerobic exercise.
	Start movement away from symptom area.
	Progress to tension neural movement before and/or after low aerobic exercise; progress tension movement toward location of symptoms.
Manual therapy	Perform neural rubbing at abnormal impulse-generating sites; start outside of nerve, then progress onto nerve. Follow with neural slider, then progress to tension using movements at site of symptoms.
Graded exposure and pacing	Build low aerobic capacity for 2 to 5 hours weekly at heart rate 55%–75% of maximum; progress to high-intensity interval training (HIIT).
	Pace by adding 1 to 5 minutes every day to every other day.
Container-dependent dysfunction	
Container	Treat first.
Muscle	Perform soft tissue mobilization, stretching, and strengthening for muscle.
	Perform eccentric strengthening for tendon.
Joint	Apply overpressure, mobilization, manipulation, and range of motion restoration in three planes.
Spine	Identify preferred direction mechanical problems that have centralization.
Neural movement	Prescribe slider neural movement following container treatment, progressing to tension neural movement if necessary.

KEY MESSAGES

- Peripheral neurogenic pain results from alterations in nerve structure, nerve dynamics, or the interface with other tissues in the anatomical path of the peripheral nerve.

- Both the nociceptive:inflammatory and nociceptive:ischemia pain mechanisms may occur with the PNPM.

- Neurodynamics is the study of how the mechanics and physiology of the nervous system relate to each other and to the patient's symptoms. Neurodynamic tests assess the mechanics and physiology of a part of the nervous system.

- Peripheral nerve is made up of connective tissue that is continuous with the dura mater and epidural tissues in the spinal cord canal and extends into the brain representing a continual flow of tissue and movement.

- Elongation is an important part of nerve dynamics, as is the ability to absorb pressure.

- Peripheral nerve can generate pain in the following ways: direct injury or trauma, immobilization, indirect injury or trauma to connective tissue surrounding nerve, double crush syndrome (two or more separate injuries involving nerve), and AIGSs in nerve that become demyelinated and can spontaneously generate signals.

- Features of central sensitization can accompany the PNPM and may dominate different treatment sessions. The clinician's ongoing assessment of the dominating mechanism guides treatment.

- The subjective clinical evaluation for PNPM, as with other pain mechanisms, includes gathering of information on pain location; description; frequency; onset or mechanism of injury; 24-hour behavior of symptoms; aggravating and alleviating factors; thoughts, beliefs, and cultural responses; and past and current treatments.

- The goal of the objective examination is to ascertain whether the pain is related to the nerve and/or to the tissue that surrounds the nerve. The mechanical examination has two parts: the nerve conduction examination and the neurodynamic examination.

- The nerve conduction examination consists of sensory tests and motor tests.

- The neurodynamic examination involves mechanical movements that challenge the compression, tensile load acceptance, and transference properties of neural tissues and their surrounding connective tissues interfaces. Dysfunction of the nerve itself is termed *neural dependent*, and movement quality, dysfunction, or derangement impairments of the surrounding tissues is termed *container dependent*.

- Management of PNPM patients has two main goals: reduce the mechanosensitivity and restore the normal movement ability of the nervous system. Patient education and active and passive treatment are the key components of intervention.

References

1. Bloodworth D, Calvillo O, Smith K, et al. Chronic pain syndromes: Evaluation and treatment. In: Braddom RL, ed. *Physical Medicine and Rehabilitation*. 2nd ed. Philadelphia, PA: Saunders; 2001:913-933.
2. Scholz J, Mannion RJ, Hord DE, et al. A novel tool for the assessment of pain: Validation in low back pain. *PLoS Med*. 2009;6(4):e1000047.
3. Jensen TS, Baron R. Translation of symptoms and signs into mechanisms in neuropathic pain. *Pain*. 2003;102:1-8.
4. Bennett MI, Attal N, Backonja MM, et al. Using screening tools to identify neuropathic pain. *Pain*. 2007;127:199-203.

5. Woolf CJ, Mannion RJ. Neuropathic pain: Aetiology, symptoms, mechanisms, and management. *Lancet.* 1999;353:1959-1964.
6. Shacklock, M. Neurodynamics. *Physiotherapy.* 1995;81:9-16.
7. Breig A. *Adverse Mechanical Tension in the Central Nervous System.* Stockholm, Sweden: Almqvist and Wiskell; 1978.
8. Elvey RL. Treatment of arm pain associated with abnormal brachial plexus tension. *Aust J Physiother.* 1986;32:225-230.
9. Maitland G. The slump test: Examination and treatment. *Aust J Physiother.* 1985;31:215-219.
10. Butler DS. *Mobilization of the Nervous System.* Melbourne, Australia: Churchill Livingstone; 1991.
11. Gifford LS. Factors influencing movement — neurodynamics. In: Pitt-Brooke J, Reid H, Lockwood J, et al, eds. *Rehabilitation of Movement.* London, England: W.B. Saunders; 1998:159-195.
12. Butler DS. *The Sensitive Nervous System.* Adelaide, Australia: Noigroup; 2000.
13. Smith JW. Factors influencing nerve repair. *Arch Surg.* 1966:93:335-341.
14. Millesi H, Zoch G, Riehsner R. Mechanical properties or peripheral nerves. *Clin Orthop.* 1995:314:76-83.
15. Inman VT, Saunders JBC. The clinic-anatomical aspects of the lumbosacral region. *J Radiol.* 1942;38:669-678.
16. Louis R. Vertebroradicular and vertebromedullar dynamics. *Anat Clin.* 1981;3:1-11.
17. Breig A. *Biomechanics of the Central Nervous System.* Stockholm, Sweden: Almqvist and Wiksell; 1960.
18. Beith ID, Robins EJ, Richard PR. An assessment of the adaptive mechanisms within and surrounding the peripheral nervous system, during changes in nerve bed length resulting and underlying joint movement. In: Shacklock MO, ed. *Moving in on Pain.* Sydney, Australia: Butterworth-Heinemann; 1995:194-203.
19. Zoech G, Reihsner R, Beer R, et al. Stress and strain in peripheral nerves. *Neuro-Orthopedics.* 1991;10:73-82.
20. Wright TW, Glowczewski F, Wheeler D, et al. Excursion and strain on the median nerve. *J Bone Joint Surg Am.* 1996;78:1897-1903.
21. Pechan J, Julis F. The pressure measurement in the ulnar nerve: A contribution to the pathophysiology of cubital tunnel syndrome. *J Biomechanics.* 1975;8:75-79.
22. Kleinrensink GJ, Stoeckart R, Mulder PGH, et al. Upper limb tension tests as tools in the diagnosis of nerve and plexus lesions. *Clin Biomechan.* 2000;15:9-14.
23. Weinstein JN. Pain. In: Frymoyer JW, ed. *The Adult Spine: Principles and Practice.* Philadelphia, PA: Lippincott-Raven; 1997.
24. Yuan O, Dougherty L, Margulies SS. In vivo human spinal cord deformation and displacement in flexion. *Spine.* 1998;23:1677-1683.
25. Muhle C, Wiskirchen J, Weinert D, et al. Biomechanical aspects of subarachnoid space and cervical cord in healthy individuals examined with kinematic magnetic resonance imaging. *Spine.* 1998;23:556-567.
26. Ochs S. Basic properties of axoplasmic transport. In: Dyck PJ, Thomas PK, Lambert EH, et al, eds. *Peripheral Neuropathy.* 2nd ed. Philadelphia, PA: W.B. Saunders; 1984:1459-1478.
27. Dahlin LB, McLean WG. Effects of graded experimental compression on slow and fast axonal transport in rabbit vagus nerve. *J Neurol Sci.* 1986;72:19-30.
28. Haak RA, Kleinhaus FW, Ochs S. The viscosity of mammalian nerve axoplasm measured by electron spin resonance. *J Physiol.* 1976;263:115-137.
29. Baker P, Ladds M, Rubinson K. Measurement of the flow properties of isolated axoplasm in a defined chemical environment. *J Physiol.* 1977;269:10-11.
30. Hurst LC, Weissberg D, Carroll RE. The relationship of the double crush to carpal tunnel syndrome: An analysis of 1000 cases of carpal tunnel syndrome. *J Hand Surg [Br].* 1985;10:202-205.
31. Dahlin LB, Archer DR, McLean WG. Treatment with an aldose reductase inhibitor can reduce the inhibition of fast axonal transport following nerve compression in the rat. *Diabetologia.* 1987;30:414-418.
32. Dommisse GF. The blood supply of the spinal cord and the consequences of failure. In: Boyling JD, Palastanga N, eds. *Grieve's Modern Manual Therapy.* 2nd ed. Edinburgh, Scotland: Churchill Livingstone; 1994:3-20.
33. Lundborg G. *Nerve Injury and Repair.* Edinburgh, Scotland: Churchill Livingstone; 1988.
34. Kandel ER, Schwartz JH, Jessell TM. *Essentials of Neural Science and Behavior.* Stamford, CT: Appleton & Lange; 1995.
35. Sachs F. Biophysics of mechanoreception. *Membr Biochem.* 1986:6:173-192.
36. Foster RE, Whalen CC. Reorganization of the axonal membrane of demyelinated nerve fibers. *Science.* 1980;210:661-663.
37. Devor M, Seltzer Z. Pathophysiology of damaged nerves in relation to chronic pain. In: Wall PD, Melzack R, eds. *Textbook of Pain.* 4th ed. Edinburgh, Scotland: Churchill Livingstone; 1999:129-164.
38. Asbury AK, Fields HL. Pain due to peripheral nerve damage: An hypothesis. *Neurology.* 1984;34:1587-1590.

39. Sunderland S. *Nerve Injuries and Their Repair: A Critical Appraisal*. Edinburgh, Scotland: Churchill Livingstone; 1991.
40. Takebayashi T, Cavanaugh J, Ozaktay A, Kallakuri S, Chen C. Effect of nucleus pulposus on the neural activity of dorsal root ganglion. *Spine*. 2001;26:940-945.
41. Murata Y, Rydevik B, Takahashi K, Larsson K, Olmarker K. Incision of the intervertebral disc induces disintegration and increases permeability of the dorsal root ganglion capsule. *Spine*. 2005;30:1712-1716.
42. Takahashi N, Yabuki S, Aoki Y, Kikuchi S. Pathomechanisms of nerve root injury caused by disc herniation: An experimental study of mechanical compression and chemical irritation. *Spine*. 2003;28:435-441.
43. Rempel D, Dahlin L, Lundborg G. Pathophysiology of nerve compression syndromes: Response of peripheral nerves to loading. *J Bone Joint Surg (Am)*. 1999;81:1600-1610.
44. Parke W, Whalen J. The vascular pattern of the human dorsal root ganglion and its probable bearing on a compartment syndrome. *Spine*. 2002;27:347-352.
45. Yabuki S, Onda A, Kikuchi S, Myers R. Prevention of compartment syndrome in dorsal root ganglion caused by exposure to nucleus pulposus. *Spine*. 2001;26:870-875.
46. Baron R. Peripheral neuropathic pain: From mechanisms to symptoms. *Clin J Pain*. 2000;16(suppl): S12-S20.
47. Bove G, Light A. The nervi nervorum: Missing link for neuropathic pain? *Pain Forum*. 1997;6:181-190.
48. Lundborg G. Intraneural microcirculation. *Orthop Clin North Am*. 1988;19:1-12.
49. Lundborg G, Dahlin L. The pathophysiology of nerve compression. *Hand Clin*. 1992;8:215-227.
50. Dahlin L, Nordborg C, Lundborg G. Morphologic changes in nerve cell bodies induced by experimental graded nerve compression. *Exp Neurol*. 1987;95:611-621.
51. Greening J, Lynn B. Minor peripheral nerve injuries: An underestimated source of pain? *Manu Ther*. 1998;3:187-194.
52. Mackinnon S. Double and multiple crush syndromes: Double and multiple entrapment neuropathies. *Hand Clin*. 1992;8:369-390.
53. Hall T, Elvey R. Nerve trunk pain: Physical diagnosis and treatment. *Manu Ther*. 1999;4:63-73.
54. Neary D, Ochoa RW. Sub-clinical entrapment neuropathy in man. *J Neurol Sci*. 1987;24:283-298.
55. Kuslich SD, Ulstrom CL, Michael CJ. The tissue origin of low back pain and sciatica. *Orthop Clin North Am*. 1991;22:181-187.
56. Howe JF, Loeser JD, Calvin WH. Mechanosensitivity of dorsal root ganglia and chronically injured axons: A physiological basis for radicular pain of nerve root compression. *Pain*. 1977;3:25-41.
57. Raminsky M. Ectopic generation of impulses and cross-talk in spinal nerve roots of "dystrophic" mice. *Ann Neurol*. 1978;3:351-357.
58. Sluka KA, Willis WD, Westlund KN. The role of dorsal root reflexes in neurogenic inflammation. *Pain Forum*. 1995;4:141-149.
59. Daemen MA, Kurvers HA, Kitslaar PJ, et al. Neurogenic inflammation in an animal model of neuropathic pain. *Neurol Res*. 1998;20:41-45.
60. Shacklock M. Clinical applications of neurodynamics. In: Shacklock M, ed. *Moving In on Pain*. Sydney, Australia: Butterworth-Heinemann, 1995:123-131.
61. Gifford L. Acute low cervical nerve root conditions: Symptom presentations and pathobiological reasoning. *Manu Ther*. 2001;6:106-115.
62. Matzner O, Devor M. Contrasting thermal sensitivity of spontaneously active A- and C-fibers in experimental nerve end neuromas. *Pain*. 1987;30:373-384.
63. Eliav E, Herzberg U, Ruds MA, et al. Neuropathic pain from an experimental neuritis of the rat sciatic nerve. *Pain*. 1999;83:169-182.
64. Redford EJ, Hall SM, Smith KJ. Vascular changes and demyelination induced by the intraneural injection of tumor necrosis factor. *Brain*. 1995;118:869-878.
65. Zochodne DW, Theriault M, Sharkey KA, Cheng C, Sutherland G. Peptides and neuromas: Calcitonin gene-related peptide, substance P, and mast cells in a mechanosensitive human sural neuroma. *Muscle Nerve*. 1997;20:875-880.
66. Bove G, Ransil B, Lin H, Leem J. Inflammation induces ectopic mechanical sensitivity in axons of nociceptors innervating deep tissues. *J Physiol*. 2003;90:1949-1955.
67. Bove G, Zaheen A, Bajwa Z. Subjective nature of lower limb radicular pain. *J Manip Physiol Ther*. 2005;28:12-14.
68. Moghtaderi A, Izadi, S. Double crush syndrome: An analysis of age, gender and body mass index. *Clin Neurol Neurosurg*. 2008;110:25–29.
69. Tal M, Bennett GJ. Extra-territorial pain in rats with a peripheral neuropathy: Mechano-hyperalgesia and mechano-allodynia in the territory of the uninjured nerve. *Pain*. 1994;57:375-382.

70. Sotgiu ML, Biella G. Role of input from saphenous afferents in altered spinal processing of noxious signal that follows sciatic nerve construction in rats. *Neurosci Lett.* 1997;223:101-104.
71. Woolf C. Dissecting out mechanisms responsible for peripheral neuropathic pain: Implications for diagnosis and therapy. *Life Sci.* 2004;74:2605-2610.
72. Watkins L, Maier S. Neuropathic pain: The immune connection. *Pain Clin Updates.* 2004;13:1-4.
73. Melzack R. Evolution of the neuromatrix theory of pain. *Pain Pract.* 2005;5:85-94.
74. Shacklock M. Central pain mechanisms: A new horizon in manual therapy. *Aust J Physiother.* 1999;45:83-92.
75. Moseley G. A pain neuromatrix approach to patients with chronic pain. *Manu Ther.* 2003;8:130-140.
76. Vogt B. Pain and emotion interactions in subregions of the cingulate gyrus. *Nature Rev Neurosci.* 2005;6:533-544.
77. Vlaeyen J, Linton S. Fear avoidance and its consequences in chronic musculoskeletal pain: A state of the art. *Pain.* 2000;85:317-332.
78. Dyck PJ. Quantitative severity of neuropathy. In: Dyck PJ, Thomas PK, Lambert EH, et al, eds. *Peripheral Neuropathy.* 2nd ed. Philadelphia, PA: W.B. Saunders; 1993.
79. Gifford L, Butler DS. The integration of pain sciences into clinical practice. *J Hand Ther.* 1997;10:86-95.
80. Tanaka N, Yoshinori F, An H, Ikuta Y, Yasuda M. The anatomic relation among the nerve roots, intervertebral foramina, and intervertebral discs of cervical spine. *Spine.* 2000;25:286-291.
81. Smart KM, Blake C, Staines A, Doody C. Clinical indicators of "nociceptive," "peripheral neuropathic" and "central" mechanisms of musculoskeletal pain: A Delphi survey of expert clinicians. *Manu Ther.* 2010;15:80-87.
82. Nee RJ, Butler DS. Management of peripheral neuropathic pain: Integrating neurobiology, neurodynamics, and clinical evidence. *Phys Ther Sport.* 2006;7:36-49.
83. Temple CL, Ross DC, Dunning CE, Johnson JA, King GJ. Tensile strength of healing peripheral nerves. *J Reconstr Microsurg.* 2003;19:483-488.
84. Jiang B, Zhang P, Yan J, Zhang H. Dynamic observation of biomechanic properties of sciatic nerve at the suture site in rats following repairing. *Artif Cells Blood Substit Immobil Biotechnol.* 2008;36:45-50.
85. Shy ME, Frohman EM, So YT, et al. Report of the Therapeutics and Technology Assessment Subcommitte of the American Academy of Neurology. *Neurology.* 2003;60(6):898-904.
86. Bovie J, Hansson P, Lindblom U. *Touch, Temperature, and Pain in Health and Disease: Mechanisms and Assessment.* Seattle, WA: IASP Press; 1994.
87. Omer GE, Bell-Krotoski J. Sensibility testing. In: Omer GE, Spinner M, Van Beck AL, eds. *Management of Peripheral Nerve Problems.* 2nd ed. Philadelphia, PA: W.B. Saunders; 1998.
88. Merskey H, Bogduk N. *Classification of Chronic Pain.* 2nd ed. Seattle, WA: IASP Press; 1994.
89. Nitta H, Tajima T, Sugiyama H, et al. Study of dermatomes by means of selective lumbar spinal nerve block. *Spine.* 1993;10:1782-1786.
90. Kerr RS, Cadoux-Hudson TS, Adams CB. The value of accurate clinical assessment in the surgical management of the lumbar disc protrusion. *J Neurol Neurosurg Psychiatry.* 1988;51:169-173.
91. Nolan FM. *Introduction to the Neurological Examination.* Philadelphia, PA: FA Davis; 1996.
92. Medical Research Council. *Aids to the Examination of the Peripheral Nervous System.* London, England: HMSO; 1976. Memorandum No. 45.
93. Kendall FP, McCreary EK. *Muscles, Testing and Function.* 3rd ed. Baltimore, MD: Williams & Wilkins; 1983.
94. Sherrington, CS. *The Integrative Action of the Nervous System.* New Haven, CT: Yale University Press; 1906.
95. Stam J, van Crevel H. Reliability of the clinical and electromyographic examination of tendon reflexes. *J Neurol.* 1990;237:427-431.
96. Noigroup Team. *The Neurodynamic Techniques: A Definitive Guide from the Noigroup Team.* Adelaide, Australia: Noigroup Publications; 2005.
97. Rempel D, Keir P, Smutz WP, et al. Effects of static fingertip loading on carpal tunnel pressure. *J Orthop Res.* 1997;15:422-426.
98. Rempel D, Bach JM, Richmond CA, et al. Effects of forearm pronation and supination on carpal tunnel pressures. *J Hand Surg Am.* 1998;23:38-42.
99. Kleinrensink GJ, Stoeckart R, Vleeming A, et al. Mechanical tension in the median nerve: The effects of joint position. *Clin Biomech.* 1995;10:240-244.
100. Ogata K, Naito M. Blood flow of peripheral nerve: Effects of dissection, stretching, and compression. *J Hand Surg Br.* 1986;11:10-14.
101. Wall EJ, Massie JB, Kwan MK, et al. Experimental stretch neuropathy. *J Bone Joint Surg Br.* 1992;74:126-129.

102. Rempel D, Dahlin L, Lundborg G. Pathophysiology of nerve compression syndromes: Response of peripheral nerve to loading. *J Bone Joint Surg Am*. 1999;81:1600-1610.
103. Gelberman RH, Szabo RM, Williamson RV, et al. Sensibility testing in peripheral nerve compression syndromes: An experimental study in humans. *J Bone Joint Surg Am*. 1983;65:632-638.
104. Lundborg G, Myers R, Powell H. Nerve compression injury and increased endoneurial fluid pressure a "miniature compartment syndrome." *J Neurol Neurosurg Psychiatry*. 1983;46:1119-1124.
105. Dyck PJ, Lais AC, Giannini C. Structural alterations of nerve during cuff compression. *Proc Natl Acad Sci USA*. 1990;87:9828-9832.
106. van Meeteren NL, Brakee JH, Helders PJ, et al. Functional recovery from sciatic nerve crush lesion in the rat correlates with individual differences in responses to chronic intermittent stress. *J Neurosci Res*. 1997;48:524-532.
107. De Lorenzo RA, Olsen JE, Boska M, et al. Optimal positioning for cervical immobilization. *Ann Emerg Med*. 1996;28:301-308.
108. Weiss ND, Gordon L, Bloom T, et al. Position of wrist associated with lowest carpal tunnel pressure: Implications for splint design. *J Bone Joint Surg Am*. 1995;77:1695-1699.
109. McKenzie R, May S. *The Lumbar Spine: Mechanical Diagnosis & Therapy*. Waikanae, New Zealand: Spinal Publications; 2003.
110. Meyer J, Kulig, K, Landel R. Differential diagnosis and treatment of subcalcaneal heel pain: A case report. *J Orthop Sports Phys Ther*. 2002;32:114-124.
111. Wainner R, Fritz J, Irrgang J, Boninger M, Delitto A, Allison S. Reliability and diagnostic accuracy of the clinical examination and patient self-report measures for cervical radiculopathy. *Spine*. 2003;28:52-62.
112. Wainner R, Fritz J, Irrgang J, Delitto A, Allison S, Boninger M. Development of a clinical prediction rule for the diagnosis of carpal tunnel syndrome. *Arch Phys Med Rehabil*. 2005;86:609-618.
113. Shacklock, M. *Clinical Neurodynamics: A System of Musculoskeletal Treatment*. Edinburgh, Scotland: Elsevier/Butterworth Heinemann; 2005.
114. Sterling M, Treleaven J, Jull G. Response to a clinical test of mechanical provocation of nerve tissue in whiplash associated disorder. *Manu Ther*. 2002;7:89-94.
115. Hall T, Elvey R. Management of mechanosensitivity of the nervous system in spinal pain syndromes. In: Boyling J, Jull G, eds. *Grieve's Modern Manual Therapy: The Vertebral Column*. 3rd ed. Edinburgh, Scotland: Churchill Livingstone; 2004:413-431.
116. van der Heide B, Allison G, Zusman M. Pain and muscular responses to a neural tissue provocation test in upper limb. *Manu Ther*. 2001;6:154-162.
117. Phillips J, Smit X, DeZoysa N, Afoke A, Brown R. Peripheral nerves in the rat exhibit localized heterogeneity of tensile properties during limb movement. *J Physiol*. 2004;557:879-887.
118. Novak C, Mackinnon S. Evaluation of nerve injury and nerve compression in the upper quadrant. *J Hand Ther*. 2005;18:230-240.
119. Chong MS, Bajwa Z. Diagnosis and treatment of neuropathic pain. *J Pain Symptom Manage*. 2003;25(5 suppl):S4-S11.
120. Butler D, Gifford L. The concept of adverse mechanical tension in the nervous system part 2: Examination and treatment. *Physiotherapy*. 1989;75:629-636.
121. Moseley G. Evidence for a direct relationship between cognitive and physical change during an education intervention in people with chronic low back pain. *Eur J Pain*. 2004:8:39-45.
122. Vicenzino B, Neal R, Collins D, Wright, A. The displacement, velocity and frequency profile of the frontal plane motion produced by the cervical lateral glide treatment technique. *Clin Biomechan*. 1999;14:515-521.
123. Coppieters M, Stappaerts K, Wouters L, Janssens K. The immediate effects of a cervical lateral glide treatment technique in patients with neurogenic cervicobrachial pain. *J Orthop Sports Phys Ther*. 2003;33:369-378.
124. Kornberg C, Lew P. The effect of stretching neural structures on grade one hamstring injuries. *J Orthop Sports Phys Ther*. 1989;10:481-487.
125. Fasen J, O'Connor A, Schwartz SL, et al. A randomized controlled trial of hamstring stretching: Comparison of four techniques. *J Strength Cond Res*. 2009;23:661-667.
126. Coppieters M, Stappaerts K, Everaert D, Staes F. Incorporating nerve gliding techniques in conservative treatment of cubital tunnel syndrome. *J Manip Physiol Ther*. 2004;27:560-568.

APPENDIX 5.A Dermatomes and Cutaneous Nerve Fields

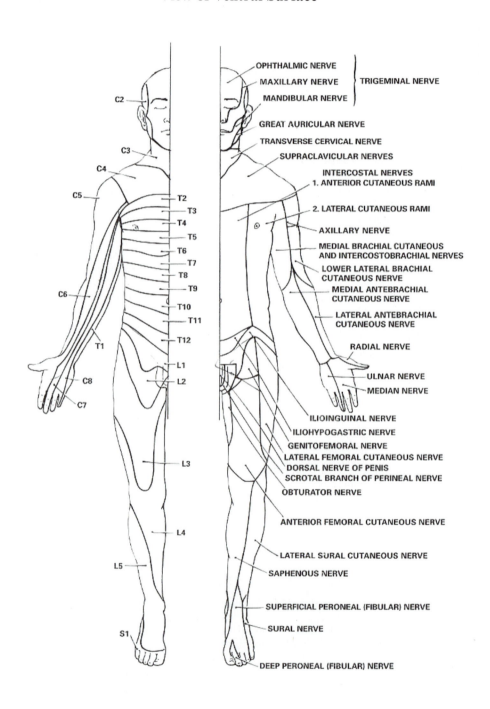

View of Dorsal Surface

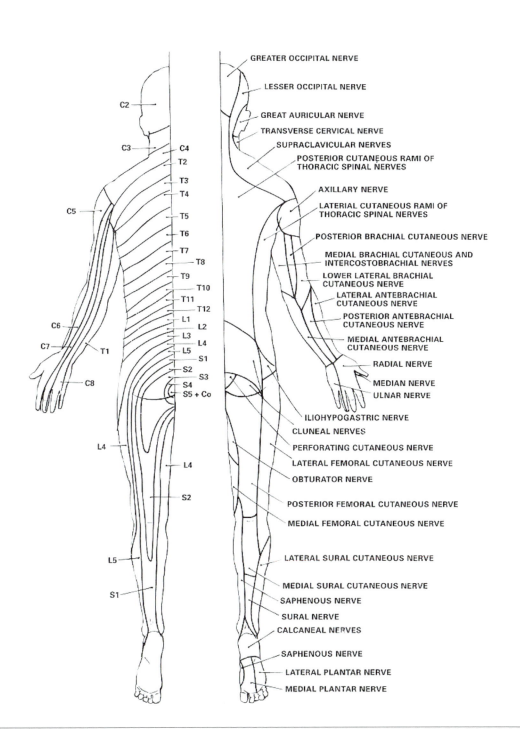

APPENDIX 5.B   Sensory Testing Guidelines and Review

Sensory Testing Guidelines

- Identify areas of sensory changes to be tested. Describe for the patient the tests to be performed and why.
- Use clear and concise communication. Explain to the patient that a *yes* answer indicates a normal sensation, *no* indicates a sensation considered to be a problem, and *don't know* indicates uncertainty and requires further assessment.
- Patient should have his or her eyes closed and be in a comfortable position.
- Establish the patient's normal response by testing the uninvolved limb or, when bilateral limb involvement is present, the abdomen.
- Start distally and work proximally when the entire limb or multiple locations in a limb need testing. With a defined area, start outside the area and progress into the area. When symptoms present, start away from the symptoms and progress toward them. If a patient is in severe pain, consider testing at a different time.
- Record findings, indicating the involvement and area (eg, tactile allodynia along sural cutaneous nerve field, hypoesthesia along L4 dermatome).
- Take measures to decrease the patient's fear and anxiety before and, if necessary, during testing; these emotions can affect results.

SENSORY TESTS[1]

Test	Description
Superficial: light touch	A nylon filament is applied perpendicular to the skin surface being tested with enough pressure to slightly bend the filament. When a nylon filament is not available, the clinician's finger can be used, placed lightly on skin surface to be tested.
Superficial: pain	Superficial pain testing should occur after light touch if needed. Patient's answers include *nothing*, *dull*, *sharp*, or *don't know*. Patient's pain appreciation may be delayed or heightened with repeated testing, so the clinician should allow time between each stimulus for the patient to answer.
Superficial: hot and cold	Hot and cold testing is not necessary if superficial pain is intact. If patient describes symptoms related to temperature, the clinician should use this test. Fill test tubes with the hottest and coldest tap water available so as to easily distinguish between the two temperatures and carefully place them on the patient's skin.
Deep sensation: proprioception and coordination	Proprioception impulses related to the sense of passive movement position and vibration pass along fibers in the posterior columns and medial lemniscus system, then are distributed to the thalamus and sensory cortex.[2] Altered proprioception and vibration are good indicators that problems are present in the columns[1] and the dorsal spinocerebellar tract.[3] Important testing procedures include keeping the patient's eyes closed, grasping the outer sides of the limb or digit with minimal pressure, and slowly moving the limb or digit in an up or down direction. While moving the limb or digit, the clinician asks the patient to identify the direction of the movement as soon as he or she feels it; the patient responds *up*, *down*, or *don't know*. Proprioception testing should be in the midrange of the extremity or joint, avoiding activation of muscle stretch receptors. A common lower body proprioception test is to have the patient slide the heel down the shin of the opposite leg; if normal, this should be done easily and without irregular deviations. A common upper body proprioception test is to have the patient use the index finger to touch the nose or to alternately touch the nose and the clinician's index finger purposely placed in different locations.

Resources
1. Butler DS. *The Sensitive Nervous System*. Adelaide, Australia: Noigroup; 2000.
2. Mayo Clinic. *Clinical Examinations in Neurology*. 6th ed. St. Louis, MO: Mosby; 1991.
3. Ross ED, Kirkpatrick JB, Lastimosa ACB. Position and vibration sensations: Functions of the dorsal spinocerebellar tract. *Ann Neurol*. 1979;5:171-177.

APPENDIX 5.C Manual Muscle Testing Guidelines and Review

Manual Muscle Testing Guidelines

- Reproducibility is important in the performance of any test and before and after repeated movement procedures to assist in ongoing clinical reasoning.
- Reassessment is needed every visit to differentiate local muscle power versus nerve-related muscle power problems.
- Establishing baselines at initial testing for muscle power allows the clinician to show cause and effect immediately after the intervention or over time.
- Often with nerve-related muscle power loss, the motor loss changes before the pain symptoms change with directional preference procedures.
- Establishing good habits in testing ensures that signs of improvement or regression are measurable.
- A maximum contraction is required.
- Apply counterforce until the muscle gives way.
- Use the midrange of a muscle for positioning. Some muscles need alternative positioning to make deficits apparent. For example, the gastrocnemius soleus, biceps, and triceps are powerful muscles at midrange; test them at the outer ranges, through ranges, and/or with load or weight bearing to appreciate deficits.
- Compare results with the patient's other side and with previous patients. It takes time and experience to get a feel for the grading system with strong, weak, and injured patients.
- Get into a routine of having the patient perform one repetition actively, looking at quality, and then having the patient perform a second repetition actively. Decide where in the range to test for maximum power.
- When testing the tendon specifically, clinicians frequently establish that tendon testing is needed throughout the range providing eccentric minimum, moderate, or maximum resistance.

UPPER LIMB TESTS

Test	Location	Description	Compensation for Weakness
Scapular retraction	C4-5, dorsal scapular nerve; rhomboids and levator scapulae	The dorsal scapular nerve muscles are responsible for stabilizing the scapula during upper limb movement. They adduct, elevate, and rotate the scapula in three planes of movement.	Elbows rising higher than hands with elevation of shoulders
Shoulder elevation	C4, spinal accessory nerve; upper trapezius assisted by levator scapulae	The trapezius is powerful as it compensates for weak scapular retraction and shoulder abduction.	Increased forward head posture and flexion of thoracic spine

Test	Location	Description	Compensation for Weakness
Shoulder abduction	C5-6, axillary nerve; deltoid and supraspinatus	It is important to clinically reason isolated rotator cuff weakness versus cervical nerve root radiculopathy. Many patients present with rotator cuff weakness that is related to an underlying cervical problem. Elbow flexion and extension manual muscle testing can help clinicians clinically reason between rotator cuff weakness and cervical radiculopathy.	Increased forward head, shoulder shrug, and scapular protraction
Shoulder adduction, internal rotators	C5, 6, and 7, upper and lower suprascapular nerve; teres major and subscapularis		
Shoulder external rotators	C4, 5, and 6, suprascapular and axillary nerve; infraspinatus and teres minor		
Elbow flexion	C5-6, musculocutaneous nerve; biceps, brachialis	If tested in less than 90°, these muscles are usually too powerful to detect weakness; consider testing in angles greater than 90° for best assessment.	Loss of erect posture, shoulder shrug, or forearm pronation
Elbow extension	C6, 7, and 8, radial nerve; triceps	Position arm above head with elbow bent below 90°, ask patient to straighten elbow as much as possible to allow assessment of strength against gravity, applying resistance at forearm just above 90° of elbow flexion.	Loss of erect posture, shoulder shrug, or forearm pronation
Thumb distal interphalange extension	C7-8, posterior interosseus nerve; extensor pollicis longus	Movement testing is important to isolate the distal interphalangeal joint and stabilize the whole thumb.	Opening of hand, wrist extension, or carpal-metacarpal extension
Finger distal interphalange flexion	C7, C8, and T1, anterior interosseus nerve; flexor digitorum profundus digits 4 and 5 innervated by ulnar nerve, digits 2 and 3 innervated by median nerve	Movement testing is important to isolate the distal interphalangeal joint and stabilize the whole finger.	Elbow and wrist flexion
Finger abduction and adduction	C8-T1, ulnar nerve; interossei and lumbricals	Movement testing is important to isolate the distal interphalangeal joint and stabilize the whole finger.	Flexion of fingers

(continues on next page)

APPENDIX 5.C Manual Muscle Testing Guidelines and Review *(continued from previous page)*

LOWER LIMB TESTS

Test	Location	Description	Compensation for Weakness
Hip flexion	L2, 3, and 4, lumbar plexus, femoral nerve; illiacus and psoas major	In seated position, have patient lift knee as high as possible, lower to comfortable height and apply resistance for test.	Hip internal or external rotation, loss of erect good posture or excessive pelvic rotation toward side being tested
Hip extension	L5, S1, inferior gluteal nerve; gluteus maximus	In prone position, have patient lift leg as high as possible with knee straight, lower to comfortable height and apply resistance for test.	Excessive lumbar lordosis or knee flexion
Knee extension	L2, 3, and 4, femoral nerve; quadriceps	In seated position, have patient extend knee as straight as possible, lower to comfortable height and apply resistance for test.	Slumping posture, hip internal and external rotation
Knee flexion	L5-S1, sciatic nerve; hamstrings	In prone position, have patient bend knee as much as possible, lower to a comfortable height and apply resistance for test.	Excessive lordosis, tibial internal and external rotation, hip internal and external rotation
Ankle dorsiflexion	L4 and 5, S1, deep peroneal nerve; tibialis anterior	There are no muscle stretch reflex tests for the L4 and L5 nerve roots, so these movement tests become very important to perform. Most patients show the inversion weakness more than the dorsiflexion.	Slumping posture, knee extension, eversion of ankle
Great toe extension	L4 and 5, S1, deep peroneal nerve; extensor hallucis longus	In seated position, have patient lift great toe as high as possible, lower to comfortable height and apply resistance.	Slumping posture, knee extension, ankle dorsiflexion
Ankle eversion	L5-S1, common peroneal nerve; peroneus longus and brevis	In seated position, have patient turn sole of foot outward as much as possible, lower to a comfortable height and apply resistance.	Slumping posture, plantarflexion of feet

Test	Location	Description	Compensation for Weakness
Ankle plantarflexion	L5, S1, and S2, tibial nerve; gastrocnemius and soleus	Considering the leverage in testing with this powerful muscle, use of the patient's body weight can provide greater insight into the muscle power deficit. The patient should be able to complete at least 6–10 repetitions. If the patient can perform 6–10 repetitions easily, then perform the test until the patient fatigues, defined as the inability to attain full range. Compare with the uninvolved side to provide additional insight into strength at each reassessment.	Partial range of plantarflexion, excessive hip hiking or mini squats with knee, excessive pronation at midfoot
Toe flexion	L5, S1, posterior tibial nerve; flexor hallucis longus, flexor digitorum longus	In seated position, have patient curl toes as much as possible, release until comfortable and apply resistance.	Slumping posture, knee flexion, ankle plantarflexion

Resources
Butler DS. *The Sensitive Nervous System*. Adelaide, Australia: Noigroup; 2000.
Kendall FP, McCreary EK. *Muscles, Testing and Function*. 3rd ed. Baltimore, MD: Williams & Wilkins; 1983.

APPENDIX 5.D Neurodynamic Test Review

PASSIVE NECK FLEXION

The passive neck flexion test mechanically loads suboccipital, cervical, upper thoracic, and cranial connective tissues, including local joints, muscles, nerves, balance organs, and eyes. The neural tissues that are stressed include the brainstem, cranial nerves, upper and lower cervical cord meninges (dura, pia, and arachnoid mater), and nerve roots. Passive neck flexion is also a loading strategy to structurally differentiate most of the upper and lower extremity peripheral nerve neurodynamic tests. Indicators for this test include symptoms located in the cranial (eg, headaches), suboccipital, cervical, upper thoracic, and upper trapezius areas and in the low back and buttocks.

Component	Description
Patient position	Patient is supine, with no pillow and with straight arms and legs. For a sensitive patient, use the unloaded neural position to perform the test.
Active test	Patient nods head toward chest. While maintaining the nod, patient lifts head, using hands to assist movement if necessary, curling chin to chest. Observe patient's ability to maintain chin tuck. To test lower cervical and upper thoracic areas, place pillows under locations where cervical flexion is needed. For structural differentiation, use hip flexion, hip internal rotation and adduction, straight leg raise, and/or dorsiflexion of foot.
Passive test, clinician action	Loading sequence from proximal to distal is as follows: 1. Perform upper cervical flexion by nodding the patient's head, with one hand guiding chin tuck and other hand cupping occipital bone. 2. Maintaining this position, complete cervical flexion to end range. 3. Maintaining this position, complete upper thoracic flexion to end range. 4. Final loading may include straight leg raise with ankle dorsiflexion to end range or cervical lateral flexion and rotation or shoulder depression and abduction to end range.
Normal response	No production or increase in symptoms. Normal stretch response near the region is associated with movement sequence, suboccipital and cervical paraspinals, cervical-thoracic junction, and upper thoracic paraspinals.
Clinical reasoning	Lhermitte's sign is a brief intermittent electric shock–like sensation that travels down the patient's legs, spine, or less commonly arms during cervical flexion or rotation or coughing. When positive, this sign indicates spinal cord damage, specifically to the dorsal columns of the cervical spinal cord.[1,2] On occasion, this test can reproduce lumbar pain or symptoms, indicating the need to include cervical movements in the lumbar neurogenic movement program.

SLUMP TEST

The slump test mechanically loads thoracic, lumbar, and coccygeal connective tissues including local joints, muscles of the spine, spinal cord, and nerves. The neural tissues stressed include thoracic and lumbar cord meninges and associated nerve roots. Indications for this test include symptoms located at the ribs; sternum; thoracic, lumbar, and sacral spinal regions; associated paraspinals; rectum; posterior buttock; hip; and ischial tuberosity regions. Symptoms following the sciatic nerve path and related to sitting and forward bending should also be considered for this test.

The slump test has two variations, short sit and long sit. The short sit variation highlights the lumbar, sacral, and posterior hip nervous tissues, whereas the long sit variation highlights the middle, lower thoracic, and upper lumbar nervous tissues. This test should not be thought of as a substitute for the straight leg raise test but as an additional and sometimes more sensitive test for spine problems and neural meninges that may be more sensitive to weightbearing positions.

Short Sit Slump Test

Component	Description
Patient position	Patient sits in an erect position with thighs together, supported to knee creases at edge of table with feet dangling. Patient clasps hands behind back to eliminate effect of upper extremities.
Active test	1. Patient slouches lumbar spine without pelvic rotation. 2. Patient nods head forward, maintaining position, and takes chin to chest. 3. Maintaining the positions, patient performs knee extension. 4. Maintaining the positions, patient performs ankle dorsiflexion. For structural differentiation, use knee extension and/or ankle dorsiflexion or neck extension to differentiate the neurogenic nature of the symptoms produced or increased.
Passive test, clinician action	Sitting next to patient, position hands at thoracic spine to guide spinal movement and lower leg to assess end feel and spring of leg movements. Loading sequence from proximal to distal is as follows: 1. Keep patient's head and neck looking forward while in spinal slump, monitoring anterior or posterior pelvic tilt. Monitor end range with gentle pressure. 2. Guide patient's head into chin tuck followed by cervical flexion to end range; monitor end range. 3. Guide knee extension to end range; maintain end range. 4. Guide ankle dorsiflexion to end range; maintain end range. 5. Additional loading includes bilateral knee extension with ankle dorsiflexion.
Normal responses	Central T8-9 area symptoms when cervical flexion is added. Anticipate a posterior thigh and knee stretch response. Neurogenic pain symptoms are typically relieved when the cervical spine is extended to end range, differentiating neurogenic symptoms from local muscle symptoms.
Clinical reasoning	Performing the test actively allows the clinician to control the situation if the patient is sensitive. If the active test causes severe, debilitating pain and leaves an almost clonus-type quadriceps contraction after the test or lasting symptoms, there is no indication to continue to passive testing.

(continues on next page)

APPENDIX 5.D Neurodynamic Test Review *(continued from previous page)*

Long Sit Slump Test
The long sit slump test can be used to begin testing for a patient who is sensitive or has difficulty with lower extremity movement.

Component	Description
Patient position	Patient sits up on table with hips and knees flexed and looks straight forward. Use pillows under knees or buttocks for patients with flexibility issues. Use more hip flexion on flexible patients.
Passive test, clinician action	Standing on one leg, clinician places knee of other leg behind lumbar spine supporting the patient's sacrum; keep hands ready to guide movement at head and lower extremity. Loading sequence from superior to inferior is as follows: 1. Keep patient's head and neck looking forward, slumping lumbar and thoracic spine; monitor for no pelvic posterior rotation; monitor end range. 2. Guide patient's head into forward nod followed by cervical flexion to end range; monitor end range. 3. Adapt the test depending on symptoms; if symptoms are unilateral in the thoracic spine, use lateral flexion and rotation away from symptoms to further load neural tissue prior to using lower extremities; maintain end range. 4. Additional spinal loading includes segmental mobilization procedures, both anterior-posterior and posterior-anterior, and lateral glides. 5. Guide knee extension to end range; maintain end range. 6. Guide ankle dorsiflexion to end range; maintain end range. 7. Final loading includes both legs extended and dorsiflexed.
Normal responses	This test has not been well researched or defined. Patients may feel hamstring, posterior knee, and upper calf stretch responses.

STRAIGHT LEG RAISE TEST

The straight leg raise (SLR) test has been shown to have good validity, especially when used with other data to diagnose disc herniation.[3,4] The SLR is the most frequently used neurodynamic test. The SLR correlates strongly with other subjective complaints of night pain, pain at rest, analgesic consumption, alleviating and aggravating movements, and objective observations of forward bending in standing. Jönsson and Strömqvist[5] suggested that an inferior surgical outcome is likely with positive postoperative SLR findings. Indications for use include symptoms located in the lumbar, sacral, and coccygeal spine; posterior hip; buttock; ischial tuberosity; and posterior knee, calf, and foot.

Component	Description
Patient position	Patient is supine with no pillow, close to edge of treatment table, with both legs extended. Sensitive patients should bend the opposite knee, especially those who are unable to lie extended because of pain, which may indicate neural load mechanosensitivity.

Component	Description
Active test	1. In supine or standing position, dorsiflex ankle. 2. Maintain ankle position. Patient keeps knee straight while lifting or kicking leg forward as far as possible. 3. For structural differentiation, use maneuvers of lumbar or cervical flexion, hip internal rotation, and hip adduction.
Passive test, clinician action	Facing the patient, cup the calcaneus with one hand to control the foot and ankle and rest other hand above patella to maintain knee extension. Loading sequence from distal to proximal is as follows: 1. Guide dorsiflexion of ankle to end range; maintain end range. 2. Guide knee extension until end range; maintain end range. 3. Guide hip flexion until end range; maintain end range. 4. Use hip adduction and internal rotation with patients who have excessive hip flexion movement. Progress movement to bilateral SLR for additional loading. 5. Use spinal lateral flexion contralateral to symptoms, posterior pelvic tilt, and assisted upper neck flexion to understand the spinal movements' effects on lower extremity symptoms indicating neural mechanosensitivity involving the spine. These movements are required to identify minor dysfunctions and frequently are used to mobilize the nervous system. Clinical reasoning for container-dependent versus neural-dependent peripheral nerve mechanical dysfunctions requires three to four load sequences.
Normal responses	Deep stretch response in posterior thigh, knee, and/or calf extending into the foot.
Clinical reasoning	The following additional ankle-foot movements can be used to place mechanical load on the sciatic nervous system below the knee, tibial, and common peroneal nerves (the distal to proximal load sequence is best when evaluating lower leg symptom location): • **Ankle dorsiflexion + eversion:** Sensitizing maneuver for the medial plantar nerve, branch of posterior tibial nerve, or neural contributions to diagnoses of piriformis syndrome, recurrent hamstring injury, plantar fasciitis, heel spur, posterior tarsal tunnel syndrome, calcaneal pain, and medial foot pain in runners. Normal responses include a stretch response at the posterior calf, posterior medial ankle, and medial border of the foot spreading to the posterior calf, knee, and thigh. • **Ankle plantarflexion + inversion:** Sensitizing maneuver for the superficial and deep peroneal nerve branch of the common peroneal nerve or neural contributions to diagnoses of lateral ankle sprains, anterior lateral compartment syndromes, superior tibiofibular joint dysfunctions or derangements, piriformis syndrome, and lower lumbar spine radiculopathy. Normal responses include a stretch response in the anterior lateral lower leg and foot that sometimes spreads to the posterior calf, knee, and thigh. • **Ankle dorsiflexion + inversion:** Sensitizing maneuver for the sural nerve branch of the tibial nerve or neural contributions to diagnoses of ankle impingement, persistent Achilles tendon problems, lateral ankle sprains, and recurrent ankle problems. Normal responses include a stretch response in the posterior calf, lateral ankle, and sometimes the lateral border of foot, occasionally spreading to the posterior knee and thigh.

(continues on next page)

APPENDIX 5.D Neurodynamic Test Review (continued from previous page)

SIDE-LYING SLUMP TEST

The side-lying slump test can differentiate neural symptoms from upper, middle, and lower lumbar neural structures.[6] Indicators for this test are symptoms located at the anterior thigh, inguinal area, anterior hip, pelvis, lower back, and abdomen. With diagnoses of inguinal ligament sprain, hip flexor strain, recurrent mechanical hip derangements, and L2-3 nerve root syndromes, this test is used to differentiate a neurogenic symptom from the local tissue.

Component	Description
Active test	1. Patient performs a backward lunge, lowering knee to floor, or a long backward step. 2. Patient maintains position; then looks down, bringing chin toward chest; then returns and looks to ceiling to allow clinician to structurally differentiate neural tissue involvement.
Passive test, patient position	Patient is in side-lying position with the symptom side up. Patient completely flexes spine by bringing head toward knee of lower leg. Patient maintains this position during test.
Passive test, clinician action	1. Brace body against posterior aspect of patient's pelvis to keep patient from rolling back; cradle top leg with knee bent. 2. Progress to end range knee flexion. 3. Grasp patient's pelvis and perform hip extension by stabilizing pelvis and guiding knee posterior. Additional sensitizing maneuvers of hip adduction and abduction can localize lateral femoral cutaneous and obturator nerve symptoms, respectively. 4. Patient extends head and cervical spine to enable clinician to structurally differentiate neurogenic symptoms from local symptoms.
Normal responses	Stretch response along anterior aspect of thigh, pelvis, and abdomen dependent on amount of hip extension.

MEDIAN NERVE TEST

The median nerve test has been around for many years and has been referred by many names. Elvey[7] first called the test the *brachial plexus tension test* in 1979, and Kenneally et al[8] used the term *upper limb tension test* in 1988 and referred to it as the "straight leg raise test of the arm." Butler[9] in 1989 and Shacklock[10] in 1995 used the term *upper limb neurodynamic test* and indicated the movement sequencing to bias the three major neural tissues of the upper limb for median, radial, and ulnar nerves. Indications for the median nerve test include symptoms specifically located in the palmar lateral aspect of the hand and fingertips following the median nerve map and any upper extremity neurogenic symptom provoked with upper extremity elevation (reaching overhead) or twisting of the forearm. Indicators to use the median nerve test include a diagnosis of carpal tunnel syndrome, post–Colles fracture symptoms, and C5-6 radiculopathy.

Component	Explanation
Active test	1. Patient stands and looks at palm of hand. 2. Patient extends elbow as far as possible behind him or her. 3. Patient reaches arm out to side until hand passes head height. It is important to get to end range, which may mean lifting higher or slightly forward or backward. Structural differentiation indicates neurogenic symptoms if adding wrist extension or cervical lateral flexion away from the reaching arm increases or reproduces symptoms. As patient performs additional loading, watch shoulder girdle for subconscious protective movements of elevation, retraction, or protraction in an effort to lessen tension on the nervous system.
Passive test, patient position	Patient is supine close to edge of bed, with legs extended and uninvolved arm extended. No pillow is used unless patient is unable to lie flat.
Passive test, clinician action	In a stride stance position, facing patient's upper body, use one hand to hold or guide patient's hand and wrist and place other hand on top of patient's shoulder to monitor elevation of shoulder girdle. The clinician, using his or her thigh of the forward leg, guides and supports patient's elbow while patient performs upper extremity movements. Movement sequencing from proximal to distal is as follows: 1. Patient performs active cervical lateral flexion away from the testing side to end range. 2. Clinician maintains patient's shoulder girdle position by placing the clinician's fist into the table at top of patient's shoulder. Make sure shoulder girdle depression is maintained mid to end range. 3. Using other hand and thigh, the clinician guides patient's shoulder into abduction, keeping neutral rotation and a flexed elbow to end range. Maintain position. Add shoulder external rotation to end range. 4. Clinician maintains all above components while allowing patient's elbow to extend to end range in forearm supination. 5. For final loading, use wrist and finger extension to end range. Assess the patient's fingers individually or as a group depending on symptom locations.
Normal responses	Stretching, pulling, tingling, and pain descriptions. Kenneally et al[8] concluded that the most common response is a deep stretch or ache in the cubital fossa extending down the anterior and radial aspect of the forearm and into the radial side of the hand. The second most common response is a tingling sensation in the thumb and first fingers; very few patients experience anterior shoulder stretch sensation.[8]
Clinical reasoning	Consider reversing the movement sequencing from distal to proximal, especially when symptoms are located in the fingers, hand, wrist, forearm, and elbow or with diagnoses of carpal tunnel syndrome, golfer's elbow, and tendonitis or tendinopathy of the elbow or wrist.

(continues on next page)

APPENDIX 5.D Neurodynamic Test Review (continued from previous page)

RADIAL NERVE TEST

Both median and radial nerve tests place tensile forces on the brachial plexus and lower cervical nerve roots and are typically performed with elbow extension. Indications for using the radial nerve test include symptoms specifically located in the dorsal aspect of the hand, especially the thumb, and the radial aspect of the forearm or radial nerve map, as well as any upper extremity neurogenic symptom provoked with upper extremity extension and abduction (reaching behind or away) or twisting of the forearm with thumb activities.

Component	Description
Active test	1. Patient stands and hangs arm at his or her side, making a fist holding the thumb. 2. Patient rotates arm inward as much as possible. 3. Patient reaches with entire arm toward floor and slightly behind back, maintaining the position. Structural differentiation indicates neurogenic symptoms if shoulder depression or cervical lateral flexion away from the reaching arm increases or produces symptoms. Because time in the position may be needed to feel the symptoms, have patient hold position 30 seconds to 2 minutes if possible.
Passive test, patient position	Patient is supine close to edge of bed, with legs extended and uninvolved arm extended. No pillow is used unless patient is unable to lie flat.
Passive test, clinician action	In a stride stance, facing patient's lower body, clinician slides enough of patient's upper body off table for clinician to place thigh of his or her back leg on top of patient's shoulder to maintain and monitor shoulder girdle depression position. Clinician uses one hand to grasp patient's lower forearm near wrist, the other cradling patient's slightly flexed elbow. The elbow hand will eventually assist with loading sequencing for wrist, hand, and thumb. Movement sequencing from proximal to distal is as follows: 1. Patient performs cervical lateral flexion away from the testing side to end range. 2. Clinician maintains patient's shoulder girdle position by placing his or her thigh at top of patient's shoulder. Make sure shoulder girdle depression is in mid to end range. Shoulder protraction can encourage further sensitizing of radial nerve if necessary. 3. Maintain above positions. Clinician uses both hands to guide shoulder internal rotation to end range. Finding end range may require extension and abduction with flexible patients. 4. Maintain above position. Clinician uses both hands to guide elbow extension and forearm pronation to end range with one hand while other hand on patient's wrist maintains internal rotation. 5. Final movements, if needed, include wrist flexion, thumb adduction, and ulnar deviation.
Normal response	Strong painful sensation or stretch over radial aspect of proximal forearm.[8] Less common responses include stretch pain in lateral aspect of upper arm or biceps areas and dorsum of wrist and hand.[8]

Component	Description
Clinical reasoning	Consider reversing the movement sequencing from distal to proximal when symptoms are located below the elbow, especially in the thumb, hand, wrist, and forearm, or with diagnoses of post–humeral fracture pain, lower cervical radiculopathy, supinator muscle pain (tennis elbow), de Quervain's tenosynovitis, and tendonitis or tendonopathy of the elbow, wrist, or thumb. If certain hand positions cause symptoms, start the test in these positions, then progress proximally with movement sequencing to differentiate neurogenic symptoms from local tissues.

ULNAR NERVE TEST

Clinicians have noticed that it is worthwhile to evaluate neurogenic symptoms with elbow flexion based on anatomical and clinical observations dating back as early as Bragard,[11] Pechan,[12] and Butler.[9] This test uses elbow flexion and pronation. Indications for using the ulnar nerve test include symptoms specifically located in the dorsal and palmar aspect of the medial hand, especially the fourth and fifth digits, including the ulnar distribution into the forearm. In addition, indications include any neurogenic symptom provoked with upper extremity elbow flexion and shoulder abduction (throwing a pitch) or twisting of the forearm with elbow flexion activities.

Component	Description
Active test	1. Patient sits or stands and places palm of hand over ear. 2. Maintaining hand on ear, patient turns fingers to point down and lift elbow up. Structural differentiation to indicate neurogenic symptoms includes shoulder depression, cervical retraction, and cervical lateral flexion away from reaching arm. Have patient sustain position for 30 seconds to 2 minutes to help identify a neurogenic component.
Passive test, patient position	Patient is supine close to edge of bed, with legs extended and uninvolved arm extended. No pillow is used unless patient is unable to lie flat.
Passive test, clinician action	In a stride position facing patient's upper body, clinician uses one hand to guide the patient's fourth and fifth fingers and wrist and places other hand on top of the patient's shoulder to monitor elevation of the shoulder girdle. Using the thigh of his or her forward leg, the clinician guides and supports patient's elbow while the patient performs upper extremity movements. Movement sequencing from proximal to distal is as follows: 1. Patient performs active cervical lateral flexion away from testing side to end range. 2. Clinician maintains patient's shoulder girdle position by placing his or her fist into table at top of patient's shoulder. Make sure shoulder girdle depression is mid to end range.

(continues on next page)

APPENDIX 5.D Neurodynamic Test Review *(continued from previous page)*

ULNAR NERVE TEST *(continued from previous page)*

Component	Description
Passive test, clinician action *(continued)*	3. Using other hand and thigh, clinician guides patient's shoulder into abduction, keeping neutral rotation and flexed elbow, to end range. Maintain position. Progress patient's shoulder external rotation toward end range.
	4. Maintaining all above components, clinician allows patient's elbow to gently flex to end range in forearm pronation.
	5. Final loading is wrist and fourth and fifth finger extension to end range. Assess fingers individually or as a group depending on symptom locations.
Normal responses	Stretch, pins and needles, and tingling sensations located in the hypothenar eminence and fourth and fifth digits.
Clinical reasoning	Consider reversing movement sequencing from distal to proximal when symptoms are located below the elbow and involve the hypothenar eminence, fourth and fifth digits of the hand, and medial wrist and forearm. Diagnoses of Guyon's canal syndrome, cubital tunnel syndrome, tendonitis or tendinopathy of the elbow or wrist, and medial hand pain require a distal to proximal movement sequence. If certain hand positions cause symptoms, start load sequencing in these positions, then progress proximally with movement sequencing.

Resources

1. Gutrecht JA, Zamani AA, Slagado ED. Anatomic-radiologic basis of Lhermitte's sign in multiple sclerosis. *Arch Neurol.* 1993;50:849-851.
2. Newton HB, Rea GL. Lhermitte's sign as a presenting symptom of primary spinal cord tumor. *J Neurooncol.* 1996;29:183-188.
3. McCombe PF, Fairbank JCT, Cockersole BC, et al. Reproducibility of physical signs in low back pain. *Spine.* 1989;14:908-918.
4. Deyo RA, Rainville J, Kent DL. What can the history and physical examination tell us about low back pain? *JAMA.* 1992;268:760-765.
5. Jönsson B, Strömqvist B. The straight leg raising test and the severity of symptoms in lumbar disc herniation. *Spine.* 1995;20:27-30.
6. Johnson B. *Mobilization of the Nervous System* [course handouts]. Chicago, IL: NOI Team; January 2012.
7. Elvey RL. Brachial plexus tension tests and the pathoanatomical origin of arm pain. In: Idezak R, ed. *Aspects of Manipulative Therapy.* Melbourne, Australia: Manipulative Physiotherapists Association of Australia; 1979.
8. Kenneally M, Rubenach H, Elvey R. The upper limb tension test: The SLR of the arm. In: Grant R, ed. *Physical Therapy of the Cervical and Thoracic Spine.* New York: Churchill Livingstone; 1988.
9. Butler DS. Adverse mechanical tension in the nervous system: A model of assessment and treatment. *Aust J Physiother.* 1989;35:227-238.
10. Shacklock M. Neurodynamics. *Physiotherapy.* 1995;81:9-16.
11. Bragard K. Die Nervendehnung als diagnostisches Prinzip ergibt eine Reihe neuer Nervenphänomene. *Münch Med Wschr.* 1929;10:1999-2003.
12. Pechan J. Ulnar nerve maneuver as diagnostic aid in its compression in the elbow region. *Cesk Neurol.* 1973;36:13-19.

Primary Resources

Butler DS. *Mobilization of the Nervous System.* Melbourne, Australia; Churchill Livingstone; 1991.
Butler DS. *The Sensitive Nervous System.* Adelaide, Australia; Noigroup; 2000.
Noigroup Team. *The Neurodynamic Techniques: A Definitive Guide from the Noigroup Team.* Adelaide, Australia: Noigroup Publications; 2005.

APPENDIX 5.E Orthopedic Outpatient: 45-Year-Old Female

Physical Therapy/Occupational Therapy Initial Evaluation

SUBJECTIVE FINDINGS

Chief complaint:	Pain located in cervical spine, right upper trapezius, lateral arm, forearm, thumb, palm, and all fingers
Descriptors:	Hand: "dead," numbness, tingling, cold feeling, weakness
	Forearm and arm: burning
	Neck: severe, sharp pain
Onset:	Recent: 3 mo ago, patient woke up with neck, shoulder, and arm pain.
	Chronic: 3 yr ago, forearm and hand symptoms were diagnosed as carpal tunnel syndrome; symptoms worsened with recent onset. Two surgeries each resulted in weaker hand and no change in symptoms; third scar tissue surgery will be scheduled once this new problem settles down.
Frequency:	Shoulder, arm, and forearm: intermittent
	Neck and hand: constant
24-hr behavior:	AM: worse (sleeping)
	PM: worse depending on activity; better during day when still
	New problem—hand symptoms unchanged
Subjective pain:	**Likert** / Faces scale: hand 3/10, arm 5/10, neck 7/10
Aggravating factors:	Sitting looking down, turning neck, any prolonged activity with arm, sleeping side lying; every 2 h needs to switch position
Relieving factors:	Holding neck still, rubbing hand, lying on back with pillows, supporting neck and elbow bent on pillows, heat, rest, medications, relaxation tapes for sleep

Pain Location

Pain Quality
Sharp
Dull
Burning
Pinching
Numbness
Tingling
Other: _____

PATIENT EDUCATION CONSIDERATIONS

Readiness to learn:	**Ready and self-motivated** Extrinsically motivated Limitations (see below)
Limitations to learning:	Cognitive Physical Language Financial Cultural **Other:** None
Teaching method preferred:	**Handout** Verbal **Demonstration** **Practice** Other:
Explain:	

(continues on next page)

APPENDIX 5.E Orthopedic Outpatient: 45-Year-Old Female *(continued from previous page)*

MEDICAL HISTORY

Past medical history:	Rates health as good
Family history:	Heart disease mother; cancer father
Surgery and invasive procedures:	2 carpal tunnel release and scar tissue release surgeries; no change in hand symptoms following surgeries
Medications:	Hydrocodone 3x daily, muscle relaxant for sleep, antidepressant daily Allergies: No known drug allergies
Previous treatments:	OT hand therapy after both surgeries; including stretching and strengthening exercises and massage; OT past 3 mo, including nerve stretching; function never returned to preexisting level after surgeries and therapy

Diagnostic tests:	X-ray:	MRI:	CT scan:	EMG:	Other:
	Degenerative changes, cervical spine	Cervical bulge C5-6, C6-7		Positive median, ulnar nerve motor and sensory findings	

PSYCHOSOCIAL FACTORS

Living situation:	Patient is single and lives with sister in a house they own; both parents are deceased.
Behavior:	Calm and cooperative
Occupation:	Consultant; travels weekly
Recreation and leisure:	Daily 2-mile walks
Functional disability:	Sustained overhead activity, carrying luggage and laptop on and off planes, very guarded with ADLs, no housework of any kind, off work past 3 mo trying to improve, has to return to work next week
Concerns:	Concern about overhead activity related to work, being able to travel for work, not participating with taking care of the house, and causing more damage to already damaged nerves

PROVISIONAL PAIN CLASSIFICATION

Peripheral neurogenic pain mechanism, mechanical inflammatory and ischemic pain; remodeling phase of healing

Provisional classification supporting information:
- Location, description, onset, surgical history, past treatments, diagnostic tests (EMG, MRI) indicating nerve pain
- Onset, frequency, aggravating and relieving factors indicating inflammatory and ischemic pain

PAIN EDUCATION TOPICS

1. Nerve pain: peripheralization and centralization, green and red lights related to return-to-work activity, pacing strategies for return to work
2. Ischemic musculoskeletal pain mechanism: need for increased blood flow to all tissues, including nerve
3. Connective tissue healing and remodeling guidelines
4. Effects of posture on arm and neck pain
5. Mechanical evaluation results and diagnostic test results confirming nerve and ischemic pain mechanisms
6. Posture and body mechanics strategies for consultant work, including prevention of forward head posturing when using phone and computer and proper lifting and carrying of luggage and laptop

(continues on next page)

APPENDIX 5.E Orthopedic Outpatient: 45-Year-Old Female *(continued from previous page)*

Physical Therapy/Occupational Therapy
Objective Evaluation

OBJECTIVE FINDINGS

Posture:	Atrophy right palmar, dorsal hand musculature; decreased right forearm girth. Forward head, minimal lateral flexion right cervical spine. Correction of posture increases symptoms but leaves patient no worse.
Active range of motion:	Cervical protrusion, full, no effect; flexion, full, increased pain; retraction, severe loss, increased pain; extension, severe loss, increased pain; right lateral flexion, moderate loss, increased pain; left lateral flexion, severe loss, increased pain; right rotation, moderate loss, increased pain; left rotation, severe loss, increased pain; 1 repetition test.
Repeated test movements:	**Visit 1** repeated exam: Cervical retraction, no effect on hand symptoms, decreased and abolished forearm, arm, and upper trapezius symptoms, centralized to neck; patient is better (increased ROM cervical left rotation, lateral flexion, extension, no effect all others; MNT decreased symptoms and increased ROM proximal to distal loading sequence but no effect distal to proximal loading sequence).
	Visit 2 repeated exam: Unloaded cervical retraction and extension, increased all symptoms, no worse, increase range of motion all directions, no effect on MNT. Therapist mobilization: Cervical traction retraction extension rotation, decrease neck, abolish arm, no effect on hand, increase range of motion all directions, no effect on MNT.
	Visit 3 repeated exam: Cervical retraction and extension, increased hand, forearm, and arm symptoms during, all symptoms worse as a result after, no effect on cervical motion and MNT; cervical retraction and lateral flexion right, decreased, all arm symptoms abolished except hand, increased but no worse. Patient is better; all cervical motions and MNT proximal to distal loading sequence, no worse left lateral flexion, rotation, and MNT distal to proximal loading sequence. Cervical flexion, all symptoms increased during and as a result worse after; symptoms, cervical motion, and MNT proximal to distal loading sequence.
Neurological and neurodynamic exam:	**Visit 1:** Sensory testing decreased in entire right hand, palm, and thumb. Motor testing right 3/5 median nerve muscles of hand, right 4/5 shoulder abduction, left 5/5 throughout. Reflex diminished right biceps reflex compared with left. MNT proximal to distal loading sequence, inconsistent production of symptoms, moderate loss of motion, apprehension with loading throughout, with repeated elbow extension, worse as a result. MNT distal to proximal loading sequence, increased symptoms with each sequence, repeated wrist and finger extension, increased symptoms in hand, no worse as a result; all other symptoms unchanged.

PROVISIONAL MECHANICAL CLASSIFICATION

Derangement: Unilateral/asymmetrical symptoms below the elbow with lateral component, active dominating mechanism

Dysfunction: Continue to rule out secondary neural, median nerve, inactive nondominating mechanism

PROVISIONAL PAIN CLASSIFICATION

Peripheral neurogenic pain mechanism, mechanical inflammatory and ischemic mechanisms; container dependent, cervical spine; secondary neural dependent, median nerve

TREATMENT

Treatment:
- Progress centralization with cervical lateral and extension procedures to reduce derangement using manual therapy lateral cervical flexion techniques followed by cervical traction, retraction, extension, and rotation techniques (first 3 wk).
- Prescribe remodeling exercises for wrist and hand flexion and extension using patient overpressure (second 4 wk).
- Progress to neural slider then tensioner exercises for median nerve, distal to proximal sequencing (second 4 wk). Full cervical motion achieved.
- Incorporate weightlifting and weightbearing exercise mimicking activities related to work (last 3 wk).
- Provide education in proper ergonomics and body mechanics specific to sleeping, computer use, lifting, prolonged sitting, and upper extremity use (last 10 wk).

Treatment summary: **15 visits over 17 wk**, 2x/wk for 3 wk, 1x/wk for 4 wk, 1x/2 wk for 10 wk. Progress desensitization of mechanical inflammatory and ischemic neural pain with progressive movement directed at cervical spine with emphasis on alignment to meet function load and ROM demands. Educate patient on the meaning of and expectations for symptoms.

Goals:

	PSFS	
	Initial	Discharge
Sit and work at computer for 1-2 hr	3	8
Sleeping through night, no interruptions	0	10
Carrying 20 lb of luggage and lifting into overhead bin	0	8
Pain limitation to function	3	8
Pain intensity rating	7	1

Abbreviations: ADLs = activities of daily living; CT = computed tomography; EMG = electromyography; MNT = median nerve test; MRI = magnetic resonance imaging; OT = occupational therapy; PSFS = Patient-Specific Functional Scale; ROM = range of motion.

APPENDIX 5.F Neurology Outpatient: 30-Year-Old Female

Physical Therapy/Occupational Therapy Initial Evaluation

SUBJECTIVE FINDINGS

Chief complaint:	Neck, shoulder, right upper arm, and low back pain
Descriptors:	Burning, numbness, tingling, dull cramping, dull ache
Onset:	8 wk ago for no apparent reason, possibly related to new wheelchair seat
Frequency:	Intermittent
24-hr behavior:	Worse in AM and PM, gets better as day goes on; activity can make worse
Subjective pain:	Likert / Faces scale: 4/10
Aggravating factors:	Excessive computer use, reading, driving, using arm overhead
Relieving factors:	Lying down, good posture, heat, medications (muscle relaxants)

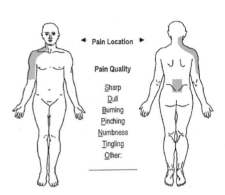

Pain Location

Pain Quality
Sharp
Dull
Burning
Pinching
Numbness
Tingling
Other:

PATIENT EDUCATION CONSIDERATIONS

Readiness to learn:	Ready and self-motivated Extrinsically motivated Limitations (see below)
Limitations to learning:	Cognitive Physical Language Financial Cultural Other: None
Teaching method preferred:	Handout Verbal Demonstration Practice Other:
Explain:	Difficulty with upper extremities in sustained overhead postures in wheelchair

MEDICAL HISTORY

Past medical history:	Cerebral palsy since a child, uses a wheelchair predominantly, otherwise healthy
Family history:	
Surgery and invasive procedures:	Epidural injection 3 wk ago was helpful for neck
Medications:	Rofecoxib works only sometimes; muscle relaxants are generally helpful Allergies: No known drug allergies
Previous treatments:	Epidural
Diagnostic tests:	X-ray: Negative MRI: Herniated nucleus pulposus C5-6 CT scan: EMG: Other:

PSYCHOSOCIAL FACTORS

Living situation:	Lives alone; parents are nearby and supportive
Behavior:	Calm and cooperative
Occupation:	Librarian
Recreation and leisure:	Participates in general fitness program at sports center 3x/wk
Functional disability:	Sustained overhead activity, prolonged sitting at computer
Concerns:	Concern about whether she should be working and doing overhead activity related to work

PROVISIONAL PAIN CLASSIFICATION

Peripheral neurogenic inflammatory pain mechanism, repair to remodeling phase of healing

Provisional classification supporting information:
- Location, description, diagnostic tests indicating nerve pain
- Onset, medication, aggravating and relieving factors indicating mechanical inflammatory pain

PAIN EDUCATION TOPICS

1. Musculoskeletal nerve pain: peripheralization and centralization
2. Use of green and red lights to guide work activities
3. Repair to remodeling phase of healing and need for increased blood flow, especially with sustained postures
4. Connective tissue healing and repair remodeling guidelines using Activity Pyramid
5. Effects of posture on arm and neck pain; confirm centralization and prescribe preferred direction–specific exercise
6. Mechanical evaluation results and diagnostic test results confirming pain mechanism and mechanical syndrome
7. Posture and body mechanics strategies for librarian work, including prevention of forward head posturing when using phone and computer, and for weightlifting at sports club

(continues on next page)

APPENDIX 5.F Neurology Outpatient: 30-Year-Old Female *(continued from previous page)*

Physical Therapy/Occupational Therapy Objective Evaluation

OBJECTIVE FINDINGS

Posture:	Forward head posture, correction decrease arm symptoms, patient better, findings relevant
Active range of motion:	Cervical flexion, nil loss, pain; cervical left rotation, side bending, nil loss, pain; cervical retraction, extension, right rotation, side bending, moderate loss, pain, 1 repetition test.
Repeated test movements:	Repeated cervical protrusion produces neck and arm pain, increases arm pain during, no worse after. Repeated cervical flexion produces neck and arm pain, increases arm pain during, remains worse as a result in arm after. Repeated cervical retraction produces neck pain, decreases and centralizes arm pain to scapula during; added patient overpressure centralizes to neck during; as a result arm and scapula pain abolish, all motions increase in loss directions, motor exam 5/5 after.
Neurological examination:	Weakness shoulder abduction right, 4/5

PROVISIONAL MECHANICAL CLASSIFICATION

Derangement: Unilateral/asymmetrical symptoms above the elbow

PROVISIONAL PAIN CLASSIFICATION

Peripheral neurogenic inflammatory pain mechanism, container dependent—cervical spine

TREATMENT

Treatment:	• Reduction of derangement using extension procedures for cervical spine, postural strategies for computer and driving to reduce forward head and maintain reduction (first 2 wk) • Lumbar roll and referral for seating and positioning for back and seat adjustment to lessen posterior dump of wheelchair (first 2 wk) • Continuous low-level heat therapy for prolonged driving and computer use to help with muscle soreness related to cervical posture (first 2 wk) • Restoration of function to include upgrade of gym program using gym ball and reciprocating upper extremity movements below, at, and above shoulders with focus on cervical, thoracic, and lumbar alignment and postural stability (last 4 wk)
Treatment summary:	**8 visits over 6 wk:** 2x/wk for 2 wk, 1x/wk for 4 wk. Progress desensitization of mechanical inflammatory neural pain mechanism with progressive movement directed at cervical spine with emphasis on alignment to meet function load and ROM demands. Provide education on meaning of and expectations for symptoms.

Goals:		PSFS	
		Initial	Discharge
	Sitting for 4 hr in wheelchair	3	10
	Computer work for 1-2 hr	3	10
	Return to fitness program 3x/wk	0	10
	Pain limitation to function	5	10
	Pain intensity rating	7	0

Abbreviations: CT = computed tomography; EMG = electromyography; MRI = magnetic resonance imaging; PSFS = Patient-Specific Functional Scale; ROM = range of motion.

> **APPENDIX 5.G** Orthopedic Outpatient: 35-Year-Old Male

Physical Therapy/Occupational Therapy Initial Evaluation

SUBJECTIVE FINDINGS

Chief complaint:	Pain in right posterior lateral lower leg with activity
Descriptors:	Numbness, tingling, deep pain
Onset:	Sprained ankle 12 wk ago, inversion sprain with pain local to ankle; in past 3 wk pain spread to lower leg
Frequency:	Intermittent
24-hr behavior:	Worse at end of day depending on activity, occasional low-level pain at night, better in AM
Subjective pain:	(Likert) / Faces scale: 4/10 with activity
Aggravating factors:	Prolonged use, sitting, initial walking, running, descending stairs, playing sports (landing, cutting)
Relieving factors:	Using heating pad, stretching calf during running, changing position

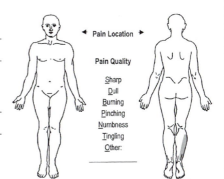

◄ Pain Location ►

Pain Quality
Sharp
Dull
Burning
Pinching
Numbness
Tingling
Other: _____

PATIENT EDUCATION CONSIDERATIONS

Readiness to learn:	(Ready and self-motivated) Extrinsically motivated Limitations (see below)
Limitations to learning:	Cognitive Physical Language Financial Cultural (Other:) None
Teaching method preferred:	Handout Verbal (Demonstration) (Practice) Other: _____
Explain:	_____

MEDICAL HISTORY

Past medical history:	Reported healthy; lot of ankle sprains in past, but this sprain different, with symptoms persisting
Family history:	No significant family history
Surgery and invasive procedures:	None
Medications:	Ibuprofen (doesn't help), as needed Allergies: No known drug allergies
Previous treatments:	Rest, no running or sports since sprain; 2 wk ago tried running and pain increased, so quit
Diagnostic tests:	X-ray: Negative MRI: _____ CT scan: _____ EMG: _____ Other: _____

(continues on next page)

APPENDIX 5.G Orthopedic Outpatient: 35-Year-Old Male *(continued from previous page)*

PSYCHOSOCIAL FACTORS

Living situation:	Single, lives alone in 3rd-floor condo; has family in area
Behavior:	Calm and cooperative
Occupation:	Trader; on feet all day
Recreation and leisure:	Runner, but no running for past 3 mo
Functional disability:	Unable to climb stairs to 3rd floor, stand on feet all day, or participate in basketball, volleyball, running
Concerns:	Concerned why pain is persisting with this ankle sprain; unable to run, play sports

PROVISIONAL PAIN CLASSIFICATION

Peripheral neurogenic pain mechanism, ischemic

PAIN EDUCATION TOPICS

1. Nerve pain education handout answering following questions: What is nerve pain? How does nerve pain behave? What treatments help nerve pain?
2. No-worse concept to establish movement guidelines with interval walk, jog, run program; symptoms during exercises permitted and goal for rehabilitation at this stage in healing; Activity Pyramid as a guide to activity
3. Benefits of movement, heat, and appropriate stress for nerve remodeling and stage of healing
4. Education regarding recurrent inversion ankle sprains and peripheral nerve relationships, including scar formation

Provisional classification supporting information:

- Location and description of symptoms, night pain, history of recurrent episodes persisting longer indicating nerve distribution and description
- Onset, frequency, 24-hr behavior of symptoms, prolonged activity aggravation, heat and movement relief, anti-inflammatory medication not helping indicating ischemic pain

Physical Therapy/Occupational Therapy
Objective Evaluation

OBJECTIVE FINDINGS

Observation:	No abnormalities or swelling noted
Manual muscle test:	Negative pain provocation, 5/5 dorsiflexion, plantarflexion, inversion, eversion
Active/passive range of motion:	Left active and passive, full all directions. Right passive dorsiflexion, eversion, inversion, minimum loss, produces pain at ankle (not patient complaint). Plantarflexion, inversion, no loss, produces pain at ankle (not patient complaint). Right active motion, same range, no pain, 1 repetition test
Repeated test movements:	Lumbar spine cleared all directions, no effect; right ankle cleared all directions, no effect.
Neurological and neurodynamic exam:	Sensory: Light touch tactile allodynia, sural distribution right
	Motor: Negative
	Reflexes: Negative
	Neurodynamic test: Positive right sural nerve test distal to proximal produces pain dorsiflexion, increases pain inversion, increases pain knee extension, increases pain SLR; minimal loss of ROM with each additional movement, no worse after.
	Repeated neurodynamic test: Sural nerve test using ankle dorsiflexion/inversion in SLR produces and increases pain during, no worse, no effect in ROM after.

PROVISIONAL MECHANICAL CLASSIFICATION
Dysfunction, neural tissue, sural nerve

PROVISIONAL PAIN CLASSIFICATION
Peripheral neurogenic ischemic pain, neural dependent, sural nerve

(continues on next page)

APPENDIX 5.G Orthopedic Outpatient: 35-Year-Old Male *(continued from previous page)*

TREATMENT

Treatment:
- Ankle ROM (dorsiflexion/eversion and dorsiflexion/inversion) using ½ foam roll, 10x each, on-off pattern (first 2 wk)
- Sural nerve slider pattern using knee extension as mobilization link in SLR test position with belt holding dorsiflexion/inversion, start 1x daily, progress to 3x daily as symptoms indicate, no worse next day (0-2 wk)
- Progress neurodynamic exercise to tensioner using ankle and foot as mobilization link with belt, continue 3x daily or before activity (2-4 wk)
- Progress to weightbearing neural slider to tensioner stretches (downward dog with ankle combined movements) maintained, 2x daily or if symptoms return (4-6 wk)
- Add sport-specific drills, including foot reach exercise (patient standing on right foot while left foot reaches) in direction of anterior lateral (or 1:00) to posterior medial rotation (or 4:00); set goals for range and speed, 4x week (6-10 wk)
- Add interval program walk to sprint, 3x/wk (8-12 wk)

Treatment summary: **1x/2 wk for 12 wk**, total 6 visits. Progress desensitization of ischemic neural pain mechanism with progressive movement directed at peripheral nervous system to meet function load and ROM demands. Provide education on meaning of and expectation for symptoms.

Goals:

	PSFS	
	Initial	Discharge
Descend 3 flights of stairs daily at condo	5	10
Basketball, 3 pickup games 2x/wk	0	7
Running 3 miles, 3x/wk	3	10
Pain limitation to function	6	10
Pain intensity rating	5	1

Abbreviations: CT = computed tomography; EMG = electromyography; MRI = magnetic resonance imaging; PSFS = Patient-Specific Functional Scale; ROM = range of motion; SLR = straight leg raise.

APPENDIX 5.H Orthopedic Outpatient: 60-Year-Old Male

Physical Therapy/Occupational Therapy Initial Evaluation

SUBJECTIVE FINDINGS

Chief complaint:	Pain in right hand from MCPs of all digits to tips and in a circular patch the size of a silver dollar on right palm
Descriptors:	Numbness, tingling, cramping weakness with prolonged activity
Onset:	>20 yr ago, initial symptoms; since last year, have gotten progressively worse
Frequency:	Reported constant; however, day of exam was able to find 10 min of relief with unloaded neural position, and after movement, symptoms returned to baseline
24-hr behavior:	Worse at night related to activity with hand, wakes up at night, change of position improves, back to baseline in AM
Subjective pain:	(Likert) / Faces scale: 5/10
Aggravating factors:	Prolonged use, golf, fly fishing, writing
Relieving factors:	No relieving factors; change of position produces temporary relief

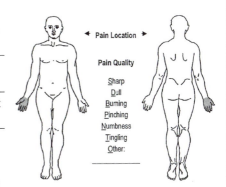

Pain Location

Pain Quality
Sharp
Dull
Burning
Pinching
Numbness
Tingling
Other: _____

PATIENT EDUCATION CONSIDERATIONS

Readiness to learn:	(Ready and self-motivated) Extrinsically motivated Limitations (see below)
Limitations to learning:	Cognitive Physical Language Financial Cultural (Other:) None
Teaching method preferred:	Handout (Verbal) (Demonstration) (Practice) Other: _____
Explain:	_____

(continues on next page)

> **APPENDIX 5.H Orthopedic Outpatient: 60-Year-Old Male** *(continued from previous page)*

MEDICAL HISTORY

Past medical history:	Reported healthy
Family history:	No significant family history
Surgery and invasive procedures:	Because of symptoms, underwent C2-C4 neck decompression 3 yr prior (no change), carpal tunnel release 2 yr prior, ulnar nerve repositioning 1 yr prior. Overall, believes that symptoms have intensified each year with each procedure.
Medications:	Duloxetine, gabapentin, celecoxib (unsure if they help; has taken for 3 yr) **Allergies:** No known drug allergies
Previous treatments:	Physical therapy postoperatively for all procedures produced no relief of symptoms but helped him return to gross motor ADLs
Diagnostic tests:	X-ray: Negative MRI: Herniated nucleus pulposus C4-5 CT scan: EMG: Negative Other:

PSYCHOSOCIAL FACTORS

Living situation:	Lives in house with his wife, has a well-established support system with 3 adult children and 4 grandchildren living in area
Behavior:	No anger about his condition, but adamantly refuses to have any additional surgery
Occupation:	Retired university professor
Recreation and leisure:	Weightlifting 3x/wk, daily cardiovascular 40 min treadmill walking; unable to golf, hunt, or fish (his passions, which he is unable to do in retirement)
Functional disability:	Unable to write checks and letters
Concerns:	Concerned about his declining function and continuing diagnosis of neural entrapments without relief from surgery or entrapments

PROVISIONAL PAIN CLASSIFICATION

Peripheral neurogenic pain mechanism, ischemic

PAIN EDUCATION TOPICS

1. Nerve pain education handout to answer following questions: What is nerve pain? How does nerve pain behave? What treatments help nerve pain?

2. No-worse concept to establish movement guidelines with check writing, fishing, and golf; symptoms during exercises permitted and goal for rehabilitation; Activity Pyramid to guide activity

3. Benefits of movement, heat, and appropriate stress for nerve remodeling

4. Change of education focus from prior treatment, in which increasing symptoms meant a worsening of the condition, to current concepts of pain biology, in which producing and increasing symptoms is the target to remodel neural tissue elasticity, strength, and function

5. Types of mechanical problems with nerve—entrapment vs neural remodeling—as a way of explaining why past surgery and therapies were not effective and the need to direct movement to the nerve

Provisional classification supporting information:
- Pain location, description, onset, history indicating nerve tissue pain
- Frequency, aggravating and alleviating factors, onset, surgical history indicating ischemic pain

Physical Therapy/Occupational Therapy Objective Evaluation

OBJECTIVE FINDINGS

Active/passive range of motion:	Full cervical ROM, 1 repetition testing, no effect on hand symptoms; full R shoulder and elbow ROM, 1 repetition testing, no effect; end range pain at R wrist, minimal loss of flexion and extension, 1 repetition testing, no effect; R digits 1-4, minimal loss of MCP extension
Repeated test movements:	Cervical spine, cleared all directions, no effect; right wrist, cleared all directions, no effect; right digits 1-4 MCP extension, increased symptoms during, no worse.
Pain-free position:	Abolish all symptoms with 3 min sustained UE neural unloaded position shoulder elevation, elbow flexion, wrist neutral; pain immediately provoked with UE neural loaded position of right elbow extension, shoulder depression
Neurodynamic testing:	**Median nerve test (MNT):** ROM loss at shoulder abduction by 30° compared with opposite UE. Effect on symptoms: Increased symptoms with neural loading distal to proximal loading sequence using finger extension, wrist extension, elbow extension and supination, shoulder external rotation and abduction. Repeated MNT movements, wrist and fingers 1-3 extension in tension position, causes an increase in symptoms during, and remains no worse after. **Ulnar nerve test (UNT):** ROM loss of elbow flexion by 40° compared with opposite UE. Effect on symptoms: Increased symptoms with neural loading distal to proximal loading sequence using finger extension, wrist extension, forearm pronation, shoulder abduction and external rotation, and elbow flexion. Repeated UNT movements, wrist and fingers 4 and 5 extension in tension position, causes an increase in symptoms during, and remains no worse after.

PROVISIONAL MECHANICAL CLASSIFICATION

Dysfunction, neural tissue, median and ulnar nerve

PROVISIONAL PAIN CLASSIFICATION

Peripheral neurogenic ischemic pain, neural dependent, median and ulnar nerve

(continues on next page)

APPENDIX 5.H Orthopedic Outpatient: 60-Year-Old Male *(continued from previous page)*

TREATMENT

Treatment:
- Establish activity baseline for check writing, fishing, and golf using driving range (0-2 wk)
- Wrist and finger ROM (extension/supination/pronation combinations) on-off, 10x each (0-2 wk)
- Median and ulnar nerve slider pattern using elbow as mobilization link in median and ulnar nerve test position, keeping wrist and fingers actively at end range, start 1x daily, progress to 3x daily as symptoms indicate, no worse next day (2-4 wk)
- Progress neurodynamic exercise to tensioner using wrist and finger as mobilization link, continue 3x daily or before activity or if symptoms increase (4-8 wk)
- Progress to weightbearing neural stretches, pushups and pull-ups, sport-specific drills for casting and golf, 2x wk (8-10 wk)

Treatment summary: **2x/wk for 2 wk, then 1x/wk for 8 wk**, total 12 visits over 10 wk. Progress desensitization of ischemic neural pain mechanism with progressive movement directed at peripheral nervous system to meet function load and ROM demands. Provide education on meaning of and expectation for symptoms.

Goals:

	PSFS Initial	PSFS Discharge
Writing 5 checks at one time	3	10
Golf, 9 holes 2x/wk	0	8
Fish, 1 hr 3x/wk	0	10
Pain limitation to function	5	10
Pain intensity rating	5	1

Abbreviations: ADLs = activities of daily living; CT = computed tomography; EMG = electromyography; MCP = metacarpophalangeal joint; MRI = magnetic resonance imaging; PSFS = Patient-Specific Functional Scale; R = right; ROM = range of motion; UE = upper extremity.

APPENDIX 5.1 Clinical Reasoning for Subjective PNS Pain Characteristics

Peripheral Nervous System Pain Mechanisms: Subjective Characteristics		
Nociceptive:Inflammatory Mechanical vs. Chemical	**Nociceptive:Ischemia**	**Peripheral Neurogenic**

Location: Localized
Frequency:
  Chemical: Constant dull ache or throb at rest
  Mechanical: Intermittent and sharp with movement
Descriptors: Swollen, throbbing, aching
Onset: Recent trauma within 3 weeks or recent flare-up of chronic pathological condition
24-hour behavior: Increased pain in the morning; gets better throughout day, then worsens at end of day and during night
Course: Improving rapidly according to expected tissue healing/pathology recovery times
Alleviating factors: Ice, responds to simple NSAIDs / analgesia medications, certain directions or positions
Aggravating factors: Heat; clearly related to certain directions or positions
Psychosocial screen: Negative
	Location: Localized
	Frequency: Intermittent
	Descriptors: Fatigue, weakness, tightness, sharp with movement
	Onset: Onset may be for no apparent reason; onset can be positional or cumulative or >21 days after connective tissue injury in a remodeling phase
	24-hour behavior: Typically better in the morning and worse in the afternoon or after maintaining an activity or position for 1-3 hours
	Course: Unchanged, plateau
	Alleviating: Heat, change position, gentle stretching/exercise, limited movement
	Aggravating: Related to prolonged movements, positions, activities
	Psychosocial screen: Negative
		Location: Localized to dermatome or cutaneous nerve field
		Intensity: High, irritable
		Frequency: Constant, intermittent, spontaneous, or paroxysmal pain
		Descriptors: Sharp, deep ache, cramp = muscle; superficial burning, parasthesia, pins and needles, shooting, electric shock like, crawling = skin; numbness, heavy, tingle, weakness = root
		Onset: History of nerve injury, pathology, or mechanical compromise
		Alleviating: Heat; antiepileptic (gabapentin, pregabalin), anti-depression (amitriptyline) medications; activities or postures associated with no movement, less tension, pressure of neural tissues
		Aggravating: Mechanical pattern involving activities and postures associated with movement; loading or compression of neural tissue; stress, mood can alter pain
		24-hour behavior: Worse at night, disturbed sleep

APPENDIX 5.J Clinical Reasoning for Objective PNS Pain Characteristics

Peripheral Nervous System Pain Mechanisms: Objective Characteristics		
Nociceptive:Inflammatory Mechanical vs. Chemical	**Nociceptive:Ischemia**	**Peripheral Neurogenic**
Objective findings: **Mechanical** • Close movement/pain relationship with active, passive, resisted repeated motion testing • Classification of mechanical diagnosis for derangement; identified preferred direction • Sprain/strain identified with pain, weakness, pain laxity, palpation • Absence of neurological signs, allodynia/hyperalgesia **Chemical** • All static/repeated movement tests increase pain; remains worse • Unable to identify position or motion to abolish symptoms • Ice temporarily eases pain with midrange position of affected area • Evidence of warmth, swelling • Antalgic posture movement pattern	**Objective findings:** Classification of mechanical diagnosis for dysfunction, posture, other • Contractile or articular tissue dysfunction: Symptoms present *during* for contractile and at *end range* for articular on repeated movement assessment; no worse as a result *after* repeated movement assessment • Patient may have a painful arc of motion or region where contractile tissue is challenged in contractile dysfunction. • **Posture syndrome:** Reproduction of symptoms is often difficult on movement exam and no loss of motion is present. Symptoms are produced with static end range posture and are abolished when stress is removed. • **Other condition:** Often this kinetic chain impairment and/or pathology affects the quality of movement or muscle activation during movement; produces symptoms and remains no worse as a result.	**Objective findings:** **Posture:** Antalgic of affected body part **Palpation:** Provoke symptoms with palpation of involved nerve **Neurological findings:** Positive for altered reflexes, sensation, muscle power, hyperalgesia/allodynia/hyperpathia in a dermatome, myotomal, cutaneous path **Repeated movement tests:** Identify preferred direction and signs of centralization with mechanical inflammation present **Repeated neurodynamic tests:** Identify nerve irritation as nerve or container dependent. **Nerve dependent:** Restriction in ROM; can produce or increase symptoms with additional movements that increase force to the neural tissues. Repeated neural tension movements *during* may increase or decrease; as a result, *after* symptoms will be no better or worse and no change in ROM will occur. **Container dependent:** May be restriction in ROM but not always; unexpected response of symptoms with additional neural tension. Latency symptom response after testing: Pain at release, decreased pain with loading. Repeated neural movements *during* increase and worsen symptoms. Symptoms change when manual muscle test or joint play test is performed in a neural tension position, which can isolate the nerve container tissue source.

APPENDIX 5.K Clinical Reasoning for PNS Pain Intervention

Peripheral Nervous System Pain Mechanism Intervention		
Nociceptive:Inflammatory Mechanical vs. Chemical	**Nociceptive:Ischemia**	**Peripheral Neurogenic**
Mechanical **Patient education:** Use pain as a guide **MICE:** Mobility, Ice, Compression, Elevation *Mobility:* Midrange motion of the involved tissue; identify directional or postural preference; use every 1–2 hours as a guideline for exercise; modify ADLs and occupational tasks. *Ice:* 30 min, 3-4x/day; light covering on skin *Compression:* Use compression garments on involved tissue during activity. *Elevation:* Typically use at end of day; may need to support involved tissue above heart. **Chemical** Patient education: Use pain as a guide **RICE:** Rest, Ice, Compression, Elevation *Rest:* Use corset or brace on involved tissue during activity; modify ADLs and occupational tasks. *Ice:* 30 min, 3-4x/day; light covering on skin *Compression:* Use compression garments on involved tissue during rest. *Elevation:* At end of day, elevate involved tissue above heart when appropriate. **Medication:** Use oral nonsteroidal medication every 4–6 hours; progress to steroid oral or injection if no effect is seen after 72 hours. **Modalities:** Use electrical stimulation to decrease edema.	**Patient education:** Repair/remodeling phase of tissue healing. Pain is no longer a guide. No worse after 20 minutes of activity is a guide. **ROM:** Progressed to end range and into pain of involved tissue in all directions; no worse as a result. **Extremity function:** Restore quality biometrics and progress from isometric to concentric to eccentric function; progress the return of ADLs, occupational tasks, and sports function. **Spine function:** Begin in antigravity position; restore neutral spine; progress through weightbearing activities with posture, body mechanics, ADLs, occupational tasks, and sports function. **Cardiovascular exercise:** Build on the patient's low aerobic capacity 2–5 hours weekly, HR at 55%–75% of max; progress to high-intensity interval training 2-3x/wk, HR at 75%–90% of max for exertion intervals (10 seconds to 1 min) followed by recovery intervals (30 seconds to 2 min) for 3–9 sets for a total of 10–30 min. **Strength training:** Weightlifting for 1-3x/wk; total body functional movement patterns **Manual therapy:** Massage, overpressure, mobilization, and manipulation applied as patient plateaus with active exercise associated with tissue dysfunction **Modalities:** Increase blood flow response before or after exercise, using hot packs, ultrasound, heat wraps (active), or electrical stimulation.	**Patient education:** Based on inflammatory or ischemic pain properties, follow previous guidelines. **Neural-dependent guidelines** *Neurodynamic movement:* Slider neural movement pre and/or post low aerobic (LA) exercise. Start movement at extremity joint away from symptom area. Progress neural movement to tension on the nerve pre and/or post LA exercise toward location of symptoms. *Manual therapy:* Neural rubbing at abnormal impulse generating site (AIGS); work away from the nerve, then move directly onto palpation of the tender region of the nerve. *Graded exposure/pacing cardiovascular exercise:* Build low aerobic capacity 2–5 hours weekly, HR at 55%–75% of max; add 1–5 min every 24–72 hours. Progress to high-intensity interval training 2-3x/wk, HR at 75%–90% of max for exertion intervals (10 seconds to 1 min) followed by recovery intervals (30 seconds to 2 min) for 3–9 sets for a total of 10–30 min. **Container-dependent guidelines** Treat container first. *Muscle:* Soft tissue massage; stretch and strengthen muscle or apply eccentric strength if tendon. *Joint:* Overpressure, mobilization, manipulation; restore ROM in 3 planes. *Neurodynamic movement:* Neural slider movement after container treatments; progress to neural tension movement if necessary.

CHAPTER 6

Central Sensitization Pain Mechanism

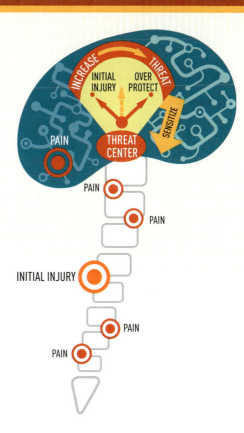

Pain is inevitable; suffering is optional.
 —Buddhist proverb

> **POINTS TO DISCUSS**
>
> - Central nervous system sensitizing processes related to the pain alarm system
> - Overview of central sensitization pain mechanism
> - Health care models in chronic pain treatment
> - Components of a subjective pain evaluation for the central sensitization pain mechanism
> - Maladaptive pain behavior
> - Objective tools and tests for central sensitization
> - Central sensitization management and intervention, including patient education and relaxation, and active movement

Central nervous system (CNS) musculoskeletal pain mechanisms are related to altered CNS circuitry and processing. These mechanisms involve pain that is referred from the CNS. The spinal cord and brain are responsible for processing input from musculoskeletal tissues and interpreting their messages. Pain that is referred from the CNS, therefore, is not from the tissues but rather is the interpretation of nociception from the tissues initially mediated by the spinal cord and the brain.

CNS cells can change their response properties when they are subjected to repeated nociceptive inputs. Clinically, this phenomenon produces heightened awareness, vigilance, and hypersensitivity in patients even without tissue impairment. These overprotective behaviors initially are useful to promote protective motor activity and therapeutic healing behavior in injured tissue; however, these behaviors become destructive if pain persists past normal connective tissue healing times.[1]

Central Nervous System Sensitizing Processes

Pain is designed to ensure survival of a species. Body responses ensure that each individual is aware of a perceived threat, and they constitute a pain alarm system. Mechanisms that sensitize nociceptors and facilitate cognitive or emotional behaviors have been linked to and are interdependent in the promotion of chronic pain.[2] These sensitizing processes of the CNS can be divided into three mechanisms: peripheral sensitization, plasticity in the spinal cord, and supraspinal modulation.[3] Plastic changes are possible at each level, from the peripheral receptor to higher level cortical structures.[4]

Peripheral Sensitization

When tissue is injured, an inflammatory response occurs. After the first wave of inflammation, inflammatory mediators are released with the processing of acute pain. In addition, a sensitization of peripheral receptors may occur subsequently that can result in an increase in central hyperexcitability.[5]

This sensitization can change the ability of primary afferent fibers to respond as usual, and the afferent fibers may activate typically inactive nociceptors.[6] For example, heat receptors can change in response to sensitized nociceptors and create spontaneous inflammation. This inflammatory response can alter genetic expression in the dorsal root ganglion and increase production of more peripheral receptors.[3]

When the CNS cells change, cells that normally would respond only to nociceptive inputs may begin to respond to inputs that are innocuous,[7] producing allodynia, or pain from a stimulus that is not normally painful. Hyperalgesia, or an increased sensitivity or response to a painful stimulus, can also occur as a result of Aβ-mediated information that stimulates a painful response in the CNS. As the pain becomes more chronic, fast-acting Aβ fibers can adopt C fiber characteristics. This hyperalgesic response can lead to sensitization of the periphery that increases the nociception transmitted to the spinal cord.[3] Some patients with hyperalgesia have demonstrated evidence of a central mechanism based on the fact that local nerve blocks did not alter sensation.[2]

Furthermore, persistent thoughts that lead the patient to focus on the injury or pain are inputs that may maintain dorsal horn cell excitability. The process can lift the descending inhibitory currents from the brain that normally prevent an increase in sensitivity. Additionally, persistent peripheral nociceptive input can induce changes in the CNS.[8] Activation of C fiber afferents releases transmitters, and repeated activation of C fibers can cause peptides to accumulate and remove the magnesium block of the N-methyl-D-aspartate (NMDA) channel. Removal of this block can create a windup phenomenon with neuronal depolarization and a baseline change in activity that increases the excitability of the neuron.[9] This receptor thereby plays a major role in the sensitivity of the nerve. Windup occurs when C fibers are repeatedly stimulated and neuronal responses in the spinal cord are enhanced. Windup results in the prolongation and amplification of neuronal responses and involves an NMDA receptor–mediated mechanism.[10]

Although peripheral sensitization is the first process that initiates central sensitization within the pain mechanism classification system (PMCS), this mechanism is classified as the peripheral neurogenic pain mechanism (PNPM; see Chapter 5). The PNPM is reviewed in this chapter to shed light on how central sensitization develops. Objectively, characteristics of peripheral sensitization present as PNPM in the PMCS because the pattern of symptoms is consistent with mechanical loads and can be subclassified using the mechanical diagnosis and therapy syndromes.

Plasticity in the Spinal Cord

Nociceptive input in the spinal cord leads to activation of NMDA receptors. Receptor field expansion occurs in the dorsal horn, and a peripheral stimulus can activate the neurons and result in hyperalgesia. Increased glial cells can contribute to the central hypersensitivity. In addition, inhibitory interneurons are destroyed, and random excitatory connections can also occur.[3] Injuries to the peripheral nerve can result in up-regulation in the dorsal root ganglion, depression of inhibitory mechanisms, and a decrease in gamma-aminobutyric acid and opioid receptors.[3] The brain and dorsal horn can be sensitized, resulting in a clinical presentation of reduced thresholds to movement and increased responses to afferent input such that normal input results in a painful response.

A characteristic common in a persistent pain state is spontaneous generation of neuronal activity in which symptoms appear to have a mind of their own, firing with no stimulus.[11] In addition, researchers agree that these characteristics indicate plasticity changes in the spinal cord when patients show heightened responses to afferent activity with repeated stimuli, increased spontaneous activity, prolonged symptoms after discharge with repeated stimulation, reduced thresholds, and expansion of receptor fields.[1,8,11]

Supraspinal Modulation

Facilitatory and inhibitory pathways can influence the spinal cord's excitability through supraspinal modulation.[3] Evidence supports the presence of descending inhibitory mechanisms of pain, but reports of facilitatory pathways from the brainstem have also been demonstrated via serotonin 5-hydroxytryptamine (5-HT) receptor pathways.[10] These pathways can be involved in emotional, sensory, autonomic, and affective components of pain. Pain responses can trigger emotional responses, and descending pathways may facilitate spinal processing of pain via brainstem and spinal cord processing loops.[10] This process supports the need to integrate pain management techniques using multiple disciplines, including physiological and psychological. Central sensitization represents changes in the properties of the neuron in the CNS in the absence of nociceptive inputs.[12] One of the most consistent predictors of developing chronic pain is the presence of another chronic pain condition.[13] With each chronic problem, the patient's CNS is sensitized further to overprotect the body.

Latremoliere and Woolf[12] described two phases in central sensitization: transcription independent and transcription dependent. The transcription-independent phase results in changes to glutamate and receptor properties dependent on NMDA, such as in the acute phase of an injury or with processes of peripheral sensitization and plasticity in the spinal cord. The transcription-dependent phase results in longer lasting changes based on synthesis of new proteins and occurs in later, chronic phases of an injury, such as in supraspinal modulation (see **Table 6.1** and **Figure 6.1**). Essentially, activation of NMDA receptors and the activation of glutamate and substance P help generate central sensitization. In addition, an increase in intracellular calcium initiates these triggers. These neurons can change and be identified as dominating through initiation of spontaneous activity, a reduced threshold for stimulation, and a larger receptive field.[12]

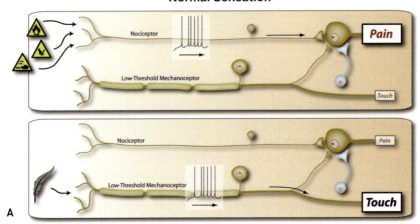

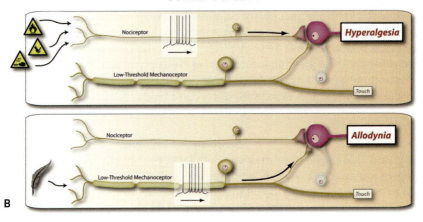

FIGURE 6.1 (**A**) Normal sensation. The somatosensory system is organized such that the highly specialized primary sensory neurons that encode low intensity stimuli only activate those central pathways that lead to innocuous sensations, while high intensity stimuli that activate nociceptors only activate the central pathways that lead to pain and the two parallel pathways do not functionally intersect. This is mediated by the strong synaptic inputs between the particular sensory inputs and pathways and inhibitory neurons that focus activity to these dedicated circuits. (**B**) Central sensitization. With the induction of central sensitization in somatosensory pathways with increases in synaptic efficacy and reductions in inhibition, a central amplification occurs enhancing the pain response to noxious stimuli in amplitude duration and spatial extent, while the strengthening of normally ineffective synapses recruits subliminal inputs such that inputs in low threshold sensory inputs can now activate the pain circuit. The two parallel sensory pathways converge. Reprinted from Woolf CJ. Central sensitization: Implications for the diagnosis and treatment of pain. *Pain.* 2011;152(3 suppl):S2-S15. The figure has been reproduced with permission of the International Association for the Study of Pain (IASP). The figure may not be reproduced for any other purpose without permission.

TABLE 6.1 Summary of Characteristics of the Transcription-Independent and Transcription-Dependent Phases

Transcription-Independent Phase	Transcription-Dependent Phase
Acute	Later stages
Increase in NMDA receptors and removal of Mg^{2+} block to NMDA channel via Ca^{2+}	Facilitation and inhibition
	Reduction in threshold
Activation of glutamate and substance P	Larger receptive field
	Long-term potentiation

Abbreviation: NMDA = *N*-methyl-D-aspartate.

Role of the Brain in the Pain Alarm System

The clinician must have a thorough understanding of the role of the brain in the interpretation of pain to be successful in treating CNS pain mechanisms. Different areas of the brain are involved in pain processing in the CNS. The frontal, premotor, primary sensory, and motor cortices, as well as the anterior cingulate and insular cortices, thalamus, posterior parietal cortex, and cerebellum, have all been shown to play a role in the interpretation of pain.[2]

Pain states can become imprinted in unique CNS pathways similar to those that produce memory.[7] Alterations in CNS cells can result in longer time frames than those that occur when C and Aδ fibers are stimulated in a mechanical nociceptive pain mechanism. Pain can increase spinal neurons and dorsal horn receptive fields when present for longer than normal healing,[2,14] producing hyperexcitability that persists and causes the tissue state to change as well. Typically the patient experiences a stimulus, and that stimulus is interpreted by the brain via the thalamus. The thalamus, as threat center and relay station, takes in information from multiple surrounding regions regarding the context and presumed threat.

If the stimulus is interpreted as a threat, then a reaction occurs. The patient's interpretation of pain is based on the perceived threat to life that then causes adaptation and finally determines how intensely the pain is perceived. All the contextual areas that contribute to pain create a neurosignature, which is the brain's association or typical pattern of neuron impulses. This neurosignature, once created, will aid the body in future experiences in which it needs to protect the body from the threat. Inherently, this threat is perceived as actual or potential tissue damage independently of whether damage or bodily injury has indeed occurred.[2]

Inactivity reduces mechanical forces and causes general deconditioning of the tissues, inevitably weakening connective tissues over time. These weakened tissues need mechanical stimuli and increasing activity to ensure proper healing and function. In addition to mechanical forces, however, social and emotional life events can decrease a patient's ability to cope with pain over time, contributing to the sensitivity of the pain alarm system. Therefore, it can be difficult to pursue an active treatment approach for tissue remodeling without first addressing the patient's pain beliefs and coping strategies. Often the affective component is dominating the patient's sensitivity to the alarm system and preventing mechanical intervention from succeeding. Without the ability or knowledge to stress tissues in an organized fashion, the patient can become fearful and misinterpret the sensation or situation as harmful or dangerous. This belief of harm can make it difficult for a clinician to remodel tissues through an active self-care approach, because the patient interprets pain as harmful rather than necessary for tissue healing.

Clinically, the ability of the tissue to inhibit pain and the ability of the patient to cope with life events are involved in both the peripheral nervous system (PNS) and CNS pain mechanisms. When psychosocial factors dominate, fears, beliefs, and concerns can make coping with the pain experience difficult. When an affective pain mechanism dominates, other physical, emotional, psychological, mental, spiritual, and holistic approaches may be needed; these approaches are discussed in Chapter 7.

Central Nervous System Pain Mechanisms

There are three CNS pain mechanisms:

1. The *central sensitization mechanism* involves the spinal cord and the brain.
2. The *affective mechanism* involves psychosocial barriers in the brain.
3. The *motor/autonomic mechanism* is characterized by cortical disinhibition and poor cortical representation in the brain.

When identifying dominating central mechanisms for pain, a clinician must consider these subclassifications because each requires different education and interventions.

For each pain mechanism involved in an individual's pain experience, multiple systems of the body can be involved. Patients who have chronic pain with high levels of somatic symptoms show increased psychological distress (eg, anxiety, depression, family-related stress).[13] The rehabilitation of patients with multiple pain mechanisms can be complex because their pain mechanisms encapsulate more body systems. For patients with CNS pain mechanisms, the problem can start with a significant tissue injury, psychological or emotional trauma, or even a benign event that happened during a stressful time. If their initial care is poorly managed or poorly explained, they may be left with more questions than answers, fueling negative thoughts and adding to the inflammatory state of all tissues. Poor medical management, patient's unwillingness to change pain-related behavior and beliefs, or genetics may allow the continued sensitization of the PNS, the CNS, and eventually the autonomic nervous system.

The way a person thinks or feels can powerfully influence sympathetic activity via circulating catecholamines, including epinephrine and norepinephrine.[15] The response to nociceptive input and CNS processing is fed back to immune, endocrine, motor, and homeostatic systems and creates long-term changes in the patient with CNS pain.[16] The road to recovery for these patients involves assessment and treatment of all systems involved. Improvement usually occurs when the patient is ready to make changes that promote efficient control of the dominating pain mechanism. The clinician notices a gradual reduction in symptoms from each pain mechanism at reassessments of pain, suffering, and function over time when the dominating mechanism is the focus of education and active care.

Many internal inputs exist, but external inputs also facilitate central pain mechanisms. Family members and support systems may unintentionally reinforce pain behaviors through patterns of enablement. Siblings, parents, or spouses may become so conditioned to the patient's disabled role that they cease to provide challenges or alternative perspectives on the patient's lifestyle and illness behaviors. Even in chronic pain states that have a genetic component, such as fibromyalgia, environmental factors can trigger symptoms.[17] The pain mechanism classification system approach helps clinicians and patients identify and lessen the inputs to the dominating pain mechanism to return control to the patient and promote freedom from pain.

Health Care Models in Chronic Pain Treatment

Different models in health care practice call for different roles and degrees of autonomy for the clinician in addressing patients with complex conditions. With a straightforward case, two pain practitioners may rely on each other as consultants or use a collaborative approach

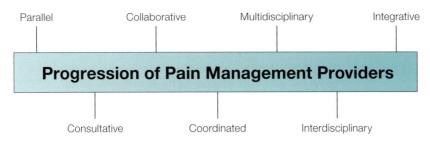

FIGURE 6.2 Pain management approaches.

to care. Patients with multisystem involvement, however, rely on multiple practitioners to work together to formulate a solution to a complex pain problem. Such patients need a health care model that has a multidisciplinary or interdisciplinary team approach.

Boon et al[18] described a continuum of pain management approaches (**Figure 6.2**) that can help providers deliver the most appropriate care when pain is complicated, multisystemic, and multidimensional. This continuum involves a progression of treatment complexity from parallel practice to consultative, collaborative, coordinated, multidisciplinary, interdisciplinary, and integrative care:

- *Parallel* practice involves two practitioners working side by side in a common setting and sharing information.
- *Consultative* practice involves clinicians consulting with other practitioners in their area of expertise.
- In *collaborative* practice, two or more clinicians share information and practice independently.
- A *coordinated* model has a formal structure, and clinicians share information and communication. Provider autonomy declines and the interests of the team's management increase, but improvements in outcome are more likely despite increased patient complexity.
- As provider decisions become more focused on the needs of the patient, practice moves from multidisciplinary care to interdisciplinary care. A *multidisciplinary* practice has a leader, and each clinician makes his or her own decisions about the patient, whereas an *interdisciplinary* group makes decisions face to face in meetings and formulates a group decision in the patient's best interest.
- *Integrative* care is an interdisciplinary model in which clinicians have a shared vision and also use complementary and alternative medicine.

An interdisciplinary pain program is often necessary to treat patients with a dominating CNS pain mechanism. Often called chronic pain care centers, these programs differ in their treatment approaches. Interdisciplinary care can be advantageous for a patient with multiple CNS pain mechanisms, because the patient's dominating mechanism is further to the right along the continuum of pain mechanisms (see **Figure 6.3**). In patients with a dominating affective or motor/autonomic pain mechanism, the relationship between pain and tissue input is complex. For example, a patient with an affective pain mechanism may experience a flare-up in the knee from being overly sensitized by more than one depressive or anxious episode in that specific week. The psychological component of the interdisciplinary approach and pain education becomes essential in rehabilitating the patient's functional loss and suffering.

As a patient lives with persisting pain, the pain begins to affect his or her entire life, from work, to sleep, to activities of daily living. It is important for the clinician to understand not

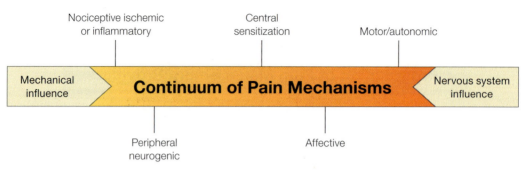

FIGURE 6.3 Continuum of pain mechanisms.

only the patient's interpretation of the pain, but also the impact that pain is having on the patient's life. Often patients with CNS mechanisms have problems coping with their pain or changes in their life and motivation after a painful episode. Interdisciplinary treatment is focused on reversing the negative impact of the pain, providing patient education from each discipline, and desensitizing the social, emotional, cognitive, and movement inputs to the central mechanisms of pain. This approach makes the best use of the patient's time and resources to gain control of all aspects of his or her suffering. It is still unclear which components of the rehabilitation of chronic pain conditions are the most efficacious and cost-effective,[19] and further research is needed regarding interventions delivered in multimodal treatment programs.

Psychology in Pain Management

Eccleston[20] discussed the psychological needs of patients with chronic pain. These patients need information and predictability. They also need to be active in their own care and to have an internal locus of control. Research has shown that patients with passive coping strategies have more distress and higher levels of disability. They tend to self-denigrate, to be angry and depressed, and to avoid painful situations. They may engage in catastrophizing thoughts and worry and may focus a high amount of attention on the pain.[20]

The clinician can use strategies in clinical practice to promote a sense of confidence, consistency, and control in chronic pain patients while acknowledging the patients' perception of the pain and discussing viable solutions to free them of it. With patients who respond with anger, hostility, and avoidance, the clinician should be clear and concise and not allow the patients to accept the notion that pain equals damage. The clinician can use active motion as a nonbiased way to assure the patients that their pain does not equal harm. If the motion is unchanged, no harm could have occurred. The patients must learn not to avoid situations of pain, but rather to use active, healthy coping strategies and accept accurate representations of clinical time frames for rehabilitation.[20] In addition, the clinician should use positive reinforcement to promote healthy behaviors, reframe negative thoughts and beliefs, and promote behaviors that do not lead to pain or fear avoidance.[20]

Patients who have an external locus of control need to understand their pain mechanisms and the brain's ability to misinterpret a signal based on the perception and context of threat. As patients take an active role in their care, they learn to understand their pain alarm system and dominating pain mechanisms, and the experience of returning to meaningful function overall lessens, controls, and abolishes pain. Fear of movement and negative, harmful cognitive processes can play as big a role in patients' pain as biomechanical or biochemical factors in mechanical tissue-related pain.[21]

Pain Evaluation for Central Sensitization

Subjective Evaluation

The central sensitization pain mechanism involves a primary maladaptive belief by the patients that pain is ongoing because the tissues have not healed. The patients may think that ongoing damage is occurring at the tissue level and that the threat of reinjury or harm is high. Enhanced sensitivity is almost always a main feature in central sensitization; the pain is normal, but the processes behind it are altered. The brain is typically thinking that there is more danger at the tissue site than is actually present. The patients may have a high level of functional disability and a history of failed interventions (medical, surgical, and therapeutic).[22]

Location

There is no familiar, textbook anatomic pattern to central sensitization symptoms (eg, dermatomal vs myotomal). The pain typically has a widespread, nonanatomical distribution. The patients may sometimes feel like the pain is spreading. They may find it difficult to localize the pain; typically it is diffuse and changes intensity in multiple areas on each visit. Clinicians may feel they are "chasing" the pain around the body, when in fact they are chasing a neurosignature around the brain. The patients may report spontaneous (ie, stimulus independent) or paroxysmal pain (ie, sudden recurrences and intensification).[22]

Frequency of Pain

The pain may have occasional periods of intermittent variation; however, patients primarily describe it as constant. The pain tends to be disproportionate relative to the nature and extent of injury or pathology.[22]

Descriptors

Patients most likely do not use consistent descriptors. They tend to use graphic terms to describe their pain and want to make sure the clinician understands how the pain feels. Patients may use multiple harmful descriptors to explain their pain, such as burning, achy, shooting, stabbing, cramping, and exploding. They may use inflammatory or ischemic descriptors, which can inform the clinician that there may be an underlying mechanical and neural tissue mechanism as well (eg, sharp, dull, achy, burning, tingling, numbness). Typically, they use vivid language when describing their pain, with phrases such as, "It feels like someone is building a wall of firecrackers on my low back. It's like an exploding, raging fire." The patients may describe the pain as having a "mind of its own" or use creative descriptors like "ants crawling on me." Pain typically is not rated below 5 out of 10. On average, patients with neuropathic pain tend to rate pain 5.7 to 7.7 out of 10.[23] Often the pain has a high level of severity and irritability, is easily provoked, and takes a long time to settle.[22]

Onset

Central sensitization pain is typically chronic, with onset greater than 3 to 4 months previously. The pain persists beyond expected tissue healing or pathology recovery times.[22] Although it can be produced in healthy individuals in experimental situations, this pain presents primarily in patients who may have an underlying vulnerability. The pain may be associated with a traumatic event or with a benign event during a stressful period, or it may start for no apparent reason.

24-Hour Behavior and Aggravating and Alleviating Factors

Patients typically report erratic patterns of pain that do not follow a diurnal pattern. They may complain of night pain or disturbed sleep.[22] Stress tends to aggravate the pain, and stressful situations change during times of the day (eg, "It gets worse when I'm at work" or "when I am in the presence of my mother-in-law"). In addition, there is a disproportionate, nonmechanical, unpredictable pattern of pain provocation in response to multiple nonspecific aggravating or alleviating factors. Pain often appears to be related to the patients' fear of activity or movements, decreasing during less feared activity or movements and increasing with the level of fear.

Medication Response

Patients are typically less responsive to simple analgesia or nonsteroidal anti-inflammatory drugs or more responsive to antiepileptic or antidepression medications.[22]

Psychological and Social Status

Patients may present with a number of yellow flags or a major dominating worry, thought, concern, misperception, or belief about pain, tissue damage, and the need to "find a cure" or "fix the problem." Anxiety, depression, or a mood or personality disorder may be a dominating factor in their pain experience, may be a side effect as a result of pain, or may not be present at all. Factors such as dissatisfaction with work or life, anxiety, frustration, and fear can all influence recovery.[24] Often patients present with a history of psychologically traumatic events that weaken overall coping capacities over time and play a significant role in maintaining ongoing pain states.[25] Simply having catastrophizing thoughts has been shown to increase levels of cortisol and proinflammatory cytokines such as interleukin-6.[26] The presence of a previous or current psychological condition (eg, depression, anxiety, posttraumatic stress disorder) that inhibits normal coping and is dominating the patient's suffering and pain experience helps the clinician identify the affective rather than central sensitization pain mechanism. A patient with central sensitization may have anxiety or depression in addition to a sensitized neurological system, but the psychological condition tends to be a by-product of the fear-avoidance behavior relative to the misinterpretation of nociception as continued harm or unhealed tissue.

In both the affective and central sensitization pain mechanisms, it is important for the clinician to address yellow flags that are dominating and contributing to pain behaviors. Understanding that yellow flags are present should lead the clinician to investigate the patients' ability to cope and recover based on their level of self-efficacy. Are the patients' pain behaviors maladaptive? Are the patients ready to make the changes necessary to get better and gain control? The clinician should address yellow flag thoughts and statements at the time the patients make them and each time after that; the longer the clinician waits to point these out, the more ingrained they become. In addressing maladaptive thoughts, the clinician reinforces to the patients, in the most respectful way possible, that these thoughts are misinterpretations.

Thoughts, Beliefs and Culture

Patients may present with maladaptive thoughts and beliefs about pain, structural damage, or instability, or the inability to find a cause or cure. They may make numerous yellow flag statements. Often it is best for the clinician to investigate the patients' readiness to change (discussed in Chapter 3), especially if they present with multiple concerns and low self-efficacy.

Maladaptive Pain Behavior

Maladaptive pain behavior is the number one predictor of a failed rehabilitation outcome. It is the most challenging state for the clinician to address and a dangerous state for the patients. Typically the clinician has doubts about the validity of the patients' experience, and no diagnostic test can identify the tissue source of the pain. The patients' belief that all pain has to be abolished or "fixed" before they can have restored function or movement is destructive to their healing process and progression of recovery.

Unnecessary surgery, injections, and manual therapy such as massage or manipulations can occur in rehabilitation programs that are focused on a tissue source of the pain.[27] Maladaptive pain behavior is challenging because pain evoked by provocation tests or patient-demonstrated tenderness may have little effect on local tissues. Normal inputs from target tissues may be processed incorrectly by the CNS and perceived as noxious, damaged, or unhealthy.

The clinician should validate that the physical findings are relevant to the impairment and functional loss perceived by the patients before engaging in specific tissue treatments. Social and emotional inputs to the pain experience can be uncontrolled and maladaptive. When managing patients with the central sensitization pain mechanism, the clinician must treat the patients' minds using cognitive–behavioral strategies and let the patients' minds treat their bodies.

Objective Evaluation

For patients with central sensitization pain, the mechanical examination shows no consistent relationship between stimulus and response. A latency effect is common with symptoms after a movement exam, and the result of a repeated movement exam is typically worse. Nonorganic tests such as Waddell's tests may show positive findings. The CNS mechanical exam, like the chemical inflammatory mechanical exam, is frequently inconclusive; the duration and location of symptoms and objective signs of chemical inflammation (warmth, redness, and swelling) usually are not present.

In healthy tissue, inputs such as light touch typically do not evoke pain. In central sensitization, however, patients may present with excessive tactile allodynia. Werneke and Hart[28] demonstrated that patients who did not demonstrate centralization had increased health care usage and chronic disability. Leg pain on intake and noncentralization were highly predictive of chronicity and more significant than psychosocial variables. In other words, in the presence of centralization, even if patients have psychosocial variables, this mechanical finding trumps sensitization. Patients with central sensitization typically complain of pain in some way with physical tests. Seldom do patients report improvement after performing a physical examination, unless a directional preference is found and a dominating mechanical derangement syndrome is presenting. The clinician must establish solid communication and rapport with the patients before and during a clinical evaluation to help alter a dominating central sensitization mechanism to a mechanical nociceptive syndrome.

In addition to a specific mechanical pain pattern, patients may display grossly abnormal movement patterns that are related to fear and their perceived need to demonstrate high pain ratings in order to be heard.[16] Sometimes patients rate their pain level as 10 out of 10. An experienced clinician understands the intensity of the patients' symptoms and help patients realize that their fear is driving their movement patterns. Once the patients' thoughts, worries, and concerns are identified, the underlying mechanical pain may become evident, dominate, and eventually be completely abolished. This use of cognitive–behavioral therapy in the mechanical assessment can promote the rapid response to treatment that can occur when the patients' thoughts are in the right direction.

Central Sensitization Screening Tools and Tests

Screening tools that can be useful in determining whether a patient has abnormal illness behaviors include Waddell's tests and the Fear-Avoidance Beliefs Questionnaire (FABQ). In addition, quantitative sensory tests include pain pressure thresholds, thermal pain thresholds, light touch, and diaphragm breathing.

Waddell's Tests

Waddell's tests are a way to determine inorganic symptoms. These tests focus on five physical signs: tenderness, simulation, distraction, regional disturbances, and overreaction.[29] *Tenderness* refers to sensitivity to palpation of a wide area on the surface of the body or pain that is not localizable. *Simulation* refers to simulating a movement without actually performing the test, such as axial loading by the clinician while the patient is seated. Another example would be rotating the patient's body passively from shoulders to trunk. *Distraction* involves changing the context of a test without alerting the patient, for instance, having the patient kick a ball with an outstretched limb or raise the leg in standing instead of performing a straight leg raise test in supine. *Regional disturbances* manifest as groups or clusters of symptoms in a large area with "giving way" on manual muscle testing for multiple dermatomes or stocking glove distributions of sensations without a neurological loss. *Overreaction* involves excessive pain behaviors or inappropriate speech responses.[29]

Waddell's tests sometimes produce false positives, but they can be effective if they are used as a screen for patients who may require more in-depth psychological assessment. Three or more positive tests identify nonorganic signs indicating that patients need further psychological screening.

Fear-Avoidance Beliefs Questionnaire

The FABQ can be used to evaluate fear-avoidance beliefs related to back pain. Evidence suggests that fear-avoidance beliefs may be a significant risk factor for recurrence in disability; fear-avoidance beliefs have been found to predict future disability and work status even after controlling for the pain factors of duration or intensity and type of treatment received.[30] Serial assessments are recommended as a possible treatment-monitoring tool.[31]

The FABQ has acceptable test–retest reliability and good internal consistency and construct and concurrent validity.[32] It can be useful in identifying elevated levels of fear and avoidance in patients with acute and chronic pain[33]; it may help clinicians identify patients with a fear-avoidance component to their pain early in treatment. Of the 16 items in the FABQ, 11 items comprise two subscales: Work (items 6, 7, 9, 10, 11, 12, and 15) and Physical Activity (items 2, 3, 4, and 5) (see **Figure 6.4**).[30] Scores are obtained by summing the responses to items within the subscales; cutoff scores suggest the treatment emphasis for lower back pain:

- A Physical Activity score of ≥14 indicates that the patient may respond better to a cognitive–behavioral approach and that the clinician should de-emphasize traditional pain-specific treatment goals.
- A Work score of <19 and other factors indicate a higher likelihood of success from joint mobilization and manipulation.[34]
- A Work score of ≥29 indicates increased risk of prolonged disability,[35] and the patient may require a multidisciplinary approach to treatment.

FIGURE 6.4 Fear-Avoidance Beliefs Questionnaire

Here are some of the things other patients have told us about their pain. For each statement, please circle any number from 0 to 6 to say how much physical activities, such as bending, lifting, walking, or driving, affect or would affect *your* back pain.

	Completely disagree			Unsure			Completely agree
1. My pain was caused by physical activity.	0	1	2	3	4	5	6
2. Physical activity makes my pain worse.	0	1	2	3	4	5	6
3. Physical activity might harm my back.	0	1	2	3	4	5	6
4. I should not do physical activities which (might) make my pain worse.	0	1	2	3	4	5	6
5. I cannot do physical activities which (might) make my pain worse.	0	1	2	3	4	5	6

The following statements are about how your normal work affects or would affect your back pain.

	Completely disagree			Unsure			Completely agree
6. My pain was caused by my work or by an accident at work.	0	1	2	3	4	5	6
7. My work aggravated my pain.	0	1	2	3	4	5	6
8. I have a claim for compensation for my pain.	0	1	2	3	4	5	6
9. My work is too heavy for me.	0	1	2	3	4	5	6
10. My work makes or would make my pain worse.	0	1	2	3	4	5	6
11. My work might harm my back.	0	1	2	3	4	5	6
12. I should not do my normal work with my present pain.	0	1	2	3	4	5	6
13. I cannot do my normal work with my present pain.	0	1	2	3	4	5	6
14. I cannot do my normal work until my pain is treated.	0	1	2	3	4	5	6
15. I do not think that I will be back to my normal work within 3 months.	0	1	2	3	4	5	6
16. I do not think that I will ever be able to go back to that work.	0	1	2	3	4	5	6

Reprinted from Waddell G, et al. A Fear-Avoidance Beliefs Questionnaire (FABQ) and the role of fear-avoidance beliefs in chronic low back pain and disability. *Pain*. 1993;52(21):132-142. This questionnaire has been reproduced with permission of the International Association for the Study of Pain (IASP). The questionnaire may not be reproduced for any other purpose without permission.

FIGURE 6.5 Algometer.

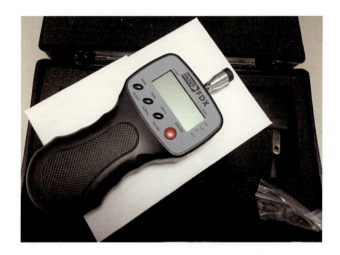

Pain Pressure Thresholds

Patients with central sensitization have hypersensitivity that is present on a quantitative sensory test known as pain pressure thresholds.[36-39] Pain pressure thresholds are measured using a handheld algometer (**Figure 6.5**). This test can reveal a lower pain threshold when a mild stimulus is applied and increased pain with painful stimuli. Central sensitization presents as hypersensitivity both in the area being tested and in healthy areas remote from the site of tissue injury. Peripheral sensitization, in contrast, is sensitized locally to the area of injury. It has been demonstrated that spinal manual therapy may be effective in reducing spinal cord hyperexcitability in the short term, perhaps by activating descending inhibitory CNS pathways. Pain pressure threshold testing showed decreases in pain at and distal to the site of injury.[36,40]

One recent systematic review and meta-analysis[41] concluded that pain pressure thresholds are a poor marker of central sensitization and that sensitization does not play a major role in patients' reporting of pain and disability. Another systematic review and meta-analysis,[42] however, found good ability to differentiate between people with osteoarthritis and healthy controls, indicating that lower pain thresholds locally may suggest peripheral sensitization and in remote areas may suggest central sensitization. Therefore, it is important to consider quantitative sensory testing as part of all subjective and objective data gathered when classifying patients with CNS pain mechanisms and not to rely solely on objective information in formulating a pain differential diagnosis.

Thermal Pain Thresholds

The ability to modulate cold temperature thresholds is thought to be a feature associated with central sensitization. Although the research reviewing thermal quantitative sensory testing parameters varies in reliability,[43] it has been suggested that hot versus cold pressure thresholds can help the clinician differentiate peripheral from central sensitization.[44,45] Cathcart and Pritchard[46] described a method of measuring cold pain threshold; they applied ice at a constant pressure to the skin and used a stopwatch to measure the time elapsed before the stimulus first became painful.

Light Touch

Light touch can be used not only to screen sensation throughout the extremities for diminished or hypersensitivity, but also to provide information about other regions of the body. Hypersensitivity has been observed in patients with central sensitization when using light touch that would not evoke a pain response in healthy people.[47] For instance, a patient with low back pain may have a midsection that does not react to light touch. Normally, a patient reacts in some way to light touch on the surface of the abdomen; the navel may wink or gently retract in a positive reflex. Often patients with central sensitization have an absence of sensation or react with increased sensitivity.[48]

Diaphragm Breathing Test

The diaphragm breathing test allows clinicians to understand not only the patients' typical respiratory pattern, but also their ability to change the breathing stereotype with the appropriate cues. Patients who have a poor respiratory stereotype with poor diaphragm activation and an inability or limited ability to change the breathing stereotype when verbally or tactilely cued are clinically more difficult to rehabilitate.[48] This test may also prompt the clinician to rule out a motor/autonomic dominating pain mechanism (discussed in Chapter 8). Poor breathing stereotypes may include excessive thoracolumbar extension on inspiration, excessive upper chest elevation, or shoulder girdle elevation. The inability to perform appropriate respiratory patterns can also inhibit patients' ability to use their brain's pain control center. Lack of relaxation and diaphragm control can limit the release of pleasure center hormones, such as serotonin, or the body's natural opiate or pain control.

To perform diaphragm breathing, the patient sits unsupported in erect posture while the clinician palpates the lower rib cage and posterolateral spine (see **Figure 6.6**). The clinician asks the patient to breathe and assesses the quality and symmetry of diaphragm activation. Preferably, the clinician sees lateral expansion of the lower ribs and widening of the intercostal spaces. There should be no superior elevation of the scapulas or shoulders, and the sternum should remain stable with anteroposterior symmetry in the upper ribs. Ideally, the patient is able to breathe posterolaterally into the clinician's fingers with appropriate support from the postural and respiratory function of the diaphragm.

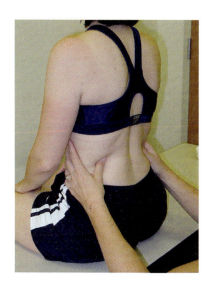

FIGURE 6.6 Diaphragm positioning test.

Selecting a Screening Tool or Test

Waddell's tests and the FABQ can be useful in assessing patients with increased need for psychological evaluations and in educating patients about areas on which to focus treatment. For instance, the FABQ allows the clinician to address work-related tasks that patients fear with controlled successful exposure to allow a change in outcome. A useful clinical reasoning tool is to perform a screening test and apply light touch and then perform a repeated movement mechanical assessment to see if any change has occurred. Sometimes patients who present with the appearance of central sensitization may just need a good mechanical examination to quantify their impairment or functional limitation and help them understand that their movements and symptoms are safe. Being able to demonstrate cause and effect to patients with dominating mechanical pain mechanisms can quickly alter their sensitivity or sense of threat related to movement and correct their misinterpretation of what those movements and symptoms mean. Screening tests such as light touch and the diaphragm positioning test can help the clinician determine how sensitive the patient is or how the patient's body adjusts to an external stimulus.

Table 6.2 summarizes the subjective and objective characteristics of central sensitization pain as a reference to guide clinical reasoning. **Appendices 6.A** and **6.B** provide a comparison among all three central pain mechanisms for subjective and objective characteristics.

TABLE 6.2 Subjective and Objective Characteristics of Central Sensitization Pain

Characteristic	Findings for Central Sensitization Pain
Subjective	
Location	Widespread, nonanatomical distribution of pain
Frequency	Constant, unremitting, spontaneous, latent, paroxysmal pain
	Easily provoked pain with all activity
Descriptors	Catastrophic terms (eg, "raging fire," "electric")
	Pain threat high
Intensity	High severity, irritability
Onset	Typically chronic, although sensitivity may occur sooner, >3 months
	Past expected tissue healing and pathology recovery times
	Pain disproportionate to the nature and extent of injury or pathology
	Potential absence of tissue injury or pathology, no apparent reason
History	Failed interventions (medical, surgical, therapeutic)
24-hour behavior	Erratic, inconsistent; night pain, disturbed sleep
Psychosocial screen	Positive for pain behaviors (maladaptive and harmful beliefs, poor self-efficacy)
	High functional disability
Aggravating and alleviating factors	Disproportionate, nonmechanical, unpredictable pattern in response to multiple nonspecific factors
	Heat typically helps
	Antiepileptic or antidepressant medications help

Characteristic	Findings for Central Sensitization Pain
Objective	
Movement testing	Easily evoked pain
	Disproportionate, inconsistent, nonmechanical anatomical pattern of pain provocation
	No relationship between stimulus and response
	Common latency effect; result is worse
Palpation	Diffuse nonanatomic areas of pain or tenderness
	Light touch elicits noxious response (allodynia) in area of symptoms
Posture	Antalgic postures or movements
	Disuse atrophy of muscles
Neurological testing	Positive for hyperalgesia, allodynia, hyperpathia
Proprioception screen	Quadruped spinal flexion and extension is performed appropriately
Breath assessment	Sitting diaphragm breathing test is positive for upper respiratory pattern
Yellow flag assessment	Positive identification of catastrophization, fear-avoidance behavior, harmful thoughts, and distress
Readiness stage	Precontemplation, contemplation, preparation
Fear-Avoidance Beliefs Questionnaire[30] score	Physical activity ≥14
Yellow flag risk score[a]	Over 55 points: Moderate risk of chronic disability
Outcome measures	Disabilities of the Arm, Shoulder and Hand; Oswestry Disability Index; Neck Disability Index; or Lower Extremity Functional Scale scores indicating moderate disability and above

[a]See Chapter 7 for a discussion of the yellow flag document that is used to assess chronic pain disability risk.

Central Sensitization Management and Intervention

People hold painful memories in the unconscious that may later emerge into consciousness when they encounter specific cues or stimuli. For example, the death of a loved one can stimulate a memory of physical pain, especially if the pain occurred at the same time as the death. The pain can reoccur at an anniversary, which acts as an unconscious trigger of the distress experienced during that time. Time is irrelevant to the unconscious mind.

Many patients with chronic pain can be taught to focus less on their pain and more on their recovery of function. Once patients understand the central sensitization pain mechanism—that internal influences such as thoughts, beliefs, worries, concerns, and fears move their pain alarm system into overprotection mode and create destructive brain changes, they are better equipped to effectively rehabilitate their functional status.[49] Moseley et al[50] demonstrated that the anticipation of experimental back pain predisposed some people with chronic pain to have an altered strategy for CNS motor control. Similarly, asymptomatic controls who merely anticipated pain were more likely to have a protective postural strategy. A patient whose physician says that forward bending can aggravate and sometimes herniate lumbar discs may visualize an image of forward bending that causes the disc to rupture. This simple thought can turn into a dominating belief that dictates the patient's postural protective strategies and movements. Even thinking about forward bending can cause the patient's pain to escalate. The fact that a simple belief can cause an altered response that generates a pain response from the CNS has implications for patients involved in ongoing litigation. The continuous legal meetings and interactions with lawyers create persistent thoughts through the perpetual focus on the initial injury or, worse, the ineffectiveness of procedures and treatments.

In the management of patients with dominating central sensitization, the main goal is graded exposure to activities that the patients perceive as being harmful to bring about a slow, progressive functional recovery. Patients are educated about their pain, their fear hierarchy, and inputs driven by their thoughts, beliefs, and cognitive misinterpretations of nociception. Recent evidence suggests benefits from the following treatments when addressing persistent pain:

- Relaxation, imagery, and hypnosis all help alter the pain experience.[51]
- Fear-reducing and -activating interventions and group interventions involving education on coping schemes and discussion have been beneficial.[52,53]
- Reducing threat via education and control of functional baselines can aid in treatment. Promotion of tissue conditioning while decreasing the activation threshold of peripheral nociceptors is important during pain management. Increasing exposure to different threats from higher order brain structures can activate regions of the brain without stimulating a harmful neurological or fear-based response, helping patients begin to progress.[2]
- Strategies to address current life adjustments also help patients who experience chronic pain.[54]
- Improving patients' self-image and social environment by building their faith in themselves is also helpful.[55]

In **Appendix 6.C**, the patient initially presented with a dominating central sensitization pain mechanism. He was evaluated on day 1 mechanically, but his mechanical examination was inconclusive. The patient needed a couple of visits and patient education before an adequate mechanical evaluation could dispel his thoughts, worries, and concerns related to movements and his lumbar disc. Once the clinician was able to get the patient to move into his end ranges following the principle of moving the tissue in a no-worse state, his mechanical presentation became more evident and eventually dominated. Although the classification was initially central sensitization, the patient quickly progressed to the peripheral neurogenic ischemic pain mechanism.

When thoughts of harm or damage can be quickly dispelled using appropriate movement strategies, mechanical therapy can function as a cognitive–behavioral therapeutic approach. Mechanical diagnosis and therapy helped this patient understand that his fear of movement had a destructive influence on his spinal-influenced behaviors and caused increased sensitivity. The patient learned that his movements were safe and positively influenced his disc problem.

Patient Education

Knowledge is a great pain liberator. Moseley[56] repeatedly demonstrated the positive impact of graded exposure to active movement and education in sensitized patients. People without any training can understand the physiology of pain.[57] Learning about pain physiology decreases the threat value of pain, reduces the power of the protective systems, and restores normal immune function.[57] Combining pain education and movement approaches increases physical capacity, reduces pain, and improves quality of life.[58]

The clinician should inform the patient that after 4 to 6 months, the tissues have been through the processes needed to heal. The tissues may have lost functional range of motion (ROM) and work capacity for certain functional demands and may be in need of blood flow and oxygen through movement, but the tissues have healed and need movement to thrive. The tissues are sensitive because of their ill health and the brain's overprotection.[16]

In the central sensitization pain mechanism, a real biological process has occurred that has the ability to magnify peripheral inputs. Inputs that normally do not hurt the person now present as noxious, and inputs that normally hurt to a small extent are now exaggerated. The patient needs to be aware that the symptoms are no longer true indicators of the health status of their tissues. Pain caused by an inflammatory or ischemic nociceptive tissue irritation mechanism is affected by a cognitive mechanism related to how the brain perceives the incoming message. This cognition increases the threat value of the pain and dictates the intensity and distress perceived. The patient's beliefs about the message and activity play a significant role in the cognitive aspects of their pain. The following sections focus on patient education to address persistent pain and to promote the benefits of relaxation.

Patient Education for Persistent Pain

Patients with persistent pain need education as the first intervention. One goal is to help them understand how persistent pain occurs. Research has shown that many people have tissue impairments but live without pain. The clinician describes the type of pain the patients are presenting with and explains how their brain may be misinterpreting the signal from the body and increasing the sensitivity of the pain alarm system. While highlighting that all pain is real, the clinician explains as often as necessary that hurt does not necessarily equal harm and that pain is caused by a perception of threat originating in the brain. The clinician helps patients identify the emotional and social triggers that increase their pain, the coping strategies they currently use, objective goals for treatment, and metrics to demonstrate functional improvement. The clinician stresses that persistent fear or concerns about diagnosis, treatments, movements, activities, being believed, and many other factors have a direct impact on the pain experience. The clinician also educates, mentors, and assists patients' self-investigation of the effects of their maladaptive beliefs about injury, activity, pain, and cultural influences.

No conclusive evidence is available about the type of educational program that works best regarding development of self-efficacy or treatment of chronic pain, but a small-group format and interactive discussions appear to be important components of educational programs.[19] **Figure 6.7** is a patient education handout that explains persistent musculoskeletal pain.

Distinguishing Good Pain from Bad Pain
It is important to help patients understand the difference between good and bad pain and challenge their application of this knowledge using their own life examples. All pain is not bad, and some pain needs to be created for patients to become free of pain.

Good pain is pain that occurs as a result of remodeling connective tissue; this pain does not worsen as a result of activity and generally gets a little better each time the activity is performed. Pain is no worse later in the day or the next morning, indicating that the tissues can handle the movement capacity. Movement or activity that makes the pain no worse has a green light, and symptoms should be interpreted as indicating that the movement or activity is safe to perform and progress. Good pain is needed for the patients to improve.

Movement or activity that produces pain when performed but leaves the patients feeling no worse (as opposed to better) has a yellow light.[21] The patients should proceed cautiously during this movement or activity to ensure that the pain is no worse 2 hours, 12 hours, and 24 hours later. In addition to feeling no worse the next day, the patients should also be able

FIGURE 6.7 Persistent Musculoskeletal Pain Patient Education Handout

Persistent Musculoskeletal Pain

WHAT IS PERSISTENT MUSCULOSKELETAL PAIN?

Persistent musculoskeletal pain is pain referred from the central nervous system (CNS). The CNS consists of the spinal cord and brain, which are responsible for processing messages from the musculoskeletal tissues (eg, muscle, ligament, bone, tendon, cartilage, peripheral nerve) and interpreting the messages. Pain referred from the CNS is not from the tissues where the pain is felt, but rather from the tissues where the message is processed and interpreted.[1] The following drawing shows how the pain message related to irritated tissues is referred to the spinal cord for processing and then to the brain for interpretation:

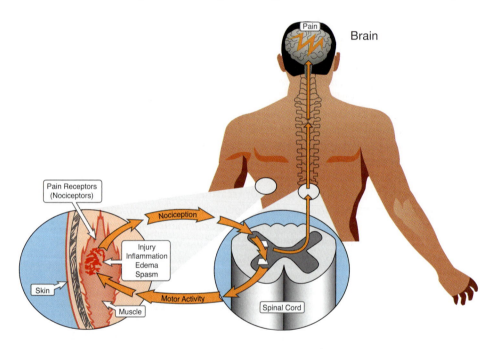

HOW DOES PERSISTENT MUSCULOSKELETAL PAIN WORK?

To understand persistent musculoskeletal pain fully, we must travel into the spinal cord and up to the brain, the command center of the pain system. When something happens in your tissues and nerves, you feel repercussions through your entire system. Remember, it is the brain that has to make the final decision as to whether or not you should be in pain. The most frequently asked question from people learning about persistent musculoskeletal pain is, "So are you saying that the pain is all in my head?" We have to be honest and say, "Yes—all pain is produced by the brain. No brain, no pain!" We do not mean, however, that the pain is imaginary or not real; much to the contrary—all pain is real. Truly understanding this simple concept is very empowering for people with persistent pain. Understanding the spinal cord and brain processes behind the pain experience can provide you with enormous control.

WHAT DOES THIS PAIN FEEL LIKE?
- Persistent musculoskeletal pain lasts longer than 4 months, which is longer than normal healing. Deconditioned healing tissues send messages indicating they have been worked. Those messages are interpreted by the spinal cord and brain as meaning that damage is still occurring, that the tissues have not healed, and that you need all the protection you can get. The brain reacts by sending severe pain to that area to protect you from moving it. This is an altered perception of the pain message and is the main feature in persistent pain.[2]
- Severe pain is always a feature in persistent pain; some people refer to this severity by saying they have a high pain threshold. Remember, the pain is normal, but the processes behind it are altered. The brain is being fed information that no longer reflects the true health and abilities of the tissues. The brain is being told that the tissues are in more danger than they actually are. This misinterpretation of the message happens in the spinal cord (the great magnifier), which sends the misinterpreted message to the brain. The brain interprets the message as a threat and creates the severity of the pain experience.[2] The concept of increased sensitivity is often challenging to grasp, but this happens in everyone when they are injured. The increased sensitivity should fade once your treatment brings the damaged structures under control, especially as you more fully understand what is going on and what you need to do to get better.
- Persistent pain may spread to areas not originally involved in the initial injury or disease process.[2]
- The pain experience can be increased by emotional or social situations and by physical movements. Common emotional and social factors that have the potential to slow down recovery from persistent pain are
    - Attitudes and beliefs about pain
    - Behaviors related to the pain
    - Financial and reimbursement problems
    - Diagnostic procedures and passive treatments
    - Emotions
    - Family stress
    - Work stress

Do these factors exist? Are they contributing to your pain experience? How are you coping to control these factors? There are treatment strategies that can help reduce these factors in the pain experience. Many times people have not been successful with previous rehabilitation because these factors were not addressed.

WHAT CAN YOU DO FOR PERSISTENT MUSCULOSKELETAL PAIN?
According to medical and scientific evidence, the combination of education, behavior management, and restoration of function gets people with persistent musculoskeletal pain back to normal.[3]

(continues on next page)

FIGURE 6.7 Persistent Musculoskeletal Pain Patient Education Handout

(continued from previous page)

- Education is the most important aspect in the treatment of persistent musculoskeletal pain. The following topics are important:
  - Explanation of the type of pain
  - Explanation of misinterpreted signals (and reassurance that the pain is real)
  - Education and identification of the emotional and social factors increasing pain
  - Identification of and education about coping strategies
  - Identification of and education about successful activities
- Behavior management is an important aspect of persistent pain rehabilitation and is guided by chronic pain psychologists. Not all patients who suffer from persistent pain need to see a psychologist; however, when emotional or social factors such as loneliness, hopelessness, anger, blame, fear, catastrophizing, and abuse are not being addressed with physical or occupational therapy, then a psychological evaluation is necessary. Sometimes a referral to a multidisciplinary pain management program may be the best comprehensive approach for you. Your psychologist can assist in the evaluation and referral.
- Restoration of function is most successful after or along with an effective education and behavioral program. As we already discussed, the brain will not allow the body to move successfully unless the messages coming in are less threatening. Once the brain interprets these messages in more positive ways, it is easier to find successful movements, function is easier, and results with training are long lasting.

Resources
1. Wall PD, Melzack R. *Textbook of Pain*. 3rd ed. Edinburgh, Scotland: Churchill Livingstone; 1994.
2. Butler DS. *The Sensitive Nervous System*. Adelaide, Australia: Noigroup; 2000.
3. Butler D. Moseley GL. *Explain Pain*. Adelaide, Australia: Noigroup Publications; 2003.

to maintain ROM in all directions as a nonbiased way of proving that the pain is good. If the patients are not able to maintain ROM, the cautionary yellow light becomes a red light, and the patients should stop that movement or activity because bad pain may be present.

Bad pain is pain related to a recent trauma or, in the case of patients with the central sensitization pain mechanism, pain that indicates that the activity level of the tissue has exceeded its tolerance, creating a flare-up. Tissue damage has not occurred; no motion or strength changes typically accompany this worsening in symptoms. Rather, the acute chemical inflammatory state created from doing too much too fast momentarily dominates. The pain appears to worsen with each repetition. When the movement or activity is completed, the spike in pain persists longer than 15 minutes, lasts into the night, and is still worse 24 hours later. On the 11-point pain rating scale, the spike is at least a three-point increase in pain from the tolerable baseline and indicates that the tissues cannot handle the movement or activity. This movement or activity has a red light, and pushing through these symptoms is unsafe and will prolong the flare-up.

Managing Flare-ups
The goal of patient education on managing flare-ups is to have the patients understand how to analyze and ultimately address incoming pain signals from the brain. Everyone overdoes activity at one time or another; most people marvel at how they used to enjoy a delayed soreness when they were young or with previous forms of exercise. Although they tolerated this soreness in healthy areas of their body, they may not tolerate it in areas they perceive as injured. Flare-ups are uncomfortable, but clinicians can instruct patients to perform safe movement and can teach them to execute the flare-up plan to help them through these episodes.

The 3 Ms of managing flare-ups should be part of the clinician's education message:

1. Modify the activity or situation that created the flare-up.
2. Manage the inflammation from the flare-up. Refer to the "Guidelines for Management of Flare-Ups" section of Chapter 4, the inflammation pain patient education handout (**Figure 4.1**), and the Activity Pyramid (**Figure 4.7**). Ensure that the patient experiences deep learning and applies the flare-up plan.
3. Move on. Refer back to the activity or situation with a new baseline (see the "Guidelines for Establishing the Activity Baseline" section in Chapter 4 and **Figures 4.5** and **4.6**) and identify a pacing strategy that leaves the pain no worse the next day.

Relaxation: Active Strategies to Activate the Brain's Pain Control Center

Negative chemical production continues in a stressed nervous system. Science has proved that the brain's pain control center is capable of modulating physical and emotional states through receptor signaling in the human brain.[59] Through the internal affective state of the patient during a pain episode, clinicians are able to modulate relief in different ways.[60] The clinician should ask how well the patients are using their own brain's pain control center. The clinician can seek to activate the patients' descending inhibitory tracts by improving the comprehension and application of education regarding pain (see **Figure 6.8**).

The clinician needs to stress diaphragmatic breathing as a "pain pill" that calms the mind and the nervous system's pain-producing tracts (see **Figure 6.9**). One pill is equal to six to 10 breaths. Prescribing breathing pills two to three times daily or when pain and stress are high assists the patient in gaining control of the descending inhibitory system. Effective ways to activate the brain's pain control center include relaxation exercises (see **Figure 6.10**) and enlisting positive thoughts during negative times.

FIGURE 6.8 Relaxation Patient Education Handout

Relaxation

HOW DOES THE BODY RESPOND TO PAIN?
The body responds to pain with a stress response. Your body considers pain a threat, and as a result your body's overall tension increases. Anxiety and tension can make dealing with the pain more difficult. When you are stressed
- Heart rate increases
- Blood pressure increases
- Respiration rate changes
- Deep stabilizing muscles lose function
- Superficial muscles become overworked

WHAT IS RELAXATION?
- A state of physical and emotional calmness
- The opposite of the stress or "fight or flight" response
- Freedom of the muscles from tension
- Little or no anxiety or irritability
- A skill that many people must learn, especially people with pain

WHAT IS THE GOAL OF RELAXATION?
- To gain control of your body and the pain process
- To change the body's state of awareness during a pain episode
- To promote quicker recovery
- To alter catastrophic thoughts

HOW CAN YOU RELAX?
- Do breathing exercises.
- Engage in biofeedback.
- Do progressive muscle relaxation.
- Use imagery.
- Practice meditation or prayer.
- Try self-hypnosis, which is focusing your attention away from your pain by making suggestions to yourself to ignore the pain or to see the pain in a different, more positive way.

GUIDELINES FOR PRACTICING RELAXATION
- The more you practice relaxation exercises, the quicker and better your body's response will be.
- Be patient and comfortable, and the skill will come with time.
- Your mind may wander during the relaxation task. Try to remain calm and focus your attention on the skill of relaxing.
- Try to remember and practice your relaxation skills during a pain episode. It is also important to practice relaxation when you are in a comfortable state.

RELAXATION EXERCISE TO RELAX MUSCLES
The following technique has been shown to help reduce tension in irritated muscles:
- Relax, and don't think about what you are doing.
- Squeeze each muscle group, starting at your toes and working up to your neck and facial muscles.
- Hold the contraction for 3 to 5 seconds. Squeeze as much as you can without increasing your pain.
- After tightening the muscles, let everything relax for 10 to 30 seconds.
- Take a deep breath in while squeezing. Exhale as you relax the muscle.
- Focus your mind on how each muscle feels as it tenses and relaxes. Note how your muscles feel with each squeeze. It may be easier or more difficult on one side of the body.
- Practice one to two times a day. Even if you don't have time to work on the technique with your whole body, work on contraction and relaxation for painful areas or the areas your therapist has indicated.

FIGURE 6.9 Diaphragm Breathing Patient Education Handout

Relaxation: Diaphragm Breathing

BREATHING AND PAIN
During times of pain or stress, people develop a rapid and shallow breathing pattern. This negative breathing pattern is often associated with increased tension in the neck, chest, and shoulders. The upper chest and shoulder muscles are overworked, increasing pain or stress.

DECREASING PAIN THROUGH BREATHING
During painful episodes, it is helpful if you take active control over your breathing pattern. Breathing in a controlled, relaxed rhythm can reduce the intensity of the pain and help you relax. Diaphragmatic breathing, sometimes called *belly breathing*, is one part of your pain control program. This type of breathing activates your brain's own pain control center, changing the stress pattern to one of relaxation and releasing natural opiates such as morphine and serotonin.

DIAPHRAGMATIC OR BELLY BREATHING EXERCISE
- Lie on your back, with pillows under your knees and your hand on your abdomen close to your belly button.
- Take a long, slow breath in through your nose. Imagine the air filling and lifting the chest, back, and especially the lower abdomen. Feel your stomach pushing up against your hand; feel your lungs in the back fill with air as well. The movement should be smooth and comfortable.
- Pause briefly, and then breathe out through your mouth. Let the pressure of your hand push your stomach down toward your spine. Think of getting rid of the "bad air" while your lower abdomen flattens.
- Stay focused on the sensation of breathing while being aware of any tension that you may be holding. The in-and-out cycles should be easy and balanced to achieve relaxation.
- Practice your breathing exercise frequently and in different positions, emotional states, and social settings. After practicing diaphragmatic breathing in the lying position, progress to practicing when sitting, standing, and walking. Practice in happy, sad, and angry emotional states. Practice at home, work, the airport, and other environments to progress this exercise and take control of your pain.
- You may get better results with practicing five times per day, approximately 2 to 5 minutes each time. Practice when you are not in pain to gain awareness and control. Perform when stress and pain are at intolerable levels to help manage your symptoms.

ADDITIONAL BREATHING EXERCISES
The following techniques will help calm you in moments of stress and anxiety and help you breathe:

Candle Imagery
1. Breathe in naturally.
2. Now breathe out, imagining a small candle a few inches in front of your mouth. Purse your lips and gently blow on the candle, making the flame flicker.
3. Don't blow it out. Instead, blow out slowly, evenly, and smoothly.

Flower Imagery
1. Breathe out naturally.
2. Now breathe in, imagining a flower a few inches in front of your mouth. Try to smell the delicate fragrance without inhaling any pollen.
3. You need to breathe in slowly and evenly to do this.

Resources
Frownfelter D, Dean E. *Principles and Practice of Cardiopulmonary Physical Therapy.* 3rd ed. St. Louis, MO: Mosby; 1996.
Kolar P, Sulc J, Kyncl M, et al. Postural function of the diaphragm in persons with and without chronic low back pain. *J Orthop Sports Phys Ther.* 2012;42:352-362.

FIGURE 6.10 Muscle Relaxation Patient Education Handout

Progressive Muscle Relaxation Exercises

WHAT IS PROGRESSIVE MUSCLE RELAXATION (PMR)?
PMR is more than just relaxation; it is about developing body awareness and learning to control each muscle group.

HOW DO YOU DO PMR?
- Practice alone in a quiet place.
- Make sure you are comfortable; remove your shoes, and wear loose-fitting clothing.
- Practice 15 minutes daily, before meals rather than after.
- Finish a session by relaxing with your eyes closed for a few seconds, and then get up slowly.
- Begin each set with a firm, solid tightening of your muscles.
- Try to target the area you are working on without contracting other, surrounding areas. (For instance, if you are supposed to contract the hand, try not to contract all the muscles of the arm.)
- Tighten the muscle for 3 to 5 seconds, then relax completely for 3 to 5 seconds.

PMR EXERCISE
1. Begin with your right hand. Turn the palm up. Relax. Turn the palm down.
2. Squeeze your right hand and make a fist. Straighten the fingers. Relax.
3. Bend your right arm. Bring the hand to your shoulder and tense the muscle. Relax. Straighten the arm and tense the muscle. Relax.
4. Turn the left palm up. Relax. Turn the palm down.
5. Squeeze your left hand and make a fist. Straighten the fingers. Relax.
6. Bend your left arm. Bring the hand to your shoulder and tense the muscle. Relax. Straighten the arm and tense the muscle. Relax.
7. Shrug your shoulders high and hold. Push the shoulders forward (hunch). Tense the muscle. Relax. Pull the shoulders back. Tense the muscle. Relax.
8. Draw your eyebrows together (frown). Raise your eyebrows, wrinkling the forehead. Tense the muscle. Relax. Squeeze the eyes tightly together. Tense the muscle. Relax.
9. Purse your lips into an O. Pull the corners of the mouth back. Tense the muscle. Relax.
10. Press your tongue against the roof of your mouth. Tense the muscle. Relax.
11. Push your head back without raising or lowering your chin, like you are trying to get away from someone who wants to kiss you or making a double chin. Tense the muscle. Relax.
12. Breathe in deeply and hold your breath, pressing the shoulders together at the back at the same time. Then let your shoulders hang. Breathe normally.
13. Tighten your abdominal muscles (draw in your belly). Tense the muscle. Relax.
14. Now arch your back. (Do *not* put strain on your spine!) Keep the rest of your body as relaxed as possible. Focus on the tension in your lower back. Tense the muscle. Relax.

15. Dig your right heel into the floor. Tense the muscle. Relax.
16. Straighten your right knee. Tense the muscle. Relax.
17. Point your right foot. Tense the muscle. Relax.
18. Flex your right foot and ankle by bringing your toes toward your nose. Tense the muscle. Relax.
19. Curl your right toes. Spread the toes apart, trying to make space between each toe. Tense the muscle. Relax.
20. Dig your left heel into the floor. Tense the muscle. Relax.
21. Straighten your left knee. Tense the muscle. Relax.
22. Point your left foot. Tense the muscle. Relax.
23. Flex your left foot and ankle by bringing your toes toward your nose. Tense the muscle. Relax.
24. Curl your left toes. Spread the toes apart, trying to make space between each toe. Tense the muscle. Relax.

Active Movement

When sensitivity appears to be centrally mediated (likely in chronic disorders), the importance of passive mobilization diminishes, and an active education-based program is more effective. A skilled physical examination is necessary when patients have been successful in reducing pain and begin to plateau, indicating that central mechanisms are reduced, mechanical mechanisms have become dominant, and it is time for a more mechanical intervention. When mechanical directional preference pain is dominating, the clinician should consider fine-tuning rehabilitation programs with remodeling exercises to address tissue dysfunctions.

A patient with mechanical pain that initially presented with central sensitization is described in **Appendix 6.D**. This patient transferred from inpatient care to outpatient care after admission secondary to a change in pain status with an acute exacerbation of cervical stenosis. The patient had negative thinking and a defeatist attitude and initially believed that surgery was the only option that would help her. Over 3 months, she gradually rehabilitated back to a cardiovascular program. The patient had a rapid response on day 3 mechanically but needed repetitive education and communication about her psychosocial yellow flags.

The central sensitization pain mechanism usually needs inputs to maintain the sensitivity, and multiple sites of altered afferent input may require treatment, especially after trauma. The key is not to offer anatomical passive treatment as the primary management option or to present it as the cure to restore function and pain control. With central sensitization, education and active exercise are the basis of the treatment approach. When central sensitization dominates, active exercise is not about directions or tissues but rather about daily graded exposure to activities that patients perceive as being harmful in order to address their fear of movement and allow them to progress to meaningful activities.

Movement is required for optimal health. A physically healthy spinal cord and brainstem are ideal for meningeal health, vascular perfusion, cerebrospinal fluid flow, lymph drainage, and distribution of transmitters and modulators throughout the extracellular fluid. A neurodynamic approach is useful in patients with the central sensitization pain mechanism, which directly affects the brain and spinal cord. The clinician can instruct patients on how to perform a slump sit slider or midrange slouch overcorrection, active movements that can stimulate neural and dural tissues while promoting awareness of posture and proprioception in sitting. A slump sit slider has been shown to maintain blood flow to the tissue sources of the CNS. Slump sit sliders can promote healthy blood flow to the brainstem and spinal cord and transition positions for spinal motions[61] (see **Figure 6.11**).

To initiate a graded exposure program, the clinician should break down movements for success, highlighting functions that the patient fears are harmful and progressing to activities that the patient has identified as being meaningful. To break down movements, the clinician starts away from the site of symptoms and progresses toward the site of symptoms. For example, if the problem is in the upper body, the clinician starts with the lower body. If the problem is in the hand, the clinician may need to start at the shoulder. In addition, integrated whole-body planned movements, such as a graded gym programs, have been successful in helping patients relearn isolated joint movement.[16]

Restoration of Function: Graded Exposure

The following are the basic principles for the clinician who is assisting patients in their return to meaningful activities:

- Decide what activities patients find meaningful to access pleasure centers. Pleasure overrides pain.
- Find patients' activity baseline, or capacity to engage in an activity without flare-up (see the "Guidelines for Establishing the Activity Baseline" section in Chapter 4 and **Figures 4.5** and **4.6**).

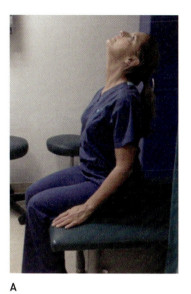 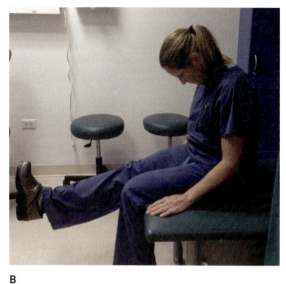

FIGURE 6.11 Slump sit slider exercises. (**A**) Cervical, thoracic, and lumbar spine extended with legs relaxed. (**B**) Cervical, thoracic, and lumbar spine flexed with knee extended and foot dorsiflexed.

- Plan and pace progression; add a minimal amount to baseline each day, such as 1% more activity or up to 5 minutes extra per day.
- Don't create a flare-up. Educate patients how to avoid and control flare-ups.

Restoration of function requires a lifestyle change, not an exercise program. The clinician should select activities that bring the patients happiness. This sounds simple, but it is difficult to support and work with patients who have been experiencing pain for a long time and may have difficulty identifying what makes them happy. The clinician must be available to validate patients' application of the education topics and tools through consultation regarding their ability to progress baselines and prevent or manage flare-ups. Education and pacing help reset the neural circuitry of pain in the brain. **Appendix 6.E** highlights the use of graded exposure to meaningful activity to treat a patient with the central sensitization pain mechanism.

The Baseline Activity Tolerance (BAT) tool (**Figures 4.5** and **4.6**) helps patients identify functional baselines to initiate graded exposure progression. The BAT was created to track patients' pain responses to activities throughout the day (worse, better, or the same). After establishing activities or times of day when the patients' pain is worse, the clinician can work with the patients on restoring their function.

As shown in this chapter's three case studies, patients present with central mechanisms that can rehabilitate slowly or quickly depending on their willingness to change, learn, and grow. If a patient is receptive to education and presents with an underlying mechanical condition, he or she can change rapidly. Patients with underlying fears or concerns must communicate and address them to allow a return to desired activities. Physiological sensitivities in the spinal cord can increase the perception of threat, and a gradual graded exposure to feared activity must take place with appropriate education about the expected response to change. Education on coping strategies, a pain journal, the Activity Pyramid (**Figure 4.7**), the BAT, and the no-worse concept can help guide the patients in managing their pain alarm system from overprotective back to normal mode. If mechanical symptoms persist and dominate, activity can progress based on a mechanical intervention of graded pacing and sound guidance to build strength and cardiovascular health. **Table 6.3** lists key intervention strategies for patients with dominating central sensitization pain. **Appendix 6.F** provides a comparison among all three central pain mechanisms for intervention strategies.

Prevention of Reoccurrence
Education should always conclude with strategies to prevent recurrence of a painful episode. There are three points to remember regarding prevention:

1. Acute flare-ups and injuries should be managed according to the flare-up plan. Patients should seek medical attention if a new injury does not improve on its own in 2 weeks.
2. All tissue health is about maintaining a balance of movement and good alignment, especially related to activity. The clinician should encourage patients to introduce motion periodically throughout the day that works in the reverse of their typical daily directions. The clinician should stress the importance of good posture when patients are working, lifting, and exercising. For example, if the patient sits and bends forward most of the day, he or she needs to take time to stand, walk, and do backward bends to keep a balance. These habits prevent minor strains and sprains.
3. The clinician should encourage patients to maintain a healthy cardiovascular system, which keeps their immune system healthy. Healthy bodies sustain fewer injuries and heal faster than unhealthy ones. We recommend 30 minutes of brisk cardiovascular activity for five to six times a week. The clinician should assist patients in selecting activities that they enjoy in order to increase compliance.

TABLE 6.3 Interventions for the Central Sensitization Pain Mechanism

Category	Interventions
Education	Explanation of the nondamaging nature of pain: Hurt vs harm, interpretation of inputs
	Pain mechanism education
	Discussion of the role of emotions, harmful and damaging thoughts, and beliefs regarding pain: Pain journal
	Training in coping strategies for loneliness, depression, fear of motion or activity: Relaxation, diaphragm breath training
	Explanation of the Activity Pyramid: Green, yellow, and red lights, flare-up management
	Identification of the activity baseline and explanation of the no-worse concept: Control to the patient
Activity	Pacing and graded exposure to activities that patient has perceived as being harmful: Build low aerobic activity, HR 55%-75% of maximum, 2 to 5 hours per week
	Weight training to build upper and lower extremity strength: Start with isolated movements, progress to function, HR 55%-75% of maximum, 2 times per week
	Deep muscle training for spine postural stabilization: Progress to function, HR 55%–75% of maximum, 2 times per week
	High-intensity interval training (HIIT): Progress to 10 to 20 minutes, HR >75% of maximum, 1 to 2 times per week
	Mechanical examination

Abbreviation: HR = heart rate.

> **KEY MESSAGES**
>
> - Pain that is referred from the central nervous system (CNS) is not from the tissues, but rather is from the interpretation of input from the tissues mediated by the spinal cord and brain.
> - The body's response to both nociceptive and CNS processing pain mechanisms feeds back to the immune, endocrine, motor, and homeostatic systems, creating long-term changes that lead to chronic pain.
> - Different team models in health care practice call for different clinician roles and degrees of autonomy when addressing patients with complex conditions.
> - For patients with chronic pain, the clinician should provide direct positive reinforcement of healthy behaviors, reframe negative thoughts and beliefs, and avoid promoting pain or fear-avoidance behaviors.
> - Maladaptive pain behavior is the primary predictor of failed rehabilitation outcomes. It is challenging for the clinician to address and dangerous for patients.
> - The clinician can begin to activate the descending inhibitory tracts by educating patients about their pain and promoting use of relaxation exercises and progressive muscle relaxation.
> - The Baseline Activity Tolerance tool can help patients establish functional baselines and track their responses to various activities throughout the day.

References

1. Melzack R, Coderre TJ, Katz J, Vaccarino AL. Central neuroplasticity and pathological pain. *Ann N Y Acad Sci*. 2001;933:157-174.
2. Moseley GL. A pain neuromatrix approach to patients with chronic pain. *Man Ther*. 2003;8:130-140.
3. Curatolo M, Arendt-Nielsen L, Petersen-Felix S. Central hypersensitivity in chronic pain: Mechanisms and clinical implications. *Phys Med Rehabil Clin N Am*. 2006;17:287-302.
4. Woolf CJ, Salter MW. Neuronal plasticity: Increasing the gain in pain. *Science*. 2000;288:1765-1769.
5. Sandkuhler J. Learning and memory in pain pathways. *Pain*. 2000;88:113-118.
6. Linley JE, Rose K, Ooi L, Gamper N. Understanding inflammatory pain: Ion channels contributing to acute and chronic nociception. *Pflugers Arch*. 2010;459:657-669.
7. Basbaum AI. Memories of pain. *Sci Med*. 1996;3(6):22-31.
8. Melzack R. Pain—An overview. *Acta Anaesthesiol Scand*. 1999;43:880-884.
9. Dickenson AH, Chapman V, Green GM. The pharmacology of excitatory and inhibitory amino acid–mediated events in the transmission and modulation of pain in the spinal cord. *Gen Pharmacol*. 1997;28:633-638.
10. Suzuki R, Rygh LJ, Dickenson AH. Bad news from the brain: Descending 5-HT pathways that control spinal pain processing. *Trends Pharmacol Sci*. 2004;25:613-617.
11. Siddall PJ, Cousins MJ. Persistent pain as a disease entity: Implications for clinical management. *Anesth Analg*. 2004;99:510-520.
12. Latremoliere A, Woolf CJ. Central sensitization: A generator of pain hypersensitivity by central neural plasticity. *J Pain*. 2009;10:895-926.
13. Von Korff M, Dworkin SF, Le Resche L, Kruger A. An epidemiologic comparison of pain complaints. *Pain*. 1988;32:173-183.
14. Woolf CJ. Central sensitization: Implications for the diagnosis and treatment of pain. *Pain*. 2011;152(3 Suppl):S2-S15.
15. Brown M, Koob GF, Rivier C. *Stress Neurobiology and Neuroendocrinology*. New York: Dekker; 1991.
16. Butler DS. *The Sensitive Nervous System*. Adelaide, Australia: Noigroup; 2000.
17. Buskila D. Genetics of chronic pain states. *Best Pract Res Clin Rheumatol*. 2007;21:535-547.
18. Boon H, Verhoef M, O'Hara D, Findlay B. From parallel practice to integrative health care: A conceptual framework. *BMC Health Serv Res*. 2004;4:15.

19. Mannerkorpi K, Henriksson C. Non-pharmacological treatment of chronic widespread musculoskeletal pain. *Best Pract Res Clin Rheumatol.* 2007;21:513-534.
20. Eccleston C. Role of psychology in pain management. *Br J Anaesth.* 2001;87:144-152.
21. McKenzie R, May S. *The Lumbar Spine: Mechanical Diagnosis & Therapy.* Waikanae, New Zealand: Spinal Publications; 2003.
22. Smart KM, Blake C, Staines A, Doody C. Clinical indicators of "nociceptive," "peripheral neuropathic" and "central" mechanisms of musculoskeletal pain: A Delphi survey of expert clinicians. *Man Ther.* 2010;15:80-87.
23. Backonja MM, Stacey B. Neuropathic pain symptoms relative to overall pain rating. *J Pain.* 2004;5:491-497.
24. Indahl A, Velund L, Reikeraas O. Good prognosis for low back pain when left untampered: A randomized clinical trial. *Spine.* 1995;20:473-477.
25. Linton SJ, Larden M, Gillow AM. Sexual abuse and chronic musculoskeletal pain: Prevalence and psychological factors. *Clin J Pain.* 1996;12:215-221.
26. Edwards RR, Kronfli T, Haythornthwaite JA, Smith MT, McGuire L, Page GG. Association of catastrophizing with interleukin-6 responses to acute pain. *Pain.* 2008;140:135-144.
27. Loeser J, Sullivan, M. Disability in the chronic low back pain patient may be iatrogenic. *Pain Forum.* 1996;4:114-121.
28. Werneke M, Hart DL. Centralization phenomenon as a prognostic factor for chronic low back pain and disability. *Spine.* 2001;26:758-764; discussion 65.
29. Waddell G, McCulloch JA, Kummel E, Venner RM. Nonorganic physical signs in low-back pain. *Spine.* 1980;5:117-125.
30. Waddell G, Newton M, Henderson I, Somerville D, Main CJ. A Fear-Avoidance Beliefs Questionnaire (FABQ) and the role of fear-avoidance beliefs in chronic low back pain and disability. *Pain.* 1993;52:157-168.
31. Werneke MW, Hart DL, George SZ, Deutscher D, Stratford PW. Change in psychosocial distress associated with pain and functional status outcomes in patients with lumbar impairments referred to physical therapy services. *J Orthop Sports Phys Ther.* 2011;41:969-980.
32. Grotle M, Brox JI, Vollestad NK. Reliability, validity and responsiveness of the Fear-Avoidance Beliefs Questionnaire: Methodological aspects of the Norwegian version. *J Rehabil Med.* 2006;38:346-353.
33. Hart DL, Werneke MW, George SZ, et al. Screening for elevated levels of fear-avoidance beliefs regarding work or physical activities in people receiving outpatient therapy. *Phys Ther.* 2009;89:770-785.
34. Flynn T, Fritz J, Whitman J, et al. A clinical prediction rule for classifying patients with low back pain who demonstrate short-term improvement with spinal manipulation. *Spine.* 2002;27:2835-2843.
35. George SZ, Fritz JM, Childs JD. Investigation of elevated fear-avoidance beliefs for patients with low back pain: A secondary analysis involving patients enrolled in physical therapy clinical trials. *J Orthop Sports Phys Ther.* 2008;38:50-58.
36. Sterling M. Testing for sensory hypersensitivity or central hyperexcitability associated with cervical spine pain. *J Manip Physiol Ther.* 2008;31:534-539.
37. Chiarotto A, Fernandez-de-Las-Penas C, Castaldo M, Villafane JH. Bilateral pressure pain hypersensitivity over the hand as potential sign of sensitization mechanisms in individuals with thumb carpometacarpal osteoarthritis. *Pain Med.* 2013;14:1585-1592.
38. Jespersen A, Amris K, Graven-Nielsen T, et al. Assessment of pressure-pain thresholds and central sensitization of pain in lateral epicondylalgia. *Pain Med.* 2013;14:297-304.
39. Finan PH, Buenaver LF, Bounds SC, et al. Discordance between pain and radiographic severity in knee osteoarthritis: Findings from quantitative sensory testing of central sensitization. *Arthritis Rheum.* 2013;65:363-372.
40. Vicenzino B, Collins D, Benson H, Wright A. An investigation of the interrelationship between manipulative therapy–induced hypoalgesia and sympathoexcitation. *J Manipulative Physiol Ther.* 1998;21:448-453.
41. Hübscher M, Moloney N, Leaver A, Rebbeck T, McAuley JH, Refshauge KM. Relationship between quantitative sensory testing and pain or disability in people with spinal pain—A systematic review and meta-analysis. *Pain.* 2013;154:1497-1504.
42. Suokas AK, Walsh DA, McWilliams DF, et al. Quantitative sensory testing in painful osteoarthritis: A systematic review and meta-analysis. *Osteoarthritis Cartilage.* 2012;20:1075-1085.
43. Moloney NA, Hall TM, Doody CM. Reliability of thermal quantitative sensory testing: A systematic review. *J Rehabil Res Dev.* 2012;49:191-207.
44. Coronado RA, Simon CB, Valencia C, George SZ. Experimental pain responses support peripheral and central sensitization in patients with unilateral shoulder pain. *Clin J Pain.* 2013;30:143-151.
45. Moseley L. *Pain* [DVD]. Aptos, CA: On Target Publications; 2013.

46. Cathcart S, Pritchard D. Reliability of pain threshold measurement in young adults. *J Headache Pain.* 2006;7:21-26.
47. Petersen-Felix S, Curatolo M. Neuroplasticity—An important factor in acute and chronic pain. *Swiss Med Wkly.* 2002;132:273-278.
48. Kolar P. Dynamic neuromuscular stabilization: A developmental kinesiology approach [course handout]. Chicago, IL: Rehabilitation Institute of Chicago; June 15-17, 2009.
49. Bradley LA. *Cognitive–Behavioral Therapy for Chronic Pain.* New York: Guilford Press; 1996.
50. Moseley GL, Nicholas MK, Hodges PW. Does anticipation of back pain predispose to back trouble? *Brain.* 2004;127:2339-2347.
51. Arnstein P. Chronic neuropathic pain: Issues in patient education. *Pain Manag Nurs.* 2004;5:34-41.
52. Von Korff M, Balderson BH, Saunders K, et al. A trial of an activating intervention for chronic back pain in primary care and physical therapy settings. *Pain.* 2005;113:323-330.
53. Christensen FB, Laurberg I, Bunger CE. Importance of the back-cafe concept to rehabilitation after lumbar spinal fusion: A randomized clinical study with a 2-year follow-up. *Spine.* 2003;28:2561-2569.
54. Gullacksen AC, Lidbeck J. The life adjustment process in chronic pain: Psychosocial assessment and clinical implications. *Pain Res Manag.* 2004;9:145-153.
55. Gustafsson M, Ekholm J, Ohman A. From shame to respect: Musculoskeletal pain patients' experience of a rehabilitation programme, a qualitative study. *J Rehabil Med.* 2004;36:97-103.
56. Moseley L. Unraveling the barriers to reconceptualization of the problem in chronic pain: The actual and perceived ability of patients and health professionals to understand the neurophysiology. *J Pain.* 2003;4:184-189.
57. Moseley GL, Nicholas MK, Hodges PW. A randomized controlled trial of intensive neurophysiology education in chronic low back pain. *Clin J Pain.* 2004;20:324-330.
58. Moseley L. Combined physiotherapy and education is efficacious for chronic low back pain. *Aust J Physiother.* 2002;48:297-302.
59. Zubieta JK, Bueller JA, Jackson LR, et al. Placebo effects mediated by endogenous opioid activity on mu-opioid receptors. *J Neurosci.* 2005;25(34):7754-7762.
60. Zubieta JK, Yau WY, Scott DJ, Stohler CS. Belief or need? Accounting for individual variations in the neurochemistry of the placebo effect. *Brain Behav Immun.* 2006;20(1):15-26.
61. Butler D. Mobilisation of the nervous system [course handouts]. Chicago, IL: Rehabilitation Institute of Chicago, September 21-22, 2004.

APPENDIX 6.A Clinical Reasoning for Subjective CNS Pain Characteristics

Central Nervous System Pain Mechanisms: Subjective Characteristics

Central Sensitization	Affective Pain Mechanism Conscious (C) vs Unconscious (U)	Autonomic/Motor Pain Mechanism
Location: Widespread, nonanatomical distribution of pain	**Location:** (C) Widespread, nonanatomical distribution; (U) axial low back pain, neck pain, headaches, knee pain (specific location)	**Location:** Widespread, nonanatomical distribution of pain to upper and/or lower extremity may include the spine, typically affects more than one nerve field
Frequency: Constant, unremitting, spontaneous, latent, paroxysmal pain; easily provoked pain with all activity	**Descriptors:** (C) Catastrophic emotional language; (U) dull, tight, weak, sharp with movement	**Frequency:** Constant unremitting, spontaneous, latent, paroxysmal pain
Descriptors: Catastrophic terms related to harm and unhealed tissue; pain threat high	**Frequency:** (C) Constant, spontaneous, latent, paroxysmal pain; (U) intermittent	**Descriptors:** Deep, dull, burning, aching, pulsating, stabbing, cold intolerance
Intensity: High severity, irritability	**Intensity:** (C) High severity, irritability; (U) low-grade irritant	**Intensity:** High severity, irritability
Onset: Chronic >3 months; past expected tissue healing & pathology recovery times; pain disproportionate to the nature and extent of injury or pathology	**Onset:** Chronic >3 months; past expected tissue healing/pathology recovery times; pain disproportionate to the nature and extent of injury or pathology	**Onset:** Chronic >3 months; past expected tissue healing/pathology recovery times; pain disproportionate to the nature and extent of injury or pathology; initial trauma managed poorly.
History: Failed interventions (medical, surgical, therapeutic)	**History:** Failed interventions (medical, surgical, therapeutic); (C) preexisting anxiety, depression, psychological trauma (ie, abuse, accident, work-related injury), CNS disorder (ie, SCI, MS, etc); (U) increased stress/repressed negative emotions regarding current life pressures, past childhood relationships with parents & siblings, characteristic of perfectionism	**History:** Immune, GI, endocrine, parasympathetic, and sympathetic systems symptoms and/or complications
24-hour behavior: Erratic, inconsistent, night pain, disturbed sleep	**24-hour behavior:** Inconsistent pain, night pain, disturbed sleep	**24-hour behavior:** Erratic, inconsistent, night pain, disturbed sleep
Psychosocial screen: Positive for pain behaviors (maladaptive and harmful beliefs/poor self-efficacy), high functional disability	**Psychosocial screen:** (C) Positive for negative emotions, altered family, work, social life, medical conflict, high functional disability; (U) appear negative on conscious level	**Psychosocial screen:** Positive for pain behaviors (maladaptive beliefs/poor self-efficacy), high functional disability
Aggravating or alleviating factors: Disproportionate, nonmechanical, unpredictable pattern in response to multiple nonspecific factors; heat helps; antiepileptic/antidepressant medications help		**Other clinical signs:** Swelling indicating lymphedema, spasticity, tone, discoloration of skin, skin and hair sensitivities, trophic changes, excessive sweating

APPENDIX 6.B Clinical Reasoning for Objective CNS Pain Characteristics

Central Nervous System Pain Mechanisms: Objective Characteristics

Central Sensitization *Spinal Cord Facilitation*	Affective Pain Mechanism Conscious (C) vs Unconscious (U) *Emotional/Social Dysfunction*	Autonomic/Motor Pain Mechanism *Cortical Disinhibition*
Objective findings: Spinal cord facilitation signs; pain evoked easily **Movement testing:** Disproportionate inconsistent nonmechanical/anatomical pattern of pain provocation; no relationship between stimulus and response; common latency effect; result is worse; absence of tissue injury/pathology **Palpation:** Diffuse nonanatomic areas of pain or tenderness; light touch elicits noxious response (allodynia) in area of symptoms. **Posture:** Antalgic postures or movements; disuse atrophy of muscles **Neurological testing:** Positive for hyperalgesia, allodynia, hyperpathia **Proprioceptive screen:** Spine and extremity tests are negative **Breath assessment:** Sitting diaphragm breathing test: upper respiratory pattern **Yellow flag assessment:** Positive identification of catastrophization, fear-avoidance behavior, harmful thoughts, distress. **Readiness stage:** Precontemplation, contemplation, preparation **Fear Avoidance Beliefs Questionnaire (FABQ) score:** Physical activity ≥ 14 **Yellow flag risk score:** Over 55 indicates moderate risk of chronic disability **Outcome measures:** Disabilities of the Arm, Shoulder and Head, Oswestry Disability Index, Neck Disability Index, Lower Extremity Function Scale, with moderate disabilities (may choose others)	**Objective findings:** (C) Similar to central sensitivity with greater emotional component; (U) similar to ischemia; treatment ineffective. Tender points: upper trapezius, lumbar paraspinals, posterior lateral aspects of the gluteus maximus, bilaterally **Yellow flag assessment:** (C) Positive for distress, negative emotions, depression, anxiety, anger, altered family/work/social life, medical conflict, reduced coping skills with life-changing events (ie, SCI, loss, amputation, neurological impairment, etc); (U) appear negative on a conscious level but positive toward increased stress & repressed negative emotions regarding current life stressors, past childhood relationships with parents & siblings, characteristic of perfectionism at the unconscious level. **Psychometric tools:** Assist referral to (C) cognitive–behavioral therapy program and/or (U) investigative psychology • Yellow Flag Risk Form: Chronic disability risk assessment (>55 points) • Anger/depression: Patient Health Questionnaire (PHQ-9) (score >10) • Anxiety: Pain Anxiety Symptom Scale (higher score) • (U) Tension myositis syndrome information document (>3 yes answers)	**Objective findings:** Same as central sensitivity; in addition signs of: • Cortical dysfunction (spasticity, tone) • Autonomic nervous system dysfunction (skin discoloration, excessive sweating, trophic changes, hair excitability, lymph edema) • Involvement of sympathetic and parasympathetic systems **General illness** may be present from immune and GI system involvement. **Proprioceptive screen:** All spine and extremity tests are positive **Palpation:** Diffuse nonanatomic areas of pain/tenderness; light touch elicits noxious response in areas with/without symptoms often within the space around the skin **2-point discrimination:** Positive findings within area of symptoms; primary sensory cortex findings **Neurological testing:** Positive findings related to loss of graphesthesia (recognition of symbols drawn on skin), incomplete drawing of body outline for area of symptoms, signs of neglect present in left–right discrimination testing; positive findings in localization and precision sensory testing

APPENDIX 6.C Chronic Pain Outpatient, 63-Year-Old Male

Physical Therapy/Occupational Therapy Initial Evaluation

SUBJECTIVE FINDINGS

Chief complaint:	LBP since 17 years old; R anterior, posterior, and lateral thigh pain
Descriptors:	Dull, throbbing, constant LBP; intermittent R thigh pain
Onset:	Injured at work 4 yr ago; 3 back fusions, the last 3 yr ago; progressively worsening pain
Frequency:	Constant LBP, intermittent R thigh and buttock pain
24-hr behavior:	Worse in PM, better as day progresses
Subjective pain:	(Likert)/ Faces scale: 6-9/10
Aggravating factors:	Prolonged activity, walking more than 4-6 blocks without a cane, sitting 30 min in poor posture, standing more than 20 min
Relieving factors:	Medications occasionally, rest, not moving "excessively"

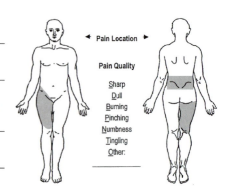

Pain Location

Pain Quality
Sharp
Dull
Burning
Pinching
Numbness
Tingling
Other:

PATIENT EDUCATION CONSIDERATIONS

Readiness to learn:	(Ready and self-motivated) Extrinsically motivated (Limitations (see below))
Limitations to learning:	Cognitive Physical Language Financial Cultural (Other:) None
Teaching method preferred:	(Handout) Verbal (Demonstration) (Practice) Other:
Explain:	Attention limited by pain

MEDICAL HISTORY

Past medical history:	Depression, cocaine addiction, "failed back" syndrome
Family history:	None
Surgery and invasive procedures:	Cervical fusion C6-C7, 4 yr prior; L4-S1 nonunion fusion, revision 1 yr later; L3-S1 revision/fusion 1 yr later
Medications:	Oxycodone, gabapentin, duloxetine, fentanyl patch Allergies: No known drug allergies
Previous treatments:	3 courses of physical therapy, without significant relief
Diagnostic tests: X-ray:	MRI: Unremarkable other than fusions and scar tissue CT scan: EMG: Other:

PSYCHOSOCIAL FACTORS

Living situation:	Patient lives with his wife but is getting a divorce after 23 yr and with 2 children, 10 and 14 yr old
Behavior:	He believes that the chronic pain program is his last hope for improvement, but he is willing to try anything. Behavior is calm and appropriate.
Occupation:	He is currently unemployed. He used to be a truck driver but is retired now.
Recreation and leisure:	Hobbies include bowling (stopped), taking walks, and watching sports
Functional disability:	He wants to return to some form of his hobbies. Now that he is retired, he wants to spend his time in leisure activities but also feels a responsibility to give back to his community.
Concerns:	Patient is concerned that he has had 4 surgeries, is on so much medication, and has an addictive personality. He wants to be able to be active again, but pain significantly limits him.

PROVISIONAL PAIN CLASSIFICATION (in order of dominance)

Visits 1–4
1. **Central sensitization**
2. **Peripheral neurogenic pain mechanism**, ischemic pain

PAIN EDUCATION TOPICS

1. Good vs bad pain, pain–brain connection
2. Postural connection to pain
3. Mechanical improvement as a sign of improvement before pain symptoms change
4. Mechanical therapy and the ability to address pain
5. Importance of a cardiovascular program

- The patient was treated based on his mechanical presentation 4 days later; treatment was not based on a fear of movement paradigm. If the patient had demonstrated more psychological undertones to his examination that indicated a need for a psychological screen, his pain may have been labeled as affective. This patient did not appear to have an affective component to his pain; rather, his depression was a side effect of his mechanical pain.

- This patient is demonstrating both central sensitization and peripheral neurogenic pain mechanisms; however, the dominating mechanism on evaluation is central sensitization. The clinician may need to educate the patient before an effective mechanical exam may occur. This education can occur immediately, and because the patient trusts the clinician and movement, he will likely then be receptive to a proper mechanical evaluation.

(continues on next page)

APPENDIX 6.C Chronic Pain Outpatient, 63-Year-Old Male *(continued from previous page)*

Physical Therapy/Occupational Therapy Objective Evaluation

OBJECTIVE FINDINGS

Repeated movement examination:	Repeated movement examination conducted after 4th day of full-day, 4-week, interdisciplinary cognitive–behavioral program including initial examination. Baseline LBP and R hip pain rated 6/10.
Active/passive range of motion:	Lumbar ROM: Maximally limited flexion and extension, Maximally limited R side glide in standing (greater on L); end range pain
	Posture in L lumbar shift (not relevant)
	Lumbar shift to L increases with walking
Repeated test movements:	Baseline symptoms: LBP and R hip pain
	Repeated flexion in standing: Increase back and leg, remains worse as a result
	Repeated extension in standing: Increase back and leg, no worse as a result
	Repeated flexion in lying: Decrease from 6/10 to 3/10, better in leg, no change in back pain and mechanically side glide better to R and L
	Repeated extension in lying: Increase in back and leg, remains worse as a result
Strength testing:	Hip abduction 3+/5 bilaterally; all other strength testing unremarkable

PROVISIONAL MECHANICAL CLASSIFICATION

Lumbar derangement: Unilateral/asymmetrical lumbar spine

PROVISIONAL PAIN CLASSIFICATION

Visit 4

Central sensitization no longer dominates; currently presents with **peripheral neurogenic pain mechanism**

TREATMENT

Treatment:	Reduction of derangement and restoration of function program. Reduction initiated with flexion in lying. Cardiovascular program with pain education and flare-up plan education. Education emphasized continuous reassessment of motion at each visit. Patient responded to flexion initially. Patient received biofeedback, OT and PT, psychotherapy, and medication monitoring with physician treatment in the full-day, 4-week, interdisciplinary cognitive–behavioral program.
Treatment summary:	**10 visits over 26 days:** 2x/wk for most weeks, with some repeat visits of pool therapy and core strengthening classes. From a functional perspective, patient doubled his sitting tolerance and tripled his standing tolerance without increased pain. He is ambulating several miles at a time without a back brace or straight cane. He is undergoing a divorce; however, they are amicable. He is off all narcotics for pain relief.

Goals:		PSFS	
		Initial	Discharge
	Return to walking 1-2 miles without assistive device	0	10
	Return to cardiovascular program 30 min 3x/wk	0	10
	Pain limitation to function	3	9
	Pain intensity rating	6	1-2

Abbreviations: CT = computed tomography; EMG = electromyography; L = left; LBP = low back pain; MRI = magnetic resonance imaging; OT = occupational therapy; PSFS = Patient-Specific Functional Scale; PT = physical therapy; R = right.

APPENDIX 6.D Inpatient, 51-Year-Old Female

Physical Therapy/Occupational Therapy
Initial Evaluation

SUBJECTIVE FINDINGS

Chief complaint:	Constant neck, R elbow numbness, 5-yr history of LBP, R posterolateral thigh and hip numbness, bilateral shoulder and arm pain
Descriptors:	Dull, constant numbness in R upper extremity; dependent in all self-care
Onset:	2 mo ago, hernia surgery; after surgery, symptoms developed in R upper extremity. MRI revealed cervical stenosis; surgery recommended, patient waiting and hoping to get stronger. Patient recently lost 100 lb. She is receiving inpatient acute rehab for a change of status.
Frequency:	Constant
24-hr behavior:	Worse in the AM, better as the day progresses, worse in the PM
Subjective pain:	Likert / Faces scale: 7-9/10
Aggravating factors:	Any movement of any kind
Relieving factors:	Medications reduce pain to 2/10

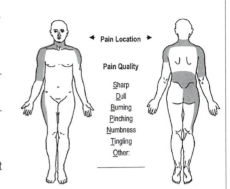

Pain Location

Pain Quality
Sharp
Dull
Burning
Pinching
Numbness
Tingling
Other:

PATIENT EDUCATION CONSIDERATIONS

Readiness to learn:	Ready and self-motivated Extrinsically motivated Limitations (see below)
Limitations to learning:	Cognitive Physical Language Financial Cultural Other: None
Teaching method preferred:	Handout Verbal Demonstration Practice Other:
Explain:	Limited by pain and decreased coping strategies

(continues on next page)

APPENDIX 6.D Inpatient, 51-Year-Old Female *(continued from previous page)*

MEDICAL HISTORY

Past medical history:	Depression, chronic pain, pleurisy, sleep apnea, 1 functioning kidney, heart murmur
Family history:	None
Surgery and invasive procedures:	Cervical fusion C5-C7 15 yr ago, hernia repair 2 mo ago, sinus repair
Medications:	Oxycodone, dexamethazone, gabapentin, methylprednisolone, metoprolol tartrate, bupropion, docusate, esomeprazole, senna tablets, miconazole, transdermal nicotine, enoxaparin **Allergies:** Iodine, sulfa, cefadroxil
Previous treatments:	No treatments reported
Diagnostic tests:	X-ray: ___ MRI: Cervical stenosis CT scan: ___ EMG: ___ Other: ___

PSYCHOSOCIAL FACTORS

Living situation:	Patient lives with her husband in a 1-level home. She is worried that he will leave her. She has a daughter and 6 siblings; she feels that her support system is not concerned about any of her feelings.
Behavior:	She believes that "nothing will ever help her." She doesn't know why the doctors even ordered PT/OT.
Occupation:	She is currently unemployed; previously she worked in accounting. She has been a housewife for the last 5 yr.
Recreation and leisure:	Her hobbies include attending Bible study and watching television.
Functional disability:	She wants to return to work but is scared because she cannot sit for long periods.
Concerns:	Patient is concerned that pain is spreading and worsening. She believes that surgery is the only thing that will help her. She is concerned about her ability to sit and to work.

PROVISIONAL PAIN CLASSIFICATION (in order of dominance)
1. **Central sensitization pain mechanism**
2. **Peripheral neurogenic pain mechanism**, ischemic pain

PAIN EDUCATION TOPICS
1. Good vs bad pain, pain–brain connection
2. Postural connection to pain
3. Mechanical therapy and the ability to address pain (to occur in outpatient therapy at the next level of care; patient to be discharged)
4. Importance of a cardiovascular program

Pain classification support
1. Type of medication that affects her symptoms
2. Level of concern and beliefs
3. Fixation on a structural fix
4. Limitations in motivation based on coping strategies
5. Location and frequency of symptoms
6. Multiple aggravating factors (any movement of any kind)
7. Medication the only relieving strategy

Focus of treatment
Education on the interpretation of pain to set up the next level of care and a potential mechanical examination

(continues on next page)

APPENDIX 6.D Inpatient, 51-Year-Old Female *(continued from previous page)*

Physical Therapy/Occupational Therapy
Objective Evaluation

OBJECTIVE FINDINGS

	Outpatient visit 1, day 3: Patient discharged from the hospital after 3 days and readmitted to outpatient spine center
Repeated movement examination:	Conducted after 3rd day in outpatient spine center; pain rated 6/10 or worse in neck and R upper extremity to elbow
Active/passive range of motion:	Cervical ROM: Severely limited extension (38°), moderately limited retraction, bilaterally moderately limited side bending (R 23°, L 25°), bilaterally moderately limited rotation (45°)
	R shoulder AROM: Limited 20° in elevation, limited 45° abduction, external rotation limited 15°, L shoulder within functional limits
Repeated test movements:	Baseline symptoms: Neck and upper trapezius pain, with R upper extremity numbness to elbow
	Repeated cervical spine retraction in sitting: End range pain, increases, no worse as a result; shoulder ROM improved approximately 10° in each plane and R upper extremity elevation fully restored
	Repeated cervical spine extension in sitting: End range pain, increases, worse as a result; no change in shoulder ROM
	Repeated cervical spine flexion repeated in sitting: No effect; no change in shoulder ROM
Strength testing:	R shoulder elevation 4/5, abduction 4/5, external rotation 3+/5; no significant strength changes after repeated movement testing

PROVISIONAL MECHANICAL CLASSIFICATION

Cervical derangement: Unilateral/asymmetrical below the elbow

PROVISIONAL PAIN CLASSIFICATION

Central sensitization no longer dominates; currently presents with **peripheral neurogenic pain mechanism**, container dependent, cervical spine

TREATMENT

Treatment: Therapy focused on debunking the notion that "nothing will ever help." Patient was educated on mechanical pain and the process of centralization. As her pain decreased, the patient's belief that surgery is the only thing that will help her also decreased. Patient was placed on a cardiovascular program with education on obtaining her target heart rate. Throughout therapy, inappropriate pain behaviors were not given attention, and positive attitudes were reinforced. Reduction of cervical spine derangement with initial retraction motion and restoration of function program. Cardiovascular program with pain education emphasizing why therapy may still be helpful and flare-up plan education. Patient has a mechanical derangement that has never been addressed.

Treatment summary: **14 visits over 12 wk:** 2x/wk for first 4 wk, decreasing to 1x/wk for 4 wk, then every other week for 4 wk. From a functional perspective, patient returns to sitting 1-2 hr to perform computer work without increased pain. She started a cardiovascular program for fitness and is more in control of her pain and flare-ups. She is performing a home exercise program independently. Patient was able to reduce the derangement in the first 8 visits and then focused on the restoration of function phase of healing to promote tissue healing and health. Her last 4 visits focused on her scapular weakness and underlying cervical extension dysfunction.

Goals:

	PSFS	
	Initial	Discharge
Return to sitting short periods (2 hr) at a computer to allow part-time work in accounting	0	6
Return to a cardiovascular program 30 min 3x/wk	0	7
Pain limitation to function	3	8
Pain intensity rating	8	3

Abbreviations: AROM = active range of motion; CT = computed tomography; EMG = electromyography; L = left; MRI = magnetic resonance imaging; OT = occupational therapy; PSFS = Patient-Specific Functional Scale; PT = physical therapy; R = right; ROM = range of motion.

APPENDIX 6.E Orthopedic Outpatient, 47-Year-Old Male

Physical Therapy/Occupational Therapy Initial Evaluation

SUBJECTIVE FINDINGS

Chief complaint:	Constant anterior trunk, low back pain, right posterior hip and thigh pain
Descriptors:	Sharp, dull, burning, pinching, numbness, tingling, cramping, "exploding in chest"
Onset:	1 yr ago, lifting child into car seat; immediate leg pain; recent worsening
Frequency:	Constant
24-hr behavior:	Worse in PM, better as day as day goes on; wakes up 2-4x/night
Subjective pain:	Likert / Faces scale: 8-10/10
Aggravating factors:	Any movement with trunk, left leg; stress from family and job
Relieving factors:	Lying down, whirlpool, walking in pool; never abolishes, just decreases

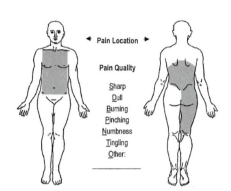

Pain Location
Pain Quality
Sharp
Dull
Burning
Pinching
Numbness
Tingling
Other:

PATIENT EDUCATION CONSIDERATIONS

Readiness to learn:	Ready and self-motivated Extrinsically motivated Limitations (see below)
Limitations to learning:	Cognitive Physical Language Financial Cultural Other: Motivational
Teaching method preferred:	Handout Verbal Demonstration Practice Other:
Explain:	A lot of PT in past, not helpful; has "tried it all," "nothing works"

MEDICAL HISTORY

Past medical history:	Depression, anxiety existed preinjury but have worsened since injury
Family history:	None
Surgery and invasive procedures:	Injections, L4/5 laminectomy 6 mo ago; neither provided expected results but lessened pain; pain is worsening and currently spreading
Medications:	Gabapentin, fluoxetine, rofecoxib, methylprednisolone dose pack 1/wk for recent flare-up Allergies: No known drug allergies
Previous treatments:	PT previously stabilization, conditioning exercise, and education to avoid extension
Diagnostic tests:	X-ray: Negative MRI: HNP L4-5 CT scan: EMG: Negative Other: Negative bone scan

PSYCHOSOCIAL FACTORS

Living situation:	Patient lives with his wife and 3 children in grade school. Wife is not involved; she views this as his problem. Wife works full-time; he stays at home.
Behavior:	Nervous and anxious
Occupation:	Consultant; works at home, stressful; lost customers because of back problems
Recreation and leisure:	Pool exercise daily
Functional disability:	Most movement; unable to perform any light household activities
Concerns:	In counseling at church; sees a psychologist for depression; is concerned that any movement keeps herniating disc; possible 2nd surgery, fusion; fears paralysis with 2nd surgery or ineffective or worse results. Believes pain needs to be gone before returning to exercises on land or any household tasks.

PROVISIONAL PAIN CLASSIFICATION

Central sensitization pain mechanism

PAIN EDUCATION TOPICS

1. Good vs bad pain, pain–brain connection
2. Strategies to activate brain's pain control center: Breathing, relaxation, motor imagery
3. Strategies to improve meaningful function and improve limitation from pain
4. Musculoskeletal nerve pain; centralization and peripheralization
5. Ischemic musculoskeletal pain mechanism; need for increased blood flow
6. Connective tissue healing and remodeling guidelines
7. Effects of posture on back and leg pain
8. Mechanical evaluation results vs diagnostic test results
9. Posture and body mechanics strategies for work, including phone and computer, and for household, including child care

(continues on next page)

> **APPENDIX 6.E Orthopedic Outpatient, 47-Year-Old Male** *(continued from previous page)*

Physical Therapy/Occupational Therapy
Objective Evaluation

OBJECTIVE FINDINGS

Visit 1:	• Tactile allodynia to light touch in all areas indicating pain • FABQ Physical Activity 30/30; FABQ Work 24/66 • Began pain education and journal; set movement guidelines based on PSFS
Visit 4:	• Mechanical evaluation performed
Posture:	Decreased lumbar lordosis sitting and standing, fully reversible lordosis, increased symptoms in both positions; no worse as a result; slow, apprehensive movements
Active range of motion:	Lumbar flexion: Nil loss, knee level (his normal) increased back pain, resting posture with increased lordosis on return
	Lumbar right and left side glide: Nil loss, increased back pain, resting posture with decreased lordosis on return
	Lumbar extension: Moderate loss (most fearful and apprehensive direction), increased leg and back pain
Neurological examination:	Sensation intact, no findings; tactile allodynia from visit 1 not present in neck, chest, or abdomen (patient remembered this and commented it might be a good thing with respect to treatment). Reflexes intact and symmetrical, 5/5 strength in bilateral knee extensor, ankle dorsiflexion, great toe extension, ankle plantar flexion. Neurodynamic test positive; slump left and straight leg raise test left with moderate loss compared to right side. Repeated slump test using ankle dorsiflexion 10x resulted in increased pain, symptoms remaining worse for remainder of session. No effect on baseline ROM measurements.
Repeated test movements:	Repeated loaded flexion and extension increase back pain and remain worse as a result.
	Repeated unloaded lumbar flexion in lying: Increased in back, no effect on leg or ROM
	Static unloaded lumbar extension: Prop on elbows 5 min, increased back pain, no effect on leg; progress to repeated press up in prone lying, 2 sets 10x, therapist overpressure with last 5, increased back pain, no effect on leg pain, no loss of motion or change in baseline motion

PROVISIONAL MECHANICAL CLASSIFICATION
Other: mechanically inconclusive

PROVISIONAL PAIN CLASSIFICATION
Central sensitization

TREATMENT

Treatment:
- Pain journaling to record intolerable episodes of 7/10 and above to identify mechanical, emotional, and social triggers
- Posture strategies for computer and driving to encourage use of slouch and overcorrect for blood flow during prolonged periods
- Review of body mechanics strategies of hip hinge for child care, household chores.
- Reinforcement of get up and move sitting strategies or stretching during day for blood flow during prolonged periods
- Reinforcement of use of deep breathing relaxation to redirect harmful interpretation when increased pain is present
- Continuous low-level heat therapy for blood flow during prolonged computer use or driving for pain management when he cannot get up and stretch
- Gradual exposure and pacing for full restoration of most meaningful activities that patient had perceived as harmful: Household chores, lifting weights, and recreation basketball
- Upgraded gym program: Improve postural awareness of lordosis using physio ball, alternating vs bilateral arm movements, and lunge rotational patterns for basketball
- Progress to sport-specific basketball drills and controlled return to play

Treatment summary: **16 visits over 16 wk:** 1x/wk for 16 wk. Progress desensitization of central and mechanical ischemic pain mechanisms with progressive movement directed at lumbar spine, with emphasis on alignment to meet function load and ROM demands; education on the meaning of and expectations for symptoms

Goals:

	PSFS	
	Initial	Discharge
Sit and work at computer for 1-2 hr	0	9
Perform regular household and child care tasks	0	9
Return to fitness and basketball program 45 min, 3x/wk	0	9
Pain limitation to function	3	9
Pain intensity rating	8	2

FABQ

Physical Activity scores	30/30	0/30
Work scores	24/66	0/66

Abbreviations: CT = computed tomography; EMG = electromyography; FABQ = Fear-Avoidance Behavior Questionnaire; HNP = herniated nucleus pulposus; MRI = magnetic resonance imaging; PSFS = Patient-Specific Functional Scale; PT = physical therapy; ROM = range of motion.

APPENDIX 6.F Clinical Reasoning for CNS Pain Intervention

Central Nervous System Pain Mechanisms: Intervention		
Central Sensitization	**Affective Pain Mechanism Conscious (C) vs Unconscious (U)**	**Autonomic/Motor Pain Mechanism**
Education: • Explanation of the nondamaging nature of pain: hurt vs harm; interpretation of inputs • Pain mechanism education • Discussion of the role of negative emotions, thoughts, and beliefs; review pain journal • Training in coping strategies for fear of motion or activity; use relaxation, diaphragm breathing training • Explanation of the Activity Pyramid: Green, yellow, and red lights, flare-up management • Identification of the activity baseline and explanation of the no-worse concept; return control to patient **Activity:** • Graded exposure to patient-identified fearful/harmful activity; build low aerobic activity, HR at 55%-75% max, for 2-5 hr/wk • Weight training to build upper and lower extremity strength; start with isolated movements and progress to function at HR 55%-75% of maximum, 2x/wk • Deep muscle training for spine postural stabilization; progress to function, 2x/wk • High-intensity interval training (HIIT); progress to 10-20 min intervals, HR >75% of max, 1-2x/wk • Mechanical exam	Same as central sensitization **(C) Education:** • Regarding readiness stage • Negative emotions' contribution to pain • Focused discussion based on psychometric tools (PHQ-9, PASS, Yellow Flag Risk Form) • Interdisciplinary cognitive–behavioral therapy program, if Yellow Flag Risk Form score >55 **(U) Education:** Tension myositis syndrome; discuss treatment progression: • Understand mechanism; brain's efforts to protect are causing tissue ischemia • Acknowledge activation of mechanism related to unconscious repressed, negative emotions • Refer to investigative psychologist if unable to self-treat with John Sarno's books (*The Mindbody Prescription: Healing the Body, Healing the Pain; Healing Back Pain: The Mind-Body Connection; The Divided Mind: The Epidemic of Mindbody Disorders*) Patients must have **psychological evaluation**, if this mechanism is classified as dominating.	Education and activity same as central sensitization **Treatment for output systems with symptoms:** Lymphedema: Lymph massage, compression stockings Tone and spasticity: Facilitatory and inhibitory techniques Immune system and metabolic disorders: Build low aerobic activity, HR 55%-75% of maximum, 2-5 hr/wk; progress to 10-20 min HIIT, HR >75% of maximum, 1-2x/wk **Treatment for cortical disinhibition:** Sensorimotor retraining approach: 5 stages to progress, 3x/day *Sensory retraining:* (1) localization training, (2) localization and precision stimulus type, (3) graphesthesia with letters & numbers, (4) graphesthesia with 3-letter words, (5) graphesthesia with simple calculations • Progress visualization, size, orientation, speed, overlapping • Progress to next stage when accuracy is 80% *Motor retraining:* (1) left–right discrimination, (2) imagined movements, (3) reflective movements, (4) local isometric bracing, (5) small-range movements with feedback, (6) full-range movements with feedback (mirrors, palpation, elastic tape, watching, imagining) • Progress therapy as patient masters exercise

CHAPTER 7

Affective Pain Mechanism

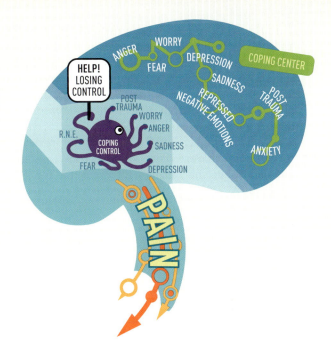

The sorrow which has no vent in tears may make other organs weep.
–Henry Maudsley, *The Pathology of Mind*

POINTS TO DISCUSS

- Connection between psychosocial factors and pain
- Affective characteristics of the conscious mind, including depression, anxiety, insomnia, anger, illness behavior, and social and cultural factors
- Affective characteristics of the unconscious mind, including current pressures of daily life, residual anger from infancy and childhood experiences and relationships, and the type A personality and characteristic trait of perfectionism
- Health care provider psychology
- Affective pain mechanism evaluation, including readiness to change education and assessment, use of psychometric screening tools, and assessment of coping strategies
- Intervention to address the affective pain mechanism, including the biopsychosocial approach, motivational interviewing, and nonpharmacy approaches to pain

---

Patients presenting with dominating central nervous system (CNS) pain mechanisms have a centralized, top-down disorder. This disorder is defined as a generalized hyperexcitability due to disturbances in serotonin and noradrenalin transmission causing mental symptoms to affect descending pain control from the brainstem to the spinal cord. In contrast, patients presenting with dominating peripheral nervous system (PNS) pain mechanisms have a bottom-up disturbance with a localized neuronal abnormality driven from the periphery.[1,2] In the context of disabling pain, psychosocial and affective characteristics (central factors) are better predictors of pain intensity, pain-related disability, and response to treatment than physical or pathophysiological (peripheral) factors,[3,4] and psychological treatments are as effective as or are more so than standard medical treatment for a variety of pain syndromes (eg, nonspecific hand and arm pain, back pain, headache, fibromyalgia).[4-8]

In the affective pain mechanism, the type and location of symptoms are not important, and the patient may not be physically disabled or functionally limited by pain. Instead, the intensity and disability of musculoskeletal pain are determined more by treatable psychological and social factors than by pathophysiological processes. This concept offers clinicians and patients hope regarding the potential for recovery. Interdisciplinary and multidisciplinary treatment teams that address CNS pain mechanisms as a biopsychosocial rather than a purely biomedical experience offer several advantages, and such teams should be more widely implemented. This chapter reviews supporting evidence regarding specific psychosocial characteristics of both conscious and unconscious aspects of chronic musculoskeletal pain and outlines interventions for patients who have dominant affective pain mechanism.

Connection Between Psychosocial Factors and Pain

The biomedical model of illness assumes a direct correlation between nociception (the pathophysiology of tissue damage) and pain (the experience of discomfort). According to this model, once the nociceptive stimulus is identified and addressed, the pain is cured. In contrast, the biopsychosocial model recognizes the limited correspondence between nociception and pain and acknowledges the complex influences of cognition, behavior, emotion, psychology, culture, beliefs, nutrition, and social variables on an individual's experience of pain. Clinicians are familiar with some of these psychosocial mediators and with the idea of secondary gain, in which behavior reflects a real or perceived benefit from the illness. They may be less familiar with the following psychosocial mediators and their dominating effect on pain:

- Unconscious or repressed negative emotions (psychosomatic disorders)
- Depression, anxiety, and anger (emotional disorders)
- Conscious tendency to misinterpret or overinterpret nociception (catastrophizing)
- Heightened concern about pain and its source (fear avoidance)
- Inability to cope with past trauma (posttraumatic stress disorder)
- Social and cultural factors that influence illness behavior
- Readiness to change (self-efficacy)

A study of patients with chronic low back pain found that psychological characteristics accounted for 26% of self-reported pain and 36% of self-reported disability.[9] Many review articles agree that conscious psychological characteristics such as coping strategies, self-efficacy beliefs, fear-avoidance behavior, and unconscious distress are relevant factors that clinicians should identify because they may lead to poorer prognosis.[4,10-12]

Pain is more likely to cause an emotional disturbance than to result from it. However, current or past psychological trauma and states can initiate a pain response. In many instances when pain persists, such trauma is the dominating reason the patient is not improving or progressing as expected. Psychological factors and psychiatric comorbidity, often unrecognized by the patient, may manifest as visits to the doctor with complaints of pain, multiple pains, or worsening pain symptoms.[13] Sarno[14] described this behavior as the *symptom imperative*, a characteristic of psychosomatic disorders that involves having one set of seemingly physical symptoms resolve and appear to be cured, only to be replaced with another set of symptoms. These psychogenic symptoms are commonly misinterpreted and treated as physical disorders.

Affective pain can present in any area of the body (eg, head, chest, back and neck, shoulder, upper and lower limbs).[15] The type and location of the symptoms are not important as long as they fulfill the purpose of diverting attention from what is transpiring in the conscious or unconscious mind. The brain chooses locations in the body based on their ability to assist in the diversion. For example, a man who likes to play tennis and experiences an acute onset of pain in his elbow naturally assumes he hurt himself during a swing but cannot identify the exact onset of the pain because it did not occur during a tennis game. The brain causes the pain by inducing mild oxygen deprivation in a tendon in the arm, causing a tissue ischemia that results in pain. This is not a nociceptive mechanism because the brain renders the lack of oxygen, not the tissue, as a protective maneuver to divert attention from escalating unconscious negative emotions.

The ego, the brain's decision maker, defends the conscious mind against painful and dangerous feelings that could jeopardize the individual's self-image. The ego conceives of a situation that stimulates the production of physical (psychosomatic) or affective symptoms automatically, without seeking approval of the thinking mind and bypassing the patient's intellect altogether. This reaction is likely subcortical; if reason were participating in the decision, then the person would likely prefer to deal with the scary feelings than suffer the pain.

Classification of Psychosocial Factors in Health Care Practice

In 1997, Kendall and colleagues[16] coined the term *yellow flags* to denote psychological, social, and environmental risk factors for prolonged disability and failure to return to work as a consequence of musculoskeletal symptoms and provided guidelines for their assessment. The impact of these guidelines on clinical practice, however, is unclear.[17] Definitions of psychosocial risk factors have been criticized as being overbroad and meaningless.[18] Identifying specific yellow flags allows timely referrals to different disciplines (eg, cognitive–behavioral psychology, primary care, interdisciplinary programs) and therefore access to different treatments. Operationalizing the subtle differences among psychosocial risk factors may thus lead to improved referral patterns and better outcomes.[4]

More recently, the recommendation has been to specify psychosocial characteristics in more detail than just calling them yellow flags. Nicholas and colleagues[4] recommended the use of multiple flag colors to indicate the importance of certain characteristics such as signs of serious pathology (red); psychiatric symptoms (orange); maladaptive beliefs, emotional responses, and pain behaviors (yellow); perceptions of the negative influence of pain on work (blue); and system or contextual obstacles (black) as a way to better guide referrals and explain treatment to patients with chronic pain. **Table 7.1** summarizes these flag colors. We use only yellow flags throughout this book to refer to psychosocial warning signs, but Nicholas et al's recommended flag colors may be useful in some settings to specify patients' characteristics.

Because pain has become an ailment of millions of Americans, experts in psychosomatic disorders have declared an epidemic of disorders associated with pain. The spread of musculoskeletal pain in recent years is partially related to underlying psychosomatic mechanisms that go unrecognized in patients who do not clearly fit a category listed in **Table 7.1**. This failure to identify psychosomatic mechanisms is caused by the misdiagnosis of pain related to both structural and mechanical abnormalities; most clinicians assume that pain is related to the periphery and lack understanding of the brain's connection to pain. In addition, clinicians may fail to recognize that pain may be related to how a patient is coping with life stresses that may be either current or distant in time.

The group of conditions termed *affective spectrum disorders* (ASDs), sometimes called *mind–body disorders*, has both physiological and psychological characteristics. These disorders can involve the conscious and unconscious mind. It is important to distinguish between

TABLE 7.1 Summary of Flag Colors to Indicate Clinically Important Information About Pain[4]

Flag Color	Meaning	Examples
Red	Signs of serious pathology	Cauda equina symptoms, fracture, and tumor
Orange	Psychiatric symptoms	Clinical depression and personality disorders
Yellow	Maladaptive beliefs, appraisals, and judgments	Belief that injury is uncontrollable or likely to worsen, expectation of poor treatment outcome, and delayed return to work
	Maladaptive emotional responses	Distress (eg, worry, fear, anxiety) that does not meet criteria for diagnosis of a mental disorder
	Maladaptive pain behavior (including pain coping strategies)	Avoidance of activities due to the expectation of increased pain and possible reinjury; overreliance on passive treatments (eg, hot or cold packs, analgesics, manual medicine)
Blue	Negative perceptions about the relationship between work and health	Belief that work is too onerous and likely to cause further injury; belief that supervisor and coworkers are unsupportive
Black	System or contextual obstacles	Legislation restricting options for return to work, conflict with insurance company over injury claim, overly solicitous family members and health care providers, and heavy work with little opportunity to modify duties

disorders that affect the conscious and unconscious mind as the psychology treatment will differ. The most common ASD related to the unconscious mind is tension myositis syndrome (TMS). In unconscious disorders, pain is created through activity of the autonomic–peptide system. The autonomic branch of the CNS controls the involuntary systems of the body, such as the circulatory, gastrointestinal, and genitourinary systems. It is active 24 hours a day and functions outside of awareness. Peptides are molecules that participate in a system of intercommunication between the unconscious mind and the body and play an important part in decreasing oxygen to tissues.[13,14]

Conscious mind ASDs include fibromyalgia, major depressive disorder, attention deficit disorder, bulimia nervosa, cataplexy, dysthymic disorder, generalized anxiety disorder, irritable bowel syndrome, migraine, obsessive–compulsive disorder, panic disorder, posttraumatic stress disorder, premenstrual dysphoric disorder, and social phobia.[8,19] It has been suggested that the conscious conditions are characterized by monoamine changes in the brain and the hypothalamic–pituitary–adrenal axis, leading to the clinical symptoms of ASD. As such, ASD may be seen as a reaction to sustained stress with high levels of cortisol production and a genetic or psychosocial vulnerability.[19] The pattern of brain atrophy is directly related to the perceptual and behavioral properties of chronic pain.[20]

Clinicians should consider the conscious and unconscious psychosocial characteristics as possible mechanisms in the manifestation and maintenance of certain chronic musculoskeletal pain conditions, especially when physical interventions have had no effect. Identifying conscious and unconscious psychosocial characteristics allows clinicians to individualize the management of the affective component of patients' pain. When dominating affective characteristics contribute to the pain experience, cognitive–behavioral psychotherapy interventions may be appropriate to address conscious characteristics, and investigative psychotherapy interventions may be appropriate to address unconscious characteristics.

Identifying the Connection Between Patients' Thoughts and Behaviors and Pain

Clinicians naturally tend to conceive of illness in biomedical terms. Even within the biomedical model, the relationship between symptoms and disease is complex. The true cognitive processes of each patient are unknowable, and clinicians can understand patients' thoughts and behaviors regarding the pain experience only through respectful questioning and observation of their body language. People appraise their bodily sensations using a preexisting cognitive schema to determine whether a particular sensation reflects underlying disease that requires attention or can safely be ignored. For example, the pain associated with the intentional stretch of a muscle before sporting activities or the pain experienced on the day after a good workout is desirable and does not trigger anxiety, withdrawal, or avoidance (ie, the pain alarm system). But pain triggered by burning one's hand on a stove triggers a different interpretation and consequences. Interpretations of pain vary widely among individuals and can vary within a particular individual over time and across situations. For example, people with similar stages of osteoarthritis may interpret pain as either a normal part of aging or as a sign of damage, with the interpretation of most individuals falling somewhere in between.

Research has established that patients' attitudes, beliefs, expectations, and coping resources can increase or diminish pain intensity and pain-related disability.[4,21,22] Pain patients may

- Misinterpret pain as tissue damage rather than a temporary problem that will improve
- Take a passive, fatalistic approach to coping or believe that the pain and disability will last forever
- Interpret pain as a sign of serious disease or a reminder of mortality
- Interpret pain as punishment for past experiences or relationships.

Cognitive errors are negatively distorted beliefs about oneself or one's situation. Common cognitive errors that affect perception of pain, distress, and disability include the following[23-25]:

- **Misinterpretation or overinterpretation of nociception.** "This pain in my arm means that my whole body is degenerating and falling apart."
- **All-or-nothing thinking.** "I can't enjoy anything until I am completely pain free."
- **Negative predictions.** "I know that learning coping techniques will not work for me."
- **Selective abstractions.** "Therapy and exercises will make me feel worse than I already do."

Self-efficacy, or the belief in one's ability to successfully achieve a desired outcome, is a cognitive factor that strongly predicts success in coping with pain and reducing disability.[26,27] Greater self-efficacy leads to reduced anxiety and its physiological concomitants, increased ability to use distraction as a coping strategy, increased determination to go on with a planned activity in spite of pain, and avoidance of rumination on the pain.[28,29] Self-efficacy can be practiced and learned. Studies have shown that active coping strategies are associated with improved functioning, whereas passive coping strategies (eg, depending on others for help in pain control, letting pain dictate and restrict one's activity level) are related to greater pain and depression levels.[24,30]

Conscious and Unconscious Psychosocial Aspects of Disabling Musculoskeletal Pain

Affective Characteristics of the Conscious Mind

Several meta-analyses and reviews have identified the most important psychosocial correlates of disabling musculoskeletal pain. Most studies have addressed lower back pain, but the findings are similar for spinal cord injury (SCI) and limb pain.[31] The psychosocial correlates of disabling musculoskeletal pain are comparable to those of other conditions causing disabling pain, such as headaches, fibromyalgia, and irritable bowel syndrome.[32] Seven psychosocial characteristics have been strongly correlated with disabling pain of all types[31]:

1. Physical or sexual abuse (current or in childhood)
2. Depression
3. Ineffective coping skills
4. Current life stress
5. Low socioeconomic status
6. Unemployment
7. Perception of a demanding employer

Depression and misinterpretation or overinterpretation of nociception have been found to be interrelated.[29,33] Pain hinders the diagnosis and treatment of depression,[34] leading to unnecessary testing, medicalization of the somatic expressions of psychological distress, increased health care costs, and poor outcomes. An intuitive sense that pain is a signal of damage, danger, or hopelessness was found to be the strongest correlate of phantom limb pain 6 months after below-the-knee amputation,[35] of nonspecific or idiopathic hand and arm pain,[36] and of a lack of improvement with physical therapy in patients with neck pain.[37] Considering the ways in which patients' conscious affect drives their interpretation of their symptoms helps clinicians understand the connection between conscious characteristics and the patients' pain experience. The sections that follow discuss the conscious characteristics of musculoskeletal pain: depression, anxiety, insomnia, anger, illness behavior, and social and cultural factors.

Depression

Epidemiologists report that rates of depression are increasing around the world. Numerous factors seem to be contributing to this worrisome situation, including war, terrorism, domestic violence, drug and alcohol abuse, displacement due to natural disasters, epidemics, and social isolation.[14] Even in comparatively stable, safe environments, an ever-increasing pace of life, information overload, and a pervasive culture of emptiness and negative attitudes are taking a heavy toll.[38] In medicine, choosing the most effective treatment requires making a correct diagnosis regarding depression.

Sadness is part of the human condition, and clinicians should not consider normal sorrow to be a depressive disorder.[38] For at least 2 decades, the medical profession, pharmaceutical companies, and the culture at large have attempted to medicate normal sadness. Human beings may feel sad when faced with heartbreak, death, natural disaster, or financial crisis. Suffering through emotional pain often helps people make better choices in future situations. In fact, normal sadness may actually improve chances for survival. Without the experience of sorrow and sadness, one cannot truly feel empathy or compassion for others. Patients typically do not like to admit that they are sad and do not tolerate depression well.

Although it is important to diagnose and treat true clinical depression, clinicians need to understand that not all sadness is pathological depression.

True clinical depression is the strongest predictor of health status across diseases and cultures.[39] Depression is characterized by sustained sadness that is severe enough to preclude normal daily functions. It is influenced by psychosocial stresses, genetic factors, neurotransmitter levels, nutritional status, sleep deprivation, disrupted neuroendocrine responses, alcohol and medication use, and multiple medical conditions. A summary of the literature on depression[24,29,33,34,38-41] recommends that clinicians make a referral to rule out clinical depression in patients in whom five or more of the following symptoms are present nearly every day over at least 2 weeks:

- Feelings of persistent sadness, anxiety, or empty mood
- Feelings of helplessness and pessimism
- Feelings of hopelessness, worthlessness, and excessive or inappropriate guilt
- Anhedonia (ie, loss of ability to feel interest or pleasure)
- Decreased energy and pervasive fatigue
- Difficulty concentrating or making decisions
- Sleep disturbance, including insomnia, hypersomnolence, or early morning awakening
- Change in weight or appetite
- Suicidal thinking

Depressed patients are often troubled more deeply by insomnia than by sadness. The relationship between insomnia and depression is important clinically, and insomnia should be considered a potential precursor to depression.

Chronic pain and depression frequently co-occur: People with pain are at increased risk for depression, and those with depression are at increased risk for pain.[40] Patients in chronic pain with depression report more severe pain, greater disability, lower functioning in work and activities of daily living, and poorer treatment outcomes for their pain.[42] For patients with dominating affective pain mechanism, clinicians need to understand the differences between those with and without depression to develop tailored interventions to effectively manage both pain and depressive mechanisms. Understanding the context of patients' lives is important to understanding their depressive symptoms. Pain may be associated with increased stress and reduced resilience and coping capability in patients who face stressful and traumatic life events.[41] **Appendix 7.A** describes a patient whose pain is related to depression associated with posttraumatic stress disorder. (The education provided to the patient in **Appendix 7.A** is discussed later in this chapter in the section "Intervention to Address the Affective Pain Mechanism.")

Research on depression in populations with several conditions has revealed the pervasiveness of this condition in patients with chronic musculoskeletal pain: A review article addressing the process of adjustment to life changes following SCI concluded that no psychological factor has received greater attention than depression, because it is thought to mediate most adjustment difficulties and to play a major role in problematic pain.[43-45] It appears that in SCI, patients at risk for depression have moderately high levels of depressive symptom intensity over time that may interfere with their ability to experience or express pain relief.[44] In acute traumatic SCI, the presence of pain was found to affect depression more than the presence of depression affected pain.[45] Patients with fibromyalgia had significantly higher scores than patients with peripheral neurogenic pain on measures of depression, anxiety, somatization, and obsession–compulsion.[46] Patients with fibromyalgia had lower functional scores than patients with neuropathic pain despite similar pain scores of intensity and duration, indicating the disabling effects when pain is dominated by CNS rather than PNS mechanisms.[46] Health-related quality of life was lower in patients with chronic pain than in healthy controls of the same cohort,[47] suggesting that pain may be the leading cause of low health-related quality of life.[48]

Regardless of preexisting comorbidities, patients with multiple sclerosis and pain had lower scores than multiple sclerosis patients without pain.[49] Thus, positive outcomes for patients in pain with affective components may be difficult to achieve because health-related quality of life is predictive of treatment success, and this factor may not always be the focus of care.[47,48]

Changes in pain affect depression symptom intensity more than changes in depression affect reports of pain intensity. Assessment of both pain and depression is easier if clinicians establish baselines before boundaries become obscured. Such assessment may help prevent acute mechanical pain from transitioning into chronic affective pain because depression can be identified and a referral recommended.

Living with pain can lead to social isolation, greater pain disability, interrupted ability to maintain roles such as parenting, financial insecurity, increased dependence on others for support, and unemployment. Financial security is often compromised by job loss, work disability, and high health care expenses.[50] Furthermore, depressed patients have reported significantly more psychosocial stress from every experience evaluated. Some patients become irritable, confrontational, or even combative, which can be perplexing to support systems and family members and can delay proper diagnosis. Irritability and agitation should always be viewed as a precursor to symptoms of depression and not lightly dismissed as annoying behavior, especially in patients with insomnia.

Elderly patients may become so profoundly depressed that they appear demented, and depression and dementia often coexist. Late-life depression that remains unrecognized and untreated can linger for years. It is associated with very poor quality of life, declining physical function and social interaction, poor compliance with medical therapy, exacerbation of chronic medical conditions, and increased morbidity and mortality (including suicide).

Studies have shown that suicidal ideation is an important parameter in patients with chronic pain.[51] Patients with suicidal ideation have more mental distress, depression, and anxiety than patients without this feature. The most important question a clinician treating depressed patients who have suicidal ideation can ask is whether they have a plan for their suicide, as this is indicative of someone who needs to be taken to an emergency room and not allowed to leave the clinic.

Anxiety and other psychosocial stressors have been significantly and independently associated with depression severity. The majority of depression studies focus predominantly on psychiatric symptoms and diagnoses. The real-world situations of patients' lives, such as interpersonal difficulties, financial problems, and exposure to violence, are often not taken into account. In contrast, clinicians are often aware of how patients' personal situations and stressors are relevant to their clinical presentations. Attending to psychosocial stressors in clinical settings may improve patients' ability to engage effectively in different treatment approaches, adhere to treatment recommendations, and demonstrate improvements in their psychiatric symptoms. Comprehension of the characteristics and screening tools involved in patient encounters can lead to early identification of patients with dominating affective pain mechanism that will need to be co-managed with a psychiatrist or psychologist.

Anxiety

Anxiety disorders are increasingly recognized as a significant psychological issue among patients with pain. Anxiety disorders may be present in as many as 60% of pain patients[52] and in 35% of patients with chronic pain, compared with 18% of the general population not experiencing neurogenic pain.[53] Comorbid anxiety and depression are common among patients with chronic pain,[54] and the likelihood of experiencing anxiety increases in individuals facing psychosocial stress.[55] Patients with pain who report anxiety symptoms in the context of psychosocial stress may also be more likely to report greater depressive symptoms. Health anxiety is another important risk factor for chronic pain and disability.[56-58] The research suggests that the effect of stress on depressive severity may be partly mediated by the level of anxiety.[59] Psychosocial pressures may be particularly problematic among patients with limited anxiety symptoms; pain patients with high baseline mental health functioning and perfectionism may be more vulnerable to mind–body disorders when exposed to significant social pressures.

Most people perceive nociceptive sensations as unpleasant but not catastrophic (ie, leading to permanent disability), and they engage in appropriate behavioral restriction followed by a gradual increase in activity as the sensation becomes less acute. In contrast, a significant group of individuals interpret pain-related sensations as not only threatening but also catastrophic; catastrophizing is thought to result from dispositional and situational factors. Pain catastrophizing exacerbates pain-related anxiety and behavioral avoidance and compulsions and thereby promotes and maintains activity limitations, disability, and the nociceptive sensation itself.[60]

The fear and anxiety-avoidance models of chronic pain follow patterns similar to anxiety disorder models.[60] Specifically, anxiety disorders either follow from or are exacerbated by one or more unpleasant experiences associated with catastrophic cognitions, significant distress, or behavioral avoidance and compulsions.[61] For people with an anxiety disorder, behavioral avoidance and compulsions prevent them from confronting and refuting their fearful cognitions, leading to a self-perpetuating cycle of anxiety.[62] Similarities between the patterns of chronic pain and anxiety disorder suggest that similar mechanisms or processes may be involved in their development and maintenance.[63] Moreover, researchers have found evidence of elevated levels of pain-related anxiety in samples of patients without chronic pain[64] and an inverse relationship between pain tolerance and panic disorder.[65] Anxiety disorders found to be closely related to musculoskeletal pain include panic disorder with or without agoraphobia, agoraphobia without history of panic disorder, specific phobia, social phobia, obsessive–compulsive disorder, generalized anxiety disorder, posttraumatic stress disorder, acute stress disorder, anxiety due to substance use or medical condition, anxiety disorder not otherwise specified, and anxiety sensitivity.[66] Symptoms of anxiety are frequently misinterpreted as those of medical illness because of considerable overlap in symptoms; examples include tachycardia, diaphoresis, tremor, shortness of breath, nausea, abdominal pain, and chest pain. Common sources of anxiety in medical diagnoses include fear of death or lingering impairment, fear of abandonment, loss of function, loss of control, fear of pain, and fear of dependency.

Understanding and treating the presentation of depression among pain patients entails consideration of anxiety and psychosocial stress as well. With respect to pain, understanding the differences between panic disorder, phobic disorder, and worried sickness is helpful:

- **Panic disorder** is defined by distinct episodes of intense fear and discomfort associated with physical symptoms including palpitations, diaphoresis, shortness of breath, tremulousness, chest pain, dizziness, and fear of impending doom or death. Paresthesia, gastrointestinal distress, and distorted perception of reality are also common. Diagnostic criteria require at least 1 month of concern or worry about the attacks or a change in behavior related to them. Panic attacks have a sudden onset and usually subside within an hour. Clusters of attacks may be separated by months of well-being.

Panic disorders typically have their onset in adolescence or early adulthood. However, anticipatory anxiety may develop over time with progressive avoidance of particular places, situations, or even activities.
- **Phobic disorders** are characterized by marked and persistent fear of objects, situations, pain, or activities that result in an immediate anxiety reaction. The desire to avoid the phobic stimulus eventually impedes social or professional functioning. Symptoms often date back to early childhood. Phobic disorders include (but are not limited to) claustrophobia; agoraphobia; fear of animals, insects, or reptiles; fear of flying; fear of public speaking; fear of movement; and fear of pain.
- **Worried sickness** affects people with medical conditions (eg, cardiovascular, pulmonary, endocrine, musculoskeletal, or neurological diagnoses) who present with anxiety as their chief complaint. When the history is nonspecific, a careful physical exam and focused diagnostic workup are necessary to rule out serious medical conditions before treatment for the anxiety can begin.

Appendix 7.B provides a case example of a patient with pain related to anxiety.

One factor possibly contributing to fear avoidance that has recently emerged in relation to chronic pain is anxiety sensitivity. Anxiety sensitivity can be defined as a person's fear of his or her own anxiety-related symptoms and is regarded as a predisposing factor in the development of certain anxiety-related disorders.[67] Anxiety sensitivity has been studied in the context of pain[68] and has been shown to play a role in pain created in laboratory[69] and pain-related distress in people with chronic pain.[70,71] However, anxiety sensitivity has not been considered in relation to broader aspects of physical and psychosocial functioning in patients with chronic pain or in relation to potential treatment process variables. This lack of attention is surprising given that fear of emotional experiences would be expected to lead to avoidance of the experiences and situations that evoke them, and both distressing emotions and avoidance appear to be cardinal features of chronic pain, particularly in patients who experience relatively greater suffering and disability.

Anxiety sensitivity and its components have been associated with greater pain, depression, pain-related anxiety, general practice visits related to pain, emotional distress, and disability in patients with chronic pain.[72] It appears that if patients with chronic pain are concerned about their experiences of pain and fearful of such experiences, they may have greater overall distress and greater deficits in daily functioning. Anxiety sensitivity could then be conceptualized as a type of distress amplifier, or a process that contributes additional adverse psychological meaning and influences to emotional and pain experiences.[73] Furthermore, it is likely that pain-related anxiety and anxiety sensitivity may both be key in the development and maintenance of chronic disabling pain. Together, the two constructs may explain some of the comorbidity of anxiety disorders in chronic pain.[74] The Escape/Avoidance subscale of the Pain Anxiety Symptoms Scale[75] (PASS) has questions that can help clinicians differentiate factors for the early identification of persons for whom pain is more likely to become chronic and disabling. These patients may benefit from treatments specifically targeting pain avoidance behaviors; treatment with graded exposure that desensitizes the fear may reduce pain-related anxiety and disabling chronic pain.[76]

History taking helps apprise clinicians of patients' beliefs, attitudes, behaviors, social history, decision-making capabilities, and motivation in times of stress. This information can have a profound impact on treatment recommendations and the success of outcomes. Identifying patients with characteristics that predispose them to an anxiety disorder may help confirm the need for a referral to a behavioral or investigative psychologist.

Insomnia

Insomnia is a sleep disorder characterized by problems falling or staying asleep or by waking up too early; those affected may also experience overall poor quality of sleep. An estimated 30% of adults have symptoms of insomnia.[77] Women and older adults seem to have the greatest difficulty achieving adequate amounts of good-quality sleep.

Detecting and alleviating chronic insomnia may reduce the risk of developing depression and anxiety. Dr. Dan G. Blazer, MD, PhD, from Duke University Medical Center noted, "Insomnia may predispose people to anxiety and depression, just as anxiety and depression may predispose people to insomnia."[77] For decades, clinicians have viewed insomnia as a symptom of depression and anxiety. People with depression often wake up at 3 or 4 AM and find that they cannot get back to sleep. Those with anxiety often struggle to fall asleep, tossing and turning for hours. Research conducted in Norway indicates that chronic insomnia can increase the likelihood of a person developing both depression and anxiety disorders.[77]

Sleep is a very active process regulated by the CNS and influences every organ system in the body. Sleep is a complex physiological, psychological, and behavioral state coordinated by neurons and neurotransmitters. Human sleep has five stages. Stages 1 to 4 involve non–rapid eye movement (REM) sleep, followed by stage 5, REM sleep. An adult sleep cycle requires approximately 90 minutes; a baby's sleep cycle takes about 60 minutes. Each stage of a sleep cycle reveals a specific electroencephalogram pattern and is associated with certain characteristics:

- **Wakefulness** is the stage before sleep.
- **Stage 1 sleep** is very shallow and superficial. The eyes move slowly, and little muscle activity occurs. Stage 1 sleep is fragmented, and awakening occurs easily; it is not restorative or refreshing.
- **Stage 2 sleep** is typically the longest stage of sleep. Eye movements slow down, and awakening can occur easily. Older individuals and people with chronic pain and illness may spend most of the night in stage 2 sleep.
- **Stage 3 sleep** is the beginning of slow wave sleep. The body's repair processes occur during this deeper stage of sleep. It is more difficult to wake up; awakening results in a dazed, disoriented feeling.
- **Stage 4 sleep** is the deepest stage of non-REM sleep. Neurotransmitters and growth hormones are synthesized. Slow wave sleep is most prominent and intense during childhood and declines at puberty and in the second and third decades of life. Slow wave sleep may be completely absent in old age.
- **Stage 5 or REM sleep** is when most dreaming occurs. Breathing becomes shallow, rapid, and irregular. Blood pressure and pulse rate rise; oxygen consumption and blood flow to the brain increase. Eyes move in a jerking manner, but muscle paralysis occurs in the extremities. People spend longer periods in dream sleep between 4 and 8 AM. REM sleep and sleepiness peak near the habitual wake time. REM sleep has a profound effect on consolidation of memory, daytime efficiency, fine motor skills, and creativity.

Everyone experiences stressful circumstances and emotionally upsetting or draining events. A loss or change of job, separation or divorce, the serious illness or death of a loved one, and legal problems can all interfere with sleep. Patients can become preoccupied with a perceived inability to sleep at night. Poor sleep habits and beliefs about insomnia acquired during the high-stress period may persist even after the situation has resolved; when people become hyperaroused by their persistent efforts to sleep, insomnia may evolve as a maladaptive conditional response. The following unhealthy habits can undermine sleep:

- **Inactivity.** Being mentally or emotionally drained but not physically tired enough to sleep can be frustrating. Physical activity helps relieve stress, reduces cortisol production, and helps normalize sleep stages.
- **Overeating and indigestion.** Abdominal bloating, indigestion, gas pains, and reflux symptoms may make sleep impossible. Weight loss often improves sleep quality.
- **Overstimulation.** Areas of the brain that regulate sleep do not turn on and off like a switch. The reticular activating system in the brainstem must be allowed to settle down.
- **Excessive worry.** Activation of the frontal cortices, limbic system, amygdala, autonomic nervous system, and adrenal glands severely compromises sleep as a result of a spike in adrenaline and cortisol.
- **Erratic schedules.** Good-quality sleep is dependent on circadian rhythms and requires cooperation with the rhythms of nature.
- **Overextension.** People who combine overstimulation, excessive worry, and erratic schedules are more likely to experience insomnia.
- **Caffeine, nicotine, and alcohol.** Caffeine is an adenosine receptor antagonist and should be avoided within 7 hours of bedtime. Nicotine is a stimulant and can result in severely disrupted sleep quality. Alcohol is a chemical depressant but can suppress dream sleep early in the night and provoke nightmares later on. Early morning awakening further disrupts sleep.
- **Bedroom environment.** Temperature can be too cold or hot. Even the luminescent light on an alarm clock can stimulate the reticular activating system in the brainstem. Noise and clutter, partners, and pets may disrupt sleep.
- **Napping.** An afternoon nap may be refreshing for some people. Patients should avoid napping more than 45 minutes, however, and take naps before 3 PM to avoid reducing their sleep incentive at night.
- **Medications.** Many medications patients take can cause sleep disturbance. Whenever possible, clinicians should check to see that patients are not taking medications known to compromise sleep.

Medical problems can disturb sleep at any age, but people in middle age and beyond often develop multiple medical conditions (eg, diabetes plus sleep apnea). Clinical experience and research demonstrate that sleep quality declines as more illnesses develop. According to the 2003 Sleep in America poll,[78] 36% of people over 65 with no health problems, 52% of people with one to three comorbid illnesses, and 69% of people with four or more medical conditions had problems sleeping. Musculoskeletal conditions that disrupt sleep include osteoarthritis, rheumatoid arthritis, bursitis, lumbar and cervical radiculopathy, and fibromyalgia. Clinical evidence has shown that 31% of patients with arthritis have difficulty falling asleep, 51% wake up too early in the morning, and 81% have trouble staying asleep.[79] The conclusion from the literature is that illness and pain make insomnia worse and insomnia exacerbates illness and pain.

Anger

An additional correlate of pain is anger, which may affect pain through biological mechanisms (eg, increased arousal) and may interfere with pain acceptance and adherence to treatment.[80] Anger can take the form of irritability and frustration related to the persistence of symptoms, lack of an established etiology, treatment failures, workers' compensation or other disability claims, and problems with finances and family relationships. Anger is an emotional state that can range in intensity from mild irritation to extreme rage and includes other closely related states such as the following[81]:

- **Hostility.** An attitude toward others that includes seeing specific individuals or groups as enemies; a readiness to become angry.
- **Aggression.** Behavior intended to remove obstacles and dangers in the environment; results can be positive or negative.
- **Chronic anger.** A pattern of thinking, acting, and feeling in which a person seeks, embraces, and prolongs anger experiences.
- **Rage.** An experience of excessive anger characterized by partial or complete loss of conscious awareness or a normal sense of self- and behavioral control.

Anger is a multicausal state, and the treatment must be multimodal. Problematic anger and aggression are related to genetics, brain development, experience, and current circumstances, just like chronic pain. There may be no single treatment for an individual with problematic anger and aggression problems because many pathways may contribute. No single center in the brain produces anger and aggression. Anger can be compared to a river fed by streams that sometimes cause it to overflow. The clinical questions to ask are: Is the anger associated with the person's pain symptoms? How many streams (triggers) feed the anger? Is the river low (ie, the person is coping well) or overflowing (ie, the person is coping poorly)? The focus of anger management treatment is on identifying anger triggers, developing coping strategies, and redirecting the responses. **Appendix 7.C** describes a patient experiencing anger mixed with depression.

Fear and anger are closely connected. Patients can be angry in their unconscious mind and not consciously know it. Emotions can be described as a physiological state and feelings as the subjective awareness of that state. The emotion of anger may be expressed in feelings of fear. The following types of anger are innate in all animals[82]:

- Predatory anger is the urge to kill and consume.
- Intermale anger is a result of competition for access to females.
- Maternal anger is directed against intruders.
- Sex-related anger is involved in aggressive courtship.
- Fear-induced anger is felt in the face of inescapable threat.
- Irritable anger is elicited by frustration, pain, or deprivation (eg, of food, water, sleep, social contact).

Fear-induced and irritable anger are the types of anger that most anger management programs address.

Illness Behavior

Given that normal responses to pain include both the cognitive (eg, uncertainty, misperception of danger) and physiological (eg, autonomic arousal) aspects of anxiety, it is not surprising that an excessive pain response often exacerbates both pain intensity and pain-related disability.[83] Anxiety in the context of disabling chronic pain often takes the form of fear- and harm-avoidance behaviors (ie, pain anxiety). A principle of operant conditioning is that behaviors that are reinforced are maintained and those that are not reinforced are extinguished. For example, behaviors such as grimacing to communicate pain or protectively cradling an arm are maintained if they are reinforced by a doting spouse or sympathetic health care provider.[84] Behaviors may also be maintained and reinforced by the rewards of avoiding the pain sensation, obtaining narcotic pain medication, and avoiding undesirable activities such as work.

Pain avoidance behaviors can exacerbate pain intensity and pain-related disability.[85] Avoidance of activity leads to anticipatory anxiety about pain (eg, muscle tension, other symptoms associated with the fight-or-flight response or sympathetic activation), which may act as a conditioned stimulus for pain that is maintained after healing. Over time, the person perceives more activities as dangerous or aversive and avoids them, leading to deconditioning and less effective coping strategies.[86] Avoiding painful activities perpetuates and reinforces the belief that pain is an indicator of tissue damage and therefore retards healing. Avoidance also prevents the opportunity to have a corrective experience and the chance to discover that many types of musculoskeletal pain eventually subside regardless of activity level. Avoiding situations perceived as dangerous and anxiety provoking is a common mechanism in the maintenance of anxiety disorders and probably of disabling pain, with patients increasingly avoiding activities they anticipate will cause pain.[86]

Social and Cultural Factors

Intuition and beliefs about illness and health care providers are influenced by prior experiences and social and cultural norms.[87-89] There are ethnic and sex-related differences in beliefs about pain and response to pain.[90] Social factors influence how families respond to pain and interact with members experiencing pain.[91] For example, children acquire attitudes and perceptions about health and health care and cognitive and behavioral responses to injury not only from their parents, but also from cultural stereotypes and the social environment.[91] The most recent medium for sociocultural influences on illness behavior is the Internet. Advertisements, articles, and blogs, particularly those about commercial treatments for pain, offer cures and imply that miraculous results are possible. As a result, patients come to expect miracle cures in a variety of contexts, often with little effort on their part. In addition, normal aspects of human development, such as the effects of aging on appearance (eg, wrinkles, gray hair, hair loss), are stigmatized. Promoting the desire to stay young forever gives people a sense of well-being and puts them at ease as they age; however, it interferes with their adaptation to the appearance-related and painful aspects of aging. Clinicians should not underestimate the impact of such marketing on disabling musculoskeletal pain and should investigate its effects through respectful questioning.

Affective Characteristics of the Unconscious Mind

The genesis of a psychosomatic disorder is thought to be related to the unconscious mind repressing negative emotions associated with current, past, or future life pressures or relationships. The unconscious mind distracts the conscious mind, diverting attention from what is transpiring in the unconscious, which might threaten the self-image created in the conscious mind. Physical symptoms that are unresponsive to any intervention may thus be a means to distract the patient from awareness of negative emotions in the unconscious mind relative to current or past (eg, childhood) relationships, current life pressures, or perfectionist traits.

The affective pain mechanism is thus related to the repression of unconscious negative emotions, including primarily rage but also shame, guilt, sadness, fear, loss of control, vulnerability, and feelings of inferiority, as well as to the trait of perfectionism. In contrast to conscious characteristics, the patient is often unaware of the role of these negative emotions in contributing to, triggering, and dominating their pain experience. Many patients with unconscious pain characteristics continue to work and exercise and are not functionally limited by their pain but believe the pain originates in the body and have pursued physiological interventions in search of a cure. Patients may become aware of the influence of unconscious mechanisms only after attempts to obtain relief through surgery, injection, manipulation, massage, exercise, and cognitive–behavioral and other psychology interventions have produced no resolution of or change in their pain.

People unconsciously repress and consciously suppress thoughts and emotions that are unpleasant, disagreeable, or unacceptable, allowing them to survive and function, but over time they may accumulate a *reservoir of rage,* another term coined by Sarno[14] to denote unconscious rage repressed over many years for many reasons. This reservoir of rage, as summarized by Sarno, involves three potential sources directly related to musculoskeletal pain:

1. Current pressures of daily life, including family (immediate and extended), work, finances, career, aging, and mortality
2. Residual anger from experiences and relationships in infancy and childhood, such as alcoholic or over- or underprotective parents; sexual, physical, or emotional abuse; or stress due to birth order roles (eg, first child as caregiver)
3. Type A personality or perfectionism, manifested in a strong inner drive to succeed, high perceived responsibility, high levels of self-motivation and discipline, a compulsion to achieve perfection, actions indicating superiority to mask feelings of inferiority, or internal conflict between the superego and id (ie, between ideal self-image and unconscious emotion).

The following sections describe in more detail the characteristics of unconscious emotions that may be linked to patients' pain experience.

Coping with Current Pressures of Daily Life

Traditionally, environmental pressures have been referred to as *stressors,* but pressures include things generally not thought of as stressors, such as being a good wife or husband, a good parent, a good son or daughter, or a good coworker. Pressure on the psyche and the disparity between conscious and unconscious reactions to life events contribute to the reservoir of rage. For example, people caring for infants or elderly parents may have negative feelings about having to care for the family member, even if they consciously do so lovingly and willingly. They repress their anger and resentment, and the nicer they are, the greater their unconscious negative reaction and the higher the possibility of psychosomatic symptoms. The unconscious mind, the narcissistic part of our emotional makeup, experiences rage in the face of illness, aging, disability, and death. These unconscious feelings are as real as conscious feelings. The altered physiology and chemistry at the tissue level (ie, lack of oxygen and blood flow) created by the brain's emotional centers distract the conscious mind from the unconscious feelings of rage.

Residual Anger from Infancy and Childhood Experiences and Relationships

The developing child needs warmth, approval, role models, and guidance. Child-raising patterns that are neglectful or hurtful wound the child's self-regard and promote low self-esteem, creating emotional needs that persist through life. Adults may yearn for what they did not get as children; the resulting sadness, hurt, and anger may accumulate in the unconscious mind and be demonstrated in their attachment patterns (ie, how they create and experience relationships). This residual anger provides a ripe environment for psychosomatic symptoms.

Physical, emotional, psychological, and social effects of childhood abuse and neglect can be triggered and become operant at any time because the unconscious does not recognize the passage of time. Repressing negative experiences and feelings and storing them in the unconscious mind may be the best coping mechanism when one cannot actively change a situation or when "good" behavior resulting from repression and self-denial is positively reinforced. When feelings of sadness, unhappiness, fear, or anger are forbidden in childhood, that prohibition can last a lifetime. The feelings stay in the unconscious, accumulating until the reservoir of rage is full and threatens the conscious mind. The more threatening these unconscious feelings are to the person's conscious self-image, the more severe the psychosomatic reaction.

Type A Personality and the Trait of Perfectionism

The drive to be perfect is a reaction to feelings of inferiority, which are predominantly unconscious. Tendencies to achieve and be nice are typical of people trying to demonstrate through performance that they are worthwhile and not inferior. These tendencies are among the most important contributors to the reservoir of rage and can be a primary factor in the genesis of psychosomatic symptoms. Although most patients deny they are perfectionists, they may admit to qualities typical of perfectionism; they may describe themselves as hardworking, conscientious, responsible, driven, success oriented, perpetual seekers of new challenges, sensitive to criticism, and their own worst critic. The drive to perfection is a life pressure and a primary contributor to the accumulation of unconscious negative emotions. In a survey of 104 patients, Sarno[14] found that perfectionism, which he called the "perfect-good drive," was a dominating or significant contributor in 94% of cases of TMS, the most common unconscious mind–body disorder:

- In 32% of cases, the perfect-good drive was the primary contributor to TMS.
- In 37%, the perfect-good drive and life pressures contributed equally.
- In 17%, the perfect-good drive and childhood abuse contributed equally.
- In 8%, all three factors (perfect-good drive, life pressures, and childhood abuse) contributed equally.
- In 4%, childhood abuse was the primary contributor.
- In 3%, life pressures were the primary contributor.

Striving to be good is not a sickness, and the psychology that triggers psychosomatic disorders is not pathological or neurotic, but rather is worthy of being ruled out when nothing else seems to help. **Figure 7.1** is a patient education handout on TMS. **Appendix 7.D** describes a patient whose pain was related to TMS.

Clinician Psychology

The psychology of clinicians may be as important as the psychology of patients in the management of disabling musculoskeletal pain. In spite of strong research support for the biopsychosocial model of illness, many clinicians persist in taking a biomedical approach. They may believe that the psychosocial dimensions of illness are not within their domain or will resolve after nociception is addressed. Even clinicians who do appreciate the psychosocial dimensions may have difficulty addressing them because of societal stigmatization of psychological illness and an exaggerated belief in their own ability to heal. Musculoskeletal clinicians often prefer intuition (ie, a combination of experience, beliefs, and habits) over evidence.[92,93] Furthermore, many prefer a paternalistic model of decision making, even though patients, by assuming a passive role, may lose an opportunity to develop self-efficacy. A passive approach to treatment has been shown to increase disability and distress in many pain conditions.[3]

FIGURE 7.1 Tension Myositis Syndrome Patient Education Handout

Tension Myositis Syndrome

Tension myositis syndrome (TMS), also known as *tension myoneural syndrome,* is pain that is attributed not to mechanical or physical factors, but rather to patients' feelings, personality, and unconscious issues. People who are most susceptible to this type of pain experience unconscious anger and rage and have a type A personality. These unconscious emotional issues initiate a process that causes physical pain and other symptoms in your body.

The theory is that the unconscious mind uses the autonomic nervous system, which regulates the internal organs, to decrease blood flow to muscles, nerves, tendons, and organs, resulting in oxygen deprivation that is experienced as pain in affected tissues. The physical pain is the mind's defense mechanism to distract the person from unconscious mental emotions such as anger, anxiety, rage, and type A stress. The emotions and stress are contained in the unconscious and thereby prevented from entering conscious awareness. Relief comes when patients recognize that the symptoms are only a distraction and not the real issue; the symptoms then serve no purpose, and they go away.

DO YOU HAVE TMS?
How can you tell if you have TMS? Circle yes or no for the following questions:

1. Do you have a strong inner drive to succeed?   Yes   No
2. Do you have a great sense of responsibility?   Yes   No
3. Are you self-motivated and disciplined?   Yes   No
4. Are you your own severest critic?   Yes   No
5. Are you a perfectionist or compulsive about being good?   Yes   No

If you circled yes for three or more questions, and if the interventions you have received have not improved your pain, your clinician may recommend an evaluation for TMS.

SYMPTOMS OF TMS
TMS is a condition characterized by psychosomatic musculoskeletal and nerve symptoms. The most common locations are the back, neck, head, and knee, but the pain may also affect other locations. TMS symptoms have a tendency to move around the body, an important diagnostic indicator.

CRITERIA FOR DIAGNOSIS
- **Lack of known physical cause.** Physical examinations have been unable to correlate pain to a physical or mechanical structure or pathology, and tests and imaging studies have ruled out serious pathology.
- **Tender points present in six locations.** Two tender points are found in the upper trapezius muscles, two in the lumbar paraspinal muscles, and two in the lateral upper buttocks. (The criteria for fibromyalgia include 11 of 18 tender points.)

(continues on next page)

FIGURE 7.1 Tension Myositis Syndrome Patient Education Handout

(continued from previous page)

- **History of other psychosomatic disorders.** Examples include irritable bowel syndrome and tension headaches.
- **History of failed interventions.** Medical interventions such as surgery, injections, manipulation, and exercise have been ineffective.

PSYCHOLOGY TREATMENT PROTOCOL

- **Education regarding psychological and physiological mechanisms.** Office visits, lectures, and written and audio materials are used to help patients understand that their physical condition is benign and that any disability is caused by pain-related fear and deconditioning, not an actual risk of further injury.
- **Writing about emotional issues.** To identify the repressed negative emotions that might exist in the patients' unconscious mind, they should consider the following: problematic childhood experiences and relationships, such as abuse or lack of love; personality traits such as perfectionism, conscientiousness, and a strong need to be liked by everyone; current life pressures (eg, family, financial, job); worries about aging and mortality; and situations that cause anger that cannot be expressed.
- **Resumption of a normal lifestyle.** Patients should discontinue all physical treatments that address a supposed structural cause of their chronic pain and that have been unable to improve their condition. Patients should discontinue precautions they take to protect their "damaged" body part. They should gradually become more involved in activities that have meaning for them.
- **Support groups and psychotherapy.** If patients do not recover quickly, the protocol also includes participation in a support group to help them explore emotional issues that may be causing their symptoms and review concepts learned during earlier education. Psychotherapy is needed by about 20% of patients; treatment is typically short term (six to 10 sessions), dynamic, and analytically oriented.

Resources
Sarno JE. *Healing Back Pain: The Mind-Body Connection.* New York: Warner Books; 1991.
Sarno JE. *The Divided Mind: The Epidemic of Mindbody Disorders.* New York: HarperCollins; 2007.
Sarno JE. *The Mindbody Prescription: Healing the Body, Healing the Pain.* New York: Warner Books; 1998.
Schechter D. *The MindBody Workbook: A Thirty Day Program of Insight and Awareness for People With Back Pain and Other Disorders.* Culver City, CA: MindBody Medicine Publications; 2008.

Patients may communicate their distress to the clinician in the form of depression and anxiety, misconceptions about nociception, and heightened concern about illness. Their reports of pain and disability may lead the clinician to believe that their pathophysiology is worse than it is, even though the evidence does not support this line of thinking.[94,95]

Clinicians frequently underestimate patients' capacity to understand the neurophysiology of pain. For this reason, they may fail to use current, accurate information about the neurophysiology of pain in forming the theoretical basis of treatment and educating patients as a part of their management approach.[96] The failure to address the neurophysiology of pain in detail is the primary barrier to reconceptualization of the problem of chronic musculoskeletal pain within the clinical and lay arenas.[96] Clinicians often feel pressured to curtail the time they spend with patients and may believe that they do not have sufficient time to understand and address their patients' feelings and expectations in detail. They may also be frustrated when treating patients with complex pain conditions that are diffuse, vague, ambiguous, and of disproportionate intensity and disability.[97,98] Not understanding and addressing these clinician barriers and beliefs adds to the misuse of procedures and diagnostic testing and to the misinterpretation of findings, enabling the affective pain mechanism to persist in dominating patients' pain experience.

Affective Pain Mechanism Evaluation

The clinician's evaluation of patients with a dominating affective pain mechanism occurs at every session, not just the initial session. Building respect and trust in the provider–patient relationship helps the clinician understand the patient's psychosocial irritants and pressures as they become more apparent with time. Understanding and appropriately classifying relevant psychosocial barriers in a timely manner can be challenging. The evaluation for the affective pain mechanism consists of questions and tools that assist the clinician's clinical reasoning toward understanding, recognizing, and communicating the relevance of psychosocial issues. This effort supports the clinician in advocating for additional team members (eg, psychologists) or patient participation in a cognitive–behavioral interdisciplinary team program, both of which will make the best use of the patient's emotional and financial resources.

The primary difference between evaluating a patient with a dominating affective pain mechanism versus other mechanisms is the psychosocial evaluation and the focus on the presence and relevance of conscious and unconscious thoughts and emotions. The clinician must ensure that patients with a dominating affective pain mechanism use effective strategies to cope with conscious suppressed emotions, unconscious repressed emotions, traumatizing psychological events, and emotional disorders that may have precipitated or initiated their pain experience. It is also imperative that the patients demonstrate awareness of the connections between negative emotions and thoughts and pain and their willingness and readiness to change how they cope when these thoughts and emotions rise. Many patients with persistent pain do not receive a psychosocial evaluation and are not offered a cognitive–behavioral approach to treatment. Those who do may not be ready to accept a pain approach that addresses cognitions, emotions, and behaviors or to make the changes necessary to gain control of their thoughts and emotions and improve function and ultimately relieve their pain. The psychosocial evaluation for a dominating affective pain mechanism consists of three parts: (1) education on and assessment of readiness to change, (2) use of screening tools, and (3) assessment of coping strategies.

Readiness to Change Education and Assessment

Clinicians generally agree that patients' taking responsibility for their recovery is critical to their success. Some patients admit they are not ready to assume responsibility, and others hide their lack of readiness behind many facets of their lives and behaviors. Patients may vocalize that they are ready to get better but are unwilling to make the changes necessary to do so. Recovery from musculoskeletal pain requires patients to change their habits, which involves acceptance of the need to do things differently.

Evaluation of the patients' readiness to change precedes all further evaluation and intervention. The section "Readiness for Treatment" in Chapter 3 reviews the six stages of readiness to change—precontemplation, contemplation, preparation, action, maintenance, and termination—and outlines evaluation strategies and associated clinician responses. The clinician asks questions and uses tools to help better understand each patient's readiness for change. If a patient is in the contemplation, preparation, or action stage of readiness to change his or her behavior, the clinician's use of psychosocial screening tools can help ensure that essential aspects of treatment and referrals for care occur.

Use of Psychosocial Screening Tools

Once the clinician has established the patients' level of readiness for change, the psychosocial evaluation can proceed. The clinician's first step is to assist patients in recognizing the relationship between negative emotions and thoughts and pain by introducing pain journaling. The negative emotions of anger, blame, hopelessness, sadness, shame, guilt, fear, anxiety, and depression trigger the nervous system to produce pain; however, patients rarely recognize these emotions and thoughts as contributing to their pain experience. The clinician may be able to coach patients in active coping strategies for some negative emotions, but he or she should be sensitive to the patients' need for additional psychological help and make referrals when necessary.

As noted in Chapter 3 (**Figure 3.2**), the patient can record in a journal when the pain is at its worst and best in three dimensions:

- **Mechanical.** What is the patient doing? Examples: sitting, standing, walking, reaching, cleaning, work tasks
- **Emotional.** How is the patient feeling? Examples: anxious, depressed, angry, hopeless, shameful, guilty, fearful, sad
- **Social.** Where is the patient, and whom is he or she with? Examples: at school, at home, at work, traveling to see mother-in-law, with an ex-spouse

The practical pain journal is not only an evaluation tool, but is also a form of treatment as patients begin to recognize the links between their symptoms and the mechanical, emotional, and social dimensions surrounding them. The goal of pain journaling is to clarify how the patients' pain connects to movement, negative emotions and thoughts, and social situations and to identify areas in which they can take more control. The practical pain journal can also be useful in identifying when pain is at its best; clinicians and patients often are surprised at the mechanical, emotional, and social triggers for feeling well.

When reviewing a practical pain journal with a patient, the clinician should ask, "Did you learn anything from your journal with respect to your pain?" This question helps the clinician understand how involved the patient is in the learning process. If the patient is able to identify trends in the emotional or social dimensions, the clinician asks the next questions: "How well are you coping with these negative emotions or social situations?" "What are your strategies to cope with these negative emotions or social situations?" "Do you want or need help coping with the emotions or social pressures you identified?" The last and often most important question is one clinicians ask of themselves: "Can I help and counsel this patient?"

As the clinician understands the patient's level of readiness to change and pain journal data, the negative emotions that are dominating the pain experience will become clearer. For example, the clinician may recognize from the journal that when the patient experiences intolerable pain, the mechanical and social dimensions are not consistent, but the emotional dimension is often characterized by anger, hopelessness, anxiety, or depression. If this is the case, the clinician can use a psychosocial screening tool to further understand the patient's emotions and to aid in decisions regarding referral to psychology. Five tools provide information that aids discussions about the need for a psychology evaluation or a cognitive–behavioral interdisciplinary program: (1) the PASS,[75] (2) the Patient Health Questionnaire (PHQ-9),[99,100] (3) the Fear-Avoidance Beliefs Questionnaire (FABQ),[101] (4) the Yellow Flag Risk Form,[102-104] and (5) a region-specific functional disability outcome measure.

Fear and anxiety have been linked to greater pain behavior and disability through psychophysiological mechanisms or through avoidance. The PASS, the most widely used measure of pain-related anxiety, has been shown to be robust across clinical and nonclinical samples[105] and has been used in taxometric assessments of the pain construct for a variety of impairments.[106] Subscales include Fear, Cognitive Anxiety, Escape/Avoidance, and Physiological Anxiety. Anxious behavior in the context of chronic pain entails negative responses such as inflated expectations of pain, which can result in reduced range of motion during physical activity, greater depression and general disability, decreased coping with pain, and increased days of work loss.[107] The PASS is a self-reported measure that consists of four 10-item subscales.[108] Individuals make a frequency rating for each item on the scale using a six-point Likert scale. Their response is to rate each item from 0 (*never*) to 5 (*always*).[107] Total scores can be between 0 and 200 points, and each subscale can range from 0 (*no pain-related anxiety*) to 50 (*maximum pain-related anxiety*). Higher scores reflect more symptoms of pain anxiety.[109] The Cognitive Anxiety subscale evaluates symptoms such as the inability to concentrate and the frequency of unwanted thoughts when the patient is in pain.[110] The Fear of Pain subscale measures frequency of thoughts provoking fear and a profound dread of negative consequences when the patient is in pain.[110] The Escape Avoidance subscale rates the frequency of behaviors aimed at minimizing the severity and duration of pain.[110] The Physiological-Anxiety subscale measures the patient's physical responses to pain, such as sweating or feeling dizzy.[110] No research has indicated a cutoff point for a total score or subscale scores as an indicator of various anxiety levels.

The PHQ-9 assists in the initial diagnosis and treatment of depression and the reassessment of the overall effectiveness of treatment. In addition, this tool can aid the clinician in understanding when normal sadness and clinical depression require formal treatment. The PHQ-9 helps the clinician assess symptoms and functional impairment to make a tentative diagnosis of major depressive disorder and derive a severity score to aid in selecting and monitoring treatment. The PHQ-9 is a self-administered version of the PRIME-MD diagnostic instrument for common mental disorders. PRIME-MD was an instrument developed and validated in the early 1990s to efficiently diagnose five of the most common types of mental disorders presenting in the medical population.[111] PHQ consists of five modules covering five common types of mental disorders: depression, anxiety, somatoform, alcohol, and eating.[111]

The purpose of the PHQ-9 is to improve the detection of major depressive disorder and as an assessment of severity of major depression in guiding treatment decisions.[99,111] The PHQ-9 has been validated for use in a variety of medical settings and the general population.[99,100,111] It consists of two components: assessing symptoms and functional impairment to make a tentative major depressive disorder diagnosis, and deriving a severity score to help select and monitor treatment.[99,111] The severity scores are interpreted as 0 to 4, none; 5 to 9, mild depression; 10 to 14, moderate depression (10 is the cutoff score for major depressive disorder); 15 to 19, moderately severe depression; 20 to 27, severe depression.[99] Recommendations for treatment vary based on total scores: 0 to 4, provide education; 5 to 9, provide support and education, recommend that the patient call if symptoms worsen, and recommend that patient return in 1 month for re-screening or re-screen in 2 weeks at physical therapy appointment; 10+, provide support and education, offer to refer the patient to an appropriate resource, determine the patient's preference for evaluation for counseling, medications, or both. If the patient declines the referral, the clinician should advise the patient to call if symptoms worsen and screen again in 2 weeks at the physical therapy appointment.[99]

The last item in the PHQ-9 asks the patients to rate whether within the past 2 weeks, they had thoughts that they would be better off dead or of hurting themselves.[99] If the patients respond positively, the clinician should follow up with the following questions: "Have you done anything to hurt yourself or have you tried to kill yourself?" "Do you feel like killing yourself now?" "Have you thought about how you might try to hurt yourself?" The clinician should use these questions to determine the patients' intent, their plans to attempt suicide, their access to means, and any safety measures (when the patients have these thoughts, do they tell anyone). The patients should be referred to appropriate resources or emergency room.

Evidence suggests that fear-avoidance beliefs may be the most important risk factor for recurrence of disability. The FABQ measures patients' fear of pain and resulting avoidance of activity. Fear-avoidance beliefs have been found to be predictive of future disability and work status even after controlling for pain duration and intensity and type of treatment received.[101] **Figure 6.4** provides the FABQ tool (scoring guidelines are provided in the section "Fear-Avoidance Beliefs Questionnaire" in Chapter 6).

The Yellow Flag Risk Form aids the clinician and patients in understanding the extent to which yellow flags are contributing to the patients' pain experience and the risk of continued pain-related disability. The Yellow Flag Risk Form also helps the clinician make informed comments regarding prognosis, determine the most appropriate interventions, and document patient progress or lack thereof with a reliable and valid measure. The clinician can use this tool in screening musculoskeletal pain patients for active yellow flags on the first visit to supplement the subjective pain evaluation questions and answers related to thoughts, beliefs, and cultural attitudes toward pain; past and current treatment effectiveness; and stage of readiness for change. If it becomes apparent during subsequent visits that a patient is not recovering and a more formal measure is needed, the Yellow Flag Risk Form is also an excellent reevaluation tool. The numbers of each response are added to derive a total score. The maximum score is 130 points. The higher the number, the greater the risk. Linton and Hallden[103,104,112] suggested a cutoff score of 50% (ie, ≥65 of 130 points) to indicate a high risk of chronic pain and disability. Recommended cutoff scores are as follows: under 55 points, low risk of chronic disability; 55 to 65 points, moderate risk of chronic disability; over 65 points, high risk of chronic pain and disability.

When yellow flag risk scores are high, the clinician should focus management on reducing the patients' dependency on medication and other passive forms of treatment, developing patients' self-treatment skills and encouraging an active patient role in self-care, referring the patients for a psychology evaluation, and providing counseling regarding contributing affective components. It is important for the clinician to reassure patients that yellow flags are not their fault and to suggest the need for additional support to maximize the likelihood of recovery.

Disability is the inability to perform activities of daily living. Functional disability is an outcome of paramount importance in charting the progress of a patient undergoing treatment for pain. Region-specific functional disability outcome measures assist the clinician in understanding limitations in the patients' function, allow for ongoing reassessment of functional training programs, and aid in clinical reasoning and assessment of treatment effectiveness. The following region-specific outcome measures are recommended:

- The Oswestry Disability Index[113] measures disability resulting from lumbar spine pain.
- The Neck Disability Index[114] measures disability resulting from cervical spine pain.
- The Disabilities of the Arm, Shoulder and Hand Questionnaire[115] measures disability resulting from upper extremity problems.
- The Lower Extremity Functional Scale[116] measures disability resulting from lower extremity problems.

Assessment of Coping Strategies

An affective pain mechanism evaluation is not complete without an assessment of the patient's active and passive strategies for coping with the pain. Asking patients to describe how they cope with different emotions, thoughts, and functional loss allows clinicians to understand the patients' coping style and it effectiveness. Unhealthy forms of coping include the following:

- *Anxious coping* is the use of cognitive distortions that maintain the exaggerated apprehension seen in generalized anxiety and fear-based avoidance disorders.
- *Defensive coping* is the use of excuses and assumptions, usually by people prone to irritation, hostility, passive aggression, or anger.
- *Depressed coping* is the use of rumination, indifference, and learned helplessness to follow illogical beliefs that unsolvable problems will persist.
- *Internalization* is the direction of negative feelings inward in ways that are not evident to others, often resulting in stress-related symptoms (eg, pain, fight-or-flight reactions, immune symptoms) that interfere with healthy coping.
- *Escape* through food and substances is the use of carbohydrate-rich foods (which contain serotonin), fatty foods (which contain dopamine), or sweet foods or substances such as opiates or alcohol to forget stressors.
- *Entrapment* is the continued use of ineffective strategies for self-distraction (eg, obsessions, compulsions, excessive guilt, self-doubt, work, perfectionism) to avoid confronting key issues.

Healthy forms of coping include the following:

- *Objectifying problems* is redirecting thoughts and emotions away from personal issues to define the key issues, which aids in the development of self-awareness of the problem.
- *Identifying illogic* is recognizing automatic thoughts and thought distortions that maintain maladaptive moods.
- *Reframing beliefs* is reinterpreting automatic thoughts and the emotions they evoke.
- *Listening to the body* is connecting stress-related symptoms with the emotional triggers that initiate them and replacing low-energy with higher energy physical activity.
- *Restoring meaning* is connecting health with core beliefs and a sense of purpose and acceptance and finding the meaning in their suffering.
- *Applying positive psychology* is discovering and applying one's strengths or spiritual beliefs to find effective ways to work through key issues.

Unhealthy forms of coping can be a major limiting factor to a person's success with rehabilitation. Pain management, restoration of function, and improvement in quality of life involve changing unhealthy forms of coping to healthy forms. One cannot unlearn a motor behavior, but one can choose to change an unhealthy habit through practice. Often, patients are not aware of their unhealthy coping strategies, and when the clinician identifies a strategy as unhealthy, patients may be reluctant to change it. Challenging patients to identify and classify their own coping strategies as unhealthy or healthy can help them understand the overall effect of each strategy on their pain and help them develop solutions to enable change. Sometimes simply identifying cause and effect can be the motivation a patient needs to commit to changing. This method is called "catch and correct"; the more the patient catches and correct, the more he or she wins.

Clinician intervention begins with helping patients to identify unhealthy forms of coping and to develop healthy forms of coping. The emphasis in intervention is on recognizing unhealthy behaviors and coaching patients to embrace healthy ways of living and behaving. **Table 7.2** lists the subjective and objective characteristics of patients with the affective pain

TABLE 7.2 Subjective and Objective Characteristics of the Affective Pain Mechanism

Characteristic	Findings for Affective Pain	
	Conscious	**Unconscious**
Subjective		
Location	Widespread, nonanatomical distribution	Axial low back pain, neck pain, headaches, knee pain (specific location)
Frequency	Constant, spontaneous, latent, paroxysmal	Intermittent
Descriptors	Catastrophic, emotional language	Dull, tight, weak, sharp with movement
Intensity	High severity, irritability	Low-grade irritant
Onset	Chronic, >3 months past expected tissue healing and pathology recovery times; disproportionate to the nature and extent of injury or pathology	
History	Failed interventions (medical, surgical, therapeutic); preexisting anxiety, depression, or psychological trauma (eg, abuse, accident, work-related injury); central nervous system disorder (eg, spinal cord injury, multiple sclerosis)	Failed interventions (medical, surgical, therapeutic); increased stress or repressed negative emotions regarding current life pressures or childhood relationships with parents and siblings; perfectionism
24-hour behavior	Inconsistent; night pain and disturbed sleep are common	
Psychosocial screen	Positive for negative emotions; altered family, work, or social life; medical conflict; high functional disability	Appear negative on conscious level
Objective		
	Similar to central sensitization, with greater emotional component	Similar to ischemia; past treatment ineffective; tender points at upper trapezius, lumbar paraspinals, posterior and lateral glutei bilaterally
Yellow flag assessment	Positive for distress and other negative emotions (eg, depression, anxiety, anger); altered family, work, or social life; medical conflict; reduced coping skills with life-changing events (eg, spinal cord injury, loss, amputation, neurological impairment)	Appear negative on conscious level but positive for increased stress, repressed negative emotions regarding current life stressors and childhood relationships with parents and siblings, and characteristics of perfectionism
Screening tools	Assist referral to a cognitive–behavioral program • Yellow Flag Risk Form: Chronic disability risk assessment • Fear-Avoidance Beliefs Questionnaire score: Physical Activity • Patient Health Questionnaire: Anger/Depression • Pain Anxiety Symptom Scale: Anxiety	Assist referral to psychology • Yellow Flag Risk Form: Chronic disability risk assessment • Fear-Avoidance Beliefs Questionnaire score: Physical Activity • Patient Health Questionnaire: Anger/Depression • Pain Anxiety Symptom Scale: Anxiety • Tension myositis syndrome information (eg, Figure 7.1)

mechanism. **Appendices 7.E** and **7.F** provide a comparison among all three central pain mechanisms for subjective and objective characteristics.

Intervention to Address the Affective Pain Mechanism

The affective pain mechanism is dominated by psychosocial factors, and patients with this mechanism must change the cognitive, emotional, and behavioral dimensions of their pain to improve their quality of life. Behavior management, or changing behavior in relation to a certain problem, must come from within the person with the problem. The clinician's recommendations are beneficial only to the extent that the patients recognize them as beneficial and act on them. Three key techniques are used in interventions with patients with a dominating affective pain mechanism: (1) the biopsychosocial approach, (2) motivational interviewing, and (3) nonpharmacy approaches to pain.

Biopsychosocial Approach

The affective pain mechanism is best managed using a biopsychosocial approach. The biopsychosocial model of pain is an alternative to the predominant biomedical model, which can provide no further benefit to patients with dominating affective pain mechanism. The biomedical model of pain, which is held by many medical doctors, therapists, chiropractors, and even patients with chronic pain, views pain as explainable solely in biological, pathoanatomical, or medical terms related to the body. The biomedical model acknowledges that mental or emotional problems may result from chronic pain but maintains that the pain itself is entirely biological in origin and is referred from the body. The biomedical model also assumes that the only truly effective treatment for pain involves medical approaches directed at the body.

According to the biopsychosocial model, it is impossible to fully understand the problem of pain using physical or medical concepts alone. Unlike the biomedical model, which separates body and mind, the biopsychosocial model is a holistic perspective in which mind and body are seen as intertwined and pain is considered an output of the brain and mind with respect to perceived threats to the body. For patients with the affective pain mechanism, the clinician must take into account not only the biological, but also the cognitive, emotional, psychological, social, and nutritional factors involved. Biopsychosocial interactions of pain have been represented in the onion skin model, attributed to Loeser[117] and Waddell[118]:

- At the core of the onion is *nociception*, or the physical sensations that make up the experience of pain. Nociception can be described in four key dimensions (see "Subjective Evaluation" section of Chapter 4): (1) location (where on the body pain is experienced), (2) intensity (strength of the pain, ranging from mild to excruciating), (3) quality or description (what the sensations feel like, eg, sharp, aching, burning), and (4) time or frequency (how the sensations vary over time, ie, constant vs intermittent).
- The layer covering the core of the onion represents *attitudes and beliefs,* or the cognitive state of awareness of pain. Attitudes and beliefs involve the patients' attention to and memories of pain and other experiences. Patients' expectations regarding the pain condition and their ability to cope with it, their perceptions of ongoing life events, thoughts that accompany their emotions, decision-making processes, and attitudes toward themselves and others are intertwined. What the patients understand and believe to be true regarding the pain message and experience forms their pain

construct and answers the question, What does the pain message mean, and how threatening is it?
- The third layer from the center is *psychological distress,* or the negative emotional states that accompany the experience of pain (eg, fear, anxiety, worry, discouragement, depression, despair, shame, guilt, anger, irritability, hostility, hopelessness) and the effects of pain on the patients' lives.
- The fourth layer from the center is *illness behavior,* or actions in response to the experience of pain, ongoing emotional states, and consequences of pain in the patients' lives. Illness behavior also includes physical activities and social interactions that affect pain intensity and influence pain-related thoughts and emotions.
- The outside layer of the onion is the *physical and social environment.* The physical environment consists of all aspects of the patients' surroundings that affect their awareness of pain and ability to cope with it (eg, weather, housing, physical objects such as beds and chairs, availability of money and other material resources, means of transportation). The social environment consists of the people, entities, and places that affect and are affected by the pain condition, including family, friends, employers, coworkers, lawyers, health care settings, and the disability compensation system.

The clinician needs to consider each of these elements in every aspect of the care that he or she delivers to a patient. Each element interacts with and is influenced by all other elements. Interactions among these elements can create vicious cycles. For example, pain sensations (nociception) often result in decreased physical activity (an illness behavior). Decreased physical activity can create feelings of depression (psychological distress) and decreased self-worth (attitudes and beliefs). Depression can lead to decreased motivation, initiative, and further decreases in activity levels (illness behavior). Decreased activity and withdrawal from other people (social and physical environment) increase depression (psychological distress) and preoccupation with negative thoughts (attitudes and beliefs) and increase awareness of pain (nociception), leading to a renewed cycle of pain and negative consequences. Even though it is difficult to directly control painful physical sensations and negative emotional reactions, the clinician can help the patients recognize and understand their pain and convince them to alter thinking, change behaviors, and take appropriate actions with the help of a cognitive–behavioral pain management program or techniques.

The clinician is equipped to promote the patients' readiness to change. Evaluation starts with a mutual understanding of the patients' ability to benefit from specific, detailed education about their condition. Research has shown that both health professionals and patients are able to understand the neurophysiology of pain, but many health professionals underestimate patients' ability to understand.[96] This underestimation may be a primary barrier to patients' reconceptualization of the problem in terms of CNS pain mechanisms; clinicians who believe that their patients will not understand the information may not include it in their management or prevention approach. The same research showed that psychologists who explicitly targeted patients' reconceptualization of the problem underestimated patient ability by a greater amount than any other professional group.[96] Failure to provide accurate information probably also limits efficacy of treatment.

Conceptualization of chronic pain in terms of a biomedical, structural pathology model has been found to exacerbate patients' pain experience,[119] and provision of information based on the biomedical model increases health care consumption.[120] In contrast, providing current, accurate information about the neurophysiology of pain reduces patients' inappropriate beliefs and attitudes about pain[101] and, when combined with physiotherapy, it improves functional and symptomatic parameters in people with chronic disabling pain.[121]

Educational strategies focusing on current, accurate information about the behavioral response to pain have also demonstrated effectiveness in both a management and a prevention context for chronic musculoskeletal pain.[122-124] **Figure 6.7** provides patient education material explaining persistent pain related to CNS mechanisms. **Figure 7.2** is a patient education handout explaining the continuum of pain mechanisms from mechanical to psychological to autonomic and the need to identify the dominant mechanism to direct treatment. Often this handout helps patients understand the types of treatments they received and gives them a better explanation for why they did not work to resolve their symptoms. It also assists patients in self-diagnosis of their dominating mechanism as they rule out the interventions that did not work and why, while simultaneously explaining what mechanisms have not been addressed and their effect on the pain experience.

Motivational Interviewing

The focus of motivational interviewing is on strengthening the factors or processes that prompt behavior change. Different theoretical perspectives posit different precursors to change, with self-efficacy, social support, decisional processes, and perceived relevance or vulnerability identified as most important. In recent decades, the importance of motivation in promoting health behavior change and skills has received increased research attention.

In an important contribution to the research about health-related behavior change, Rollnick and Miller[125] investigated the impact of clinicians' behaviors on patients' motivation and participation in behavior change and developed the technique of motivational interviewing. Motivational interviewing is a directive, patient-centered counseling style for eliciting behavior change by helping patients explore and resolve ambivalence.[126] Because of its focus on preparing people for behavior change, motivational interviewing has an important role in health behavior interventions.[127] It is guided by five general principles[126]:

1. Expressing empathy through the use of reflective listening
2. Highlighting discrepancies between the client's goals and current problem behavior through the use of reflective listening and objective feedback
3. Avoiding argumentation by assuming that the client is responsible for the decision to change
4. Rolling with resistance rather than confronting or opposing it
5. Supporting the patients' self-efficacy and optimism for change

This approach influences the decision-making process by actively engaging patients in an evaluation of their behavior and exploration of ways to change the balance between the positive and negative aspects of change.[128]

Motivational interviewing varies significantly from traditional health education approaches in which facts and their interpretation are combined into a single message provided by the clinicians, who are considered the experts, to the patients, who are the targets of the advice being imparted; the patients either accept the advice or resist it consciously or unconsciously through lack of adherence to the recommendations. In contrast, the motivational interviewing approach places patients in the role of expert, and they must decide whether the information they receive is relevant to their situation and how to interpret and integrate the information. Clinicians alter their own agenda on the basis of the patients' agenda for each session and change their interviewing style from an interrogation to a meaningful conversation.

FIGURE 7.2 Musculoskeletal Pain Mechanisms Patient Education Handout

Musculoskeletal pain mechanisms occupy a continuum from mechanical mechanisms to psychological or central nervous system mechanisms:

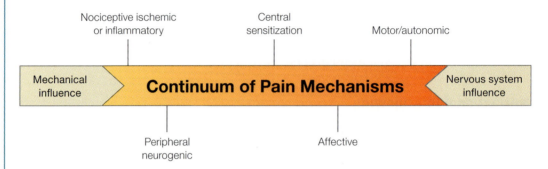

Mechanical mechanisms are structural and pathoanatomical; they originate in the body. Central mechanisms are emotional, social, cognitive, and/or behavioral; they originate in the brain.

The diagnostic tests your clinician conducts will help him or her to determine how many mechanisms of pain are present and which one is dominating before deciding on a treatment approach. For mechanical mechanisms, the treatment approach addresses the body and includes education, movement, and specific exercise. The treatment approach for psychological mechanisms addresses the brain and includes education, coping and relaxation strategies, and certain functional activities based on each patient's needs.

MECHANICAL MECHANISMS: BODY

There are two mechanical pain mechanisms: inflammation and ischemia. These mechanisms can also be directed at the peripheral nerve simultaneously and are better represented using the classification of peripheral neurogenic.

1. *Inflammation* is caused by too much fluid in the tissues. Red light activities that produce pain may worsen your condition by causing reinjury and should be avoided.
    - Chemical treatments your clinician may prescribe include rest, ice, compression, medication, and/or injections if injury has occurred. For flare-ups, which are caused by too much, too fast of certain activities resulting in pain but no reinjury, ice will help. Return to pre–flare-up activities and then attempt to progress with less vigor.
    - Mechanical treatment your clinician may perform includes establishing whether a preferred direction of movement exists that reduces your pain. If necessary, your clinician will refer you for surgery if structural mechanisms dominate your pain.

2. *Ischemia* is caused by lack of sufficient blood flow and oxygen to the tissues. Green light activities may produce pain but will leave you feeling no worse as a result. This type of pain is safe and necessary to stimulate your tissues to get better. Often clinicians prescribe movements that provoke and increase the symptoms in an effort to remodel tissue to a higher level of function and decrease its sensitivity. This may

occur at the final stages of healing following an injury or in an effort to create a more efficient environment for movement.
- Injury: Remodel tight, weak tissue back to health
- Function restoration: Apply physics to create more efficiency with movement patterns.

CENTRAL NERVOUS SYSTEM MECHANISMS: BRAIN

There are three central nervous system pain mechanisms: central sensitization, affective, and motor/autonomic.

1. *Central sensitization* occurs when the pain alarm system in your brain is stuck in overprotective mode. When you misinterpret the meaning of your pain as harmful or have negative thoughts about healing tissues (eg, I'll never get better; Pain means I'm causing tissue damage), that keeps your alarm system sensitive and is an active trigger to your pain. Thoughts of harm trigger this mechanism. Treatment includes education and the paced return of activities that cause fear or are perceived as harmful. Emphasis of education should be the fear of injury, movement, returning to life, and its contributing factors.

2. The *affective* pain mechanism is caused by psychological, social, and emotional factors that are involved in producing and maintaining pain. Both the conscious and unconscious mind may be involved and dominating, and treatment may require different psychology interventions or isolated cognitive–behavioral therapy.
    - Conscious mind refers to how pain is connected to how we think, cope, and behave—elements that we are consciously aware of. In these situations, an interdisciplinary cognitive–behavioral program is the best use of resources for intervention.
    - Unconscious mind refers to how pain is connected to feelings and emotions we may not be aware of. These repressed emotions include feelings of inferiority, sadness, anger, guilt, shame, and fear. These often stem from current and past life pressures, childhood relationships and experiences, and the trait of perfectionism or the "perfect-good drive." In these situations, an investigative psychology approach is best for helping patients become more aware of these negative emotions and to learn strategies to acknowledge and redirect them.

3. In the *motor/autonomic* pain mechanism, the brain is forgetting the body. In this mechanism, the area in the brain that represents the "body map" is in a state of dysfunction. The symptoms are related to that misrepresentation or lack or recognition occurring in the brain. The intervention involves a process of remodeling the brain's body map to recognize the body part in question.
    - Re-imaging the body image of disfigurement by using imagery, sensory, and motor exercises for the brain.
    - Re-establishing left–right discrimination using reflection in mirrors, tactile and visual awareness, and sensory and motor exercises for the brain. The intervention involves a very specific protocol.

Motivational interviewing has benefited from the concept of readiness to change, which has proved clinically useful in guiding clinicians to avoid patients' resistance: If the clinician assumes that the patient has greater readiness to change than he or she actually has, resistance will be a predictable outcome. Monitoring of readiness on an ongoing basis can thus form the platform for any derivative of motivational interviewing. Rollnick and Miller[125] argued that the quality of the patient–therapist interaction may be the key to behavior change. The spirit behind motivational interviewing involves the following concepts[127]:

- Readiness to change is not a patient trait, but a fluctuating product of interpersonal interaction.
- The therapeutic relationship functions best as a partnership rather than an expert–patient relationship.
- Motivation to change should be elicited from the patient, not imposed by the clinician.
- It is the patient's task, not the clinician's, to articulate and resolve his or her own ambivalence. But the clinician is directive in helping the patient examine and resolve ambivalence.
- Direct persuasion, in which the expert presents rational arguments for change to the patient, is not an effective method for resolving ambivalence.
- The counseling style is generally quiet and eliciting.

Figure 7.3 provides a history and overview of motivational interviewing.

Nonpharmacy Approaches to Pain

The nonpharmacy interventions to address a dominant affective pain mechanism include sleep restoration, relaxation training, active exercise, and diet. These principles are active, nonpharmaceutical ways to restore health and are typically not the first options offered in the current health care system.

Sleep Restoration

Sleep is a dynamic process. The brain is active during sleep; it responds to internal rather than external stimuli as it drifts in and out of the sleep stages. As noted in the section "Insomnia" in this chapter, the natural sleep pattern is to progress from light sleep, when one can be woken easily, through deepening non-REM sleep into the REM stage, when heavy sleep allows maximum restorative hormone flow, balancing of brain chemicals, and cellular repair.[129] The cycling of non-REM into REM sleep is repeated throughout the night, with each complete cycle lasting approximately 90 minutes.[129] Waking up naturally involves letting the stages reach completion, and after a period of REM sleep, one wakes feeling rested.

FIGURE 7.3 History and Overview of Motivational Interviewing

Motivational interviewing was developed by specialists in the addictions field who were focused on the problem of alcoholism. In traditional treatment for alcoholism, it was common for counselors and clients to disagree about the nature and extent of the clients' problems and the best course of treatment. For example, a persuasive statement from the counselor, such as, "Can't you see that your drinking is seriously damaging your marriage?" was typically met with a response like, "Yes, but it's not my drinking that's the problem; it's because my wife [or husband]…." Traditional treatment paradigms viewed this kind of interaction as a function of client characteristics such as being in denial or being resistant. Inherent in this approach were several incorrect assumptions regarding behavior change that threatened to jeopardize the quality of a therapeutic interaction.[1]

William R. Miller,[2] the originator of motivational interviewing, critically examined the causes of such disagreements between clients and counselors using a more client-centered analysis. He found that client resistance was in fact the product of interaction with a counselor who used a confrontational interviewing style. Miller suggested that rather than trying to convince clients to change, counselors would be more effective if they elicited arguments for change from the clients themselves.

A key component of such an approach is an empathic therapeutic style. Several studies have supported the contention that therapist behaviors influence treatment outcomes.[2-4] For example, one study found that the more counselors confronted clients about their drinking, the more clients drank at follow-up.[3] This work raises the hypothesis that confrontation may have a deleterious impact on self-efficacy, whereas an empathic style may support and build self-efficacy.

Miller and Rollnick[5] also observed that clinicians and trainers can become too focused on matters of technique and lose sight of the style that is central to this approach. Rollnick and Miller[6] argued that it is inappropriate to think of motivational interviewing as a technique to be applied to a group of people; rather, it is an interpersonal style shaped by the guiding principles of what triggers behavior change. A key distinction between motivational interviewing and other clinical approaches is that, in whatever form it takes, motivational interviewing will not work well if it is conceived as a cookbook approach or as a set of techniques that is applied to clients. The most important issue is whether the spirit of the method is being adhered to, particularly related to allowing clients to express their own arguments for their readiness to change.

In health care settings, clinicians are likely to encounter people with an array of problems, including those with multiple health issues and coexisting psychiatric disorders. Strategies for adapting motivational interviewing for people who have comorbidities or dual diagnoses have been proposed.[7] In particular, it has been suggested that treatment approaches with such clients may need to focus on a harm-reduction approach,[8,9] which is highly compatible with the self-determination philosophy of motivational interviewing. As suggested by social learning theory, client involvement in goal setting, regardless of the nature or number of presenting problems, is likely to be the main element in an effective therapeutic working relationship.[10]

Competence in using skills such as open- and closed-ended questions, reflective listening, and summarizing of client statements is essential to the success of motivational

(continues on next page)

> **FIGURE 7.3** History and Overview of Motivational Interviewing
>
> *(continued from previous page)*
>
> interviewing in the health care setting. It is also important to remember that motivational interviewing is directive: The clinician is both directive in focusing on particular questions and client-centered in eliciting a response to them. Specific exercises for training in these skills are described in the literature.[5]
>
> **Resources**
> 1. Rollnick S, Mason P, Butler C. *Health Behavior Change: A Guide for Practitioners*. Edinburgh, Scotland: Churchill Livingstone; 1999.
> 2. Miller W. Motivational interviewing with problem drinkers. *Behav Psychother*. 1983;11:147-172.
> 3. Miller W, Benefield R, Tonigan S. Enhancing motivation for change in problem drinking: A controlled comparison of two therapist styles. *J Consult Clin Psychol*. 1993;61:455-461.
> 4. Miller W. *The Addictive Behaviors: Treatment of Alcoholism, Drug Abuse, Smoking, and Obesity*. New York: Pergamon Press; 1980.
> 5. Miller W, Rollnick S. *Motivational Interviewing: Preparing People to Change Addictive Behaviors*. New York: Guilford Press; 1991.
> 6. Rollnick S, Miller W. What is motivational interviewing? *Behav Cog Psychother*. 1995;23:325-334.
> 7. Smyth N. Motivating persons with dual disorders: A stage approach. *Fam Soc*. 1996;77:605-614.
> 8. Carey KB. Substance use reduction in the context of outpatient psychiatric treatment: A collaborative, motivational, harm reduction approach. *Community Ment Health J*. 1996;32:291-306.
> 9. Marlatt GA. Harm reduction: Come as you are. *Addict Behav*. 1996;21:779-788.
> 10. Bandura A. *Social Foundations of Thought and Action: A Social Cognitive Theory*. Englewood Cliffs, NJ: Prentice-Hall; 1986.

The number of hours accumulated does not dictate sleeping success. Many experts report that for a person to feel refreshed, the number of complete sleep stages achieved is more important than the total sleep time.[129] Ideal sleep stages are a delicate process guided by hormone flows that can be disturbed by outside influences. Cortisol levels are reactive to light, gradually increasing in the morning to help people start their day. Melatonin release is activated by darkness, and levels of growth hormone and other restorative substances achieve their highest levels during deepest sleep. Artificial light, including light from digital screens, interrupts the circadian rhythm, as seen in the late-night habits of many patients with chronic pain, creating hormonal stresses and imbalances that interfere with metabolism, cognitive function, mood stability, and overall enjoyment of life.[129] The simple solution of regulating bed and wake times helps regulate cortisol production, which is essential for good health. Ten strategies can help patients optimize the quality of their sleep:

1. Create an ideal sleeping environment.
2. Maintain consistent bed and wake times.
3. Cool down at night and warm up while waking.
4. Make healthy food and drink choices.
5. Take early and short naps.
6. Improve sleep time to 7 to 8 hours.
7. Avoid warm baths before bedtime.
8. Exercise.
9. Take vitamins.
10. Maintain hormone balance.

Figure 7.4 is a patient education handout that provides details about each strategy.

FIGURE 7.4 Active Sleep Restoration Strategies Patient Education Handout

Sleep Restoration

Sleep cycle restoration has two components: (1) the ability to fall asleep and (2) the ability to stay asleep, allowing one to achieve the deep sleep needed for metabolic repair. *Crashing* is defined as the ability to fall asleep but not stay asleep. Crashing is an adrenaline response behavior that increases brain activity and does not allow deeper levels of sleep. Many behaviors feed a more active brain at night and do not allow deep sleep to occur.

These 10 simple strategies for sleep cycle restoration are based on behaviors needed to decrease metabolic and brain activity toward the end of the day to restore your ability to stay asleep and achieve deep sleep.

1. Create an ideal sleep environment. It is critical to make your bedroom an area of minimum stimulation and maximum relaxation. Your bedroom should be used only for sleeping, with no computer, television, or work desk present. It is desirable to have complete physical and psychological separation between your bedroom and other areas of the house where you do your work or enjoy entertainment. Eliminate clutter such as excessive clothing, books, magazines, and items on your bedside table such as car keys, cell phone, mail, or even spare change that could possibly interfere with your intention to sleep.

2. Maintain consistent bed and wake times. Structured sleepers achieve deep sleep sooner and stay in deep sleep longer than irregular sleepers. Just as with exercise, quality is more important than quantity. Establish a consistent, circadian-friendly routine to optimize hormone flows and ensure that you enjoy complete sleep stages. Melatonin floods your bloodstream on circadian cues triggered by darkness, and making your room dark (eg, when you turn out the light on your bedside table, when the sun sets if you are camping) helps you experience the highest percentage of deep sleep at the outset of the night.

If you go to bed late, sleeping in to reach your typical hourly total will not completely catch you up. If you are a night owl, however, you can probably develop some level of tolerance for a consistent, artificial light-induced late-night bedtime and late-morning awakening. A late sleeping schedule, if consistent, is less stressful to the body than the more common practice of a fluctuating bedtime. People with irregular bedtimes typically fight the natural melatonin release with various artificial stimuli (eg, TV, movies, computer, caffeine). The more artificial light and stimulation you throw into your circadian equation, the further you get from your body's natural restorative ability.

3. Cool down at night and warm up while waking. Because any time after sundown is time to prepare for sleep, it is important to wind down calmly in the hours preceding your bedtime. Minimize stimulation to your central nervous system before going to bed so you can have a smooth, relaxing transition from your busy day to downtime.

Reading is a time-tested and popular method to wind down, but choose the subject matter carefully. Avoid reading the newspaper, anything related to work, and nonfiction. Promote maximum relaxation of the mind using a self-help book, or stick with fiction for leisure reading. You may also find it helpful to decompress the busy brain by writing down your thoughts before bedtime.

(continues on next page)

FIGURE 7.4 Active Sleep Restoration Strategies Patient Education Handout

(continued from previous page)

Take 5 to 10 minutes to write out everything about your day: accomplishments, to-do tasks, stresses, and worries, but try to end on a positive thought. It is easier to arrive at solutions to problems if you don't try consciously to force them. Get them down on paper, and then let your sleeping mind do the work for you. You'll wake up feeling clearer and more positive.

In the morning, awaken gradually and naturally, coming off a complete REM-dominant sleep stage. Staying in bed a few minutes to read or talk or to do light breathing or meditation exercises or stretches is preferable to springing up after the fourth snooze alarm and rushing into action. A brief warm shower can help stimulate your central nervous system naturally and get blood circulating and is preferable to a high-carbohydrate breakfast and cup of coffee as a morning energizer.

4. Make healthy food and drink choices. What you eat and drink 2 to 3 hours before bed can have a significant impact, either positive or negative, on your ability to achieve restful sleep. In contrast to the social norm of eating sugary foods and taking a sleep medication, it is better to eat lightly before bed so that blood sugar fluctuations and potential digestive complications from lying down with a full stomach do not interfere with your sleep process. If you are a wine drinker, one glass with dinner may help you relax and unwind in the evening hours. The same goes for herbal teas; chamomile in particular is touted for its mild sedative effect. A handful of nuts can also be helpful, thanks to the ample levels of magnesium, which helps relax muscles, and L-tryptophan, which promotes the production of serotonin, the potent neurotransmitter that becomes melatonin as darkness triggers sleep. Other tryptophan-rich foods that can be eaten in moderation before bed are eggs, meat, fish, and cheese.

Avoid the conventional wisdom and social norms advising carbohydrates and ice cream as a bedtime aid. Carbohydrates and dairy overload promote an energy boost by increasing the insulin cascade that follows digestion of carbohydrates and high-sugar foods. Also avoid drinking caffeine within 8 hours before bedtime.

5. Take early and short naps. If you are able to obtain all of your required sleep at night, you'll probably have no reason to take naps during the day. However, many patients with chronic pain face obstacles (eg, job requirements, young children, noisy surroundings) to attaining adequate sleep levels. Napping can help you sustain the focus, energy, and productivity you need for an active life. Many cultures incorporate nap time into their daily schedule. Furthermore, most mammals have multiple sleep-wake sessions throughout the day. Unfortunately, the fast pace of modern life prevents napping from being a widespread lifestyle habit.

Because the rhythm of sleep stages is so critical to brain and body restoration, brief naps can produce remarkable benefits by helping you catch up on non-REM sleep stage deficiencies, shortcutting you into the deep sleep stages characterized by theta brain waves. A nap period of 20–30 minutes is sufficient to recalibrate your brain's sodium-to-potassium ratio, a critical factor in recovery from nervous system fatigue, and allows you to wake up feeling refreshed without producing the unpleasant grogginess that follows a prolonged siesta.

6. Improve sleep time to 7 to 8 hours. A large body of research has established that persons who sleep 7 to 8 hours a night live longer, healthier lives. You will discover your ideal sleep time based on how you feel the next day. If you feel rested, you achieved deep sleep for long enough; if you feel tired, you are either not sleeping enough or are sleeping too much.

7. Avoid warm baths before bedtime. If you need to relax, a lukewarm shower or bath is far more productive than a warm bath in preparing the brain to sleep. Increased warmth of water increases the temperature of the body, which increases metabolic activity. The cooler the water, the lower the metabolic activity.

8. Exercise. Exercise helps restore sleep cycles. A healthy, active body needs more than 10,000 steps per day to stimulate weight loss; the American Heart Association recommends that 2,500 to 4,000 of those steps be brisk. A pedometer that counts your accumulated steps per day can help you achieve a healthy level of exercise.

9. Take vitamins. Vitamins are necessary to aging gracefully. Staying fit and active requires supplementing the human body's essential vitamins and minerals. Consult your doctor about necessary vitamins; a multivitamin once a day is a good place to start.

10. Maintain hormone balance. Hormones change with maturity. Women may need to consult their doctors to achieve healthy estrogen levels to assist metabolic activity. Progesterone imbalance may also contribute to sleep disturbances.

Relaxation Training

The brain's pain control center is stronger than any known drug or modality. The clinical question is how well the patient is using his or her own brain's pain control center. The clinician can begin to activate the descending inhibitory tracts of patients by educating them and helping them understand their dominating pain mechanism. He or she can also promote chronic pain self-management by teaching patients how to reduce the negative thoughts and feelings that arise in response to pain and stress. Negative thoughts and feelings such as frustration, anger, resentment, irritability, sadness, discouragement, shame, guilt, anxiety, worry, fear, and general unhappiness compound the problem of chronic pain by adding to patients' suffering and misery.

One set of useful tools to increase patients' ability to self-manage both chronic pain and the negative thoughts and feelings arising from stress and life pressures is relaxation. Relaxation does not come easily; it is a creative skill similar to learning to speak a new language or play a new instrument. Practice and desire increase skill and lead to ultimate success.

Clinicians should emphasize diaphragmatic breathing, a simple form of relaxation, as a "pain pill" to rid the mind of negative thoughts and decrease pain-producing outputs. Diaphragmatic breathing can be prescribed in terms of pill dosing, with one pill equivalent to six to 10 diaphragmatic breaths. Patients should take a "breathing pill" two to three times daily or when pain and emotional pressure are at intolerable levels. Diaphragmatic breathing should be the patients' first approach to alleviating pain rather than pain medication. This technique is an active, healthy coping strategy, as opposed to the passive strategy of pain medication, and demonstrates to patients their control over their pain and negative emotions. In addition, three other types of relaxation can be taught to patients: coping relaxation, time-out relaxation, and relaxing activities.[130]

Coping relaxation helps patients cope more effectively with stressful situations, emotional upset, and intense pain episodes at the moment they occur. Patients can use coping relaxation anywhere and any time they experience physical or emotional distress. It is accomplished by using a simple but powerful technique called *deep breath*.[130] The deep breath gives the patient an immediate experience of relaxation by creating a slight increase in tension by breathing in and then letting the tension go by breathing out. The clinician instructs the patient as follows:

- Take a deep breath, and hold it in for 3 to 4 seconds. If a deep inhalation is painful, modify its depth so it is not as uncomfortable.
- Exhale slowly while saying mentally calming words such as *relax, let go, easy does it, this too shall pass*, or any other words that suggest a release of tension.
- Also while exhaling, let the jaws, shoulders, and arms go loose or limp, especially where it hurts.
- Visualize a color, smell, or image that brings comfort to enhance the activation of the deep breath and its relaxation effects. What is visualized is unique to each person.

Self-reflection following a deep breath allows the patient to change the pain-related stimulus. Self-reflection may involve asking important questions. For example, if a patient is in the middle of a stressful situation or emotional upset, he or she can ask,

- What emotions am I feeling right now?
- What is it about this situation that triggered these upset feelings?
- Am I seeing this situation clearly, or am I distorting it?
- What is the smartest and wisest thing I can do right now to manage this situation? (This question does not ask what the patient *feels* like doing, which may get him or her in more trouble.)

- Can I do anything right now to constructively change the stressful situation, or do I need to regroup emotionally and deal with it at another time after I have had a chance to think about it?

During a chronic pain flare-up, patients can ask themselves the following questions:

- Can I identify the immediate cause or trigger of this intense pain episode? Did I overdo something physically? Did I use negative thinking regarding my situation, which can be just as problematic as activity? Am I under stress or dealing with a life pressure that I am not coping well with?
- Is there anything I can learn from this pain flare-up?
- What constructive actions (physical and mental) can I take right now that will help me decrease the pain's intensity or at least get me through this temporary episode until it eases up?

By linking the deep breath to this stop-and-think process, the patient increases awareness of the situation in the here and now. The deep breath is not meant to directly solve the problem, whether it is negative emotion or severe pain. Rather, the deep breath brings attention to the situation and to the trigger of the pain and stress. With attention, patients are able to see the situation and react to it from a position of calmness, rather than simply reacting in an automatic manner, in an attempt to change the pain neurosignature. The deep breath is aimed at helping patients think more clearly, enabling them to respond to the situation more wisely and constructively. The deep breath can be more effectively used in combination with time out relaxation.

Time-out relaxation requires patients to take time out of their day (5–30 minutes) to do a special relaxation exercise or meditation in a quiet place where they cannot be disturbed so they can devote their full attention to relaxing their minds and bodies as deeply as possible.[130] It requires a comfortable position in which the patient experiences the least amount of physical strain or fear. The patient directs the mind to a specific stimulus, physical or mental, that is conducive to deep relaxation. Some patients use a visual stimulus, such as a pretty picture, photograph, burning candle, or even a spot on the wall. Others use an auditory stimulus such as the sound of ocean waves, gentle rain, wind chimes, relaxing music, or chanting; others find mental thoughts to be effective. Some immerse themselves in prayer vigils.

The benefits of time-out relaxation can aid patients with chronic pain in many ways, including relaxing tense muscles, diverting attention, increasing awareness of tension, helping with sleep problems, and revealing a new perspective on pain. To benefit from time-out relaxation, patients must practice regularly. Deep relaxation is a skill, and like any other skill, it has to be learned. For some patients it comes easily, but for others, it takes more time and practice. The clinician should emphasize to the patients not to expect immediate, significant results. Patients should start practicing when their pain is less intense, allowing them to fully immerse themselves in the technique and to do it for its own sake rather than expecting results. Later, as patients become more skilled at relaxation, they can apply it to more difficult situations, such as when they are tired, tense, emotionally upset, or experiencing severe pain.

There is no single right or best way to do time-out relaxation. What ultimately matters is what works for the individual patient. Time-out relaxation improves pain symptoms, increases enjoyment and well-being, decreases feelings of depression, and provides respite from frustration, tension, and worry.[130] Some patients prefer approaches that focus on the body (eg, focused breathing), whereas others do better with mental imagery (eg, imagining a nature walk, praying). Clinicians should take the time to discover what their patients like.

There are many examples of relaxation exercises; tools provided in Chapter 6 (**Figures 6.8, 6.9,** and **6.10**) are a small sample of what is available. Relaxing activities, although they do not typically allow the deep relaxation achieved in time-out relaxation, are nevertheless valuable because they bring pleasure and pleasure often overrides pain. Ideally, patients should have or develop a variety of relaxing activities that take place indoors and outdoors, that are done alone and with other people, and that allow their body to be in different positions. Pleasure must drive patients' choices in relaxing activities. For example, some enjoy reading, whereas others enjoy home repairs, and some enjoy fishing and find it relaxing even if they do not catch anything. Clinicians need to understand what activities are meaningful and pleasurable to their patients not only to promote relaxation, but also to aid in restoring function.

Each type of relaxation is important in the overall self-management of CNS pain. Coaching patients to make the use of relaxation techniques a lifelong habit will help patients maintain their physical, mental, and emotional well-being. Relaxation techniques must be integrated into patients' life routine and meaningful activities if they are to become a habit. Most patients cannot spend the majority of each day relaxing; in fact, some patients with chronic pain spend far too much time sitting around and doing very little. The key is for patients to achieve a healthy balance between productive activity and relaxation.

Active Exercise

When pain is caused by CNS mechanisms, as it often is in chronic disorders, the importance of passive mobilization diminishes. With chronic pain, an active, education-based program is more effective, with a skilled physical examination and manual therapy being necessary only when patients plateau or appear to be dominated by mechanical pain mechanisms. The affective pain mechanism usually needs input to maintain sensitivity, and multiple sites of altered afferent input may require treatment, especially after trauma. Passive treatment is not offered as the primary management option or presented as the cure but rather is the last line of defense in managing the affective pain mechanism.

Many patients with a dominating affective pain mechanism have an unhealthy relationship with active movement; whether patients are generally deconditioned or seriously overtraining, movement in the form of exercise is not having the positive effects they desire. Patients with the affective pain mechanism do not need skilled exercise prescription like those with mechanical mechanisms, which require the clinician to guide the remodeling of specific functions or tight, weak tissue with specific directional exercise. Patients with the affective pain mechanism need an overhaul in basic fundamentals of movement. Three general strategies are the focus with respect to exercise: (1) pacing and progress toward the return of meaningful, pleasurable activity; (2) prevention of further injury by increasing strength and muscle mass; and (3) intermittent brief periods of fast activity to restore immune system health and boost metabolism.

Pacing and Progress Toward the Return of Meaningful Activity

Exercise physiologists have described the exercise of our early ancestors as having a very low level aerobic pace, as they hunted, gathered, foraged, wandered, scouted, migrated, climbed, and crawled.[129] This low level of activity prompted our ancestors' genes to build stronger capillary networks to provide oxygen and fuel to each muscle cell and readily convert stored fat into energy (fat is the main fuel used for low-level aerobic activity).[129] This daily movement also aided the development of strong bones, joints, and connective tissue. Modern patients either are too sedentary or do workouts that are too stressful and misaligned with genetic requirements for optimum health. What human bodies crave is frequent movement at a slow, comfortable pace, like walking, hiking, easy cycling, or other light aerobic activities with a heart rate range of 55% to 75% of maximum.[129] These efforts are far less taxing than the huffing-and-puffing, struggling-and-suffering exertion levels (above 75% of maximum heart rate) that some believe leads to fitness. The specific biochemical signals created by low-level aerobic activity produce numerous health and fitness benefits[129]:

- **Improved fat metabolism.** As long as one's diet is low in insulin-producing foods, low-level aerobic exercise trains the body to effectively burn fat for fuel, increasing metabolic rate (a benefit that lasts 24 hours per day), regulating appetite, and balancing blood sugar levels nonpharmaceutically.
- **Improved cardiovascular function.** Low-level aerobic exercise increases the small vessel capillary network, muscle mitochondria, heart stroke volume, and oxygen delivery by the lungs.
- **Improved musculoskeletal system.** Aerobic exercise strengthens bones, joints, and connective tissue, especially through its reparative and recovery functions.
- **Stronger immune system.** Aerobic exercise enhances immune function by stimulating beneficial hormone flow and building a more efficient circulatory system.
- **Increased energy.** Low-level aerobic exercise boosts energy and promotes a refreshed feeling, leaving one physically tired and prepared for sleep.

To ensure these systemic changes, the clinician needs to coach patients in finding ways to move more often in their everyday activities, such as parking farther away from building entrances, taking the stairs, and walking all aisles in the grocery store, and to take on new activities that make them feel good or appear fun. Patients should strive to accumulate 2 to 5 hours per week of low-level exercise.[129] More is always better with respect to low-intensity exercise. In addition, when possible, patients should perform low-level activities barefoot frequently to develop natural balance, flexibility, and leg strength. Patients' goals over time should be as follows:

- Accumulate a minimum of 2 hours to a maximum of 5 hours per week of fun low-level activity.
- Achieve a heart rate as low as 55% and as high as 75% of maximum heart rate (target heart rate for men is 220 − age × 55%–75% and for women is 206 − [88% of age] × 55%–75%).
- Take 10,000 steps per day. Pace it, don't race it, but achieve it!

These goals are easy to set but hard to get patients to own. The best way to monitor progress toward the goal of 10,000 steps per day is to use a pedometer.[131] All steps count, and the patients can focus on increasing the number of steps by doing fun activities. Again, the focus is not on how quickly or strenuously the steps are taken, but rather on how many steps the patient takes over time. This activity helps reset the body to convert stored fat as the main fuel source. **Figure 7.5** provides patient education and a log for measuring progress in a step program.

FIGURE 7.5 Steps Program Patient Education Handout

Establishing a Steps Program

HOW MANY STEPS SHOULD YOU TAKE?
Extensive research has provided recommendations for the number of steps per day a physically active person should take based on his or her age. A smaller body of research provides recommendations for people who have a disability or chronic disease to enable them to remain physically active and maintain a well body.

RECOMMENDED AVERAGE STEPS PER DAY[1]

8- to 10-year-old children:	12,000–16,000
Healthy younger adults:	7,000–13,000
Healthy older adults:	6,000–8,000
Adults with disability or disease:	3,500–5,500
Adults desiring to lose weight:	10,000 steps per day

The average American takes only 3,000 to 5,000 steps per day! A sedentary lifestyle can put you at risk for high blood pressure, high cholesterol, arthritis, diabetes, musculoskeletal pain, and obesity. Increasing your activity can reduce your chances of stroke, heart attack, diabetes, cancer, and chronic pain. Goal setting in chronic pain should assist patients in understanding and achieving health-related fitness relative to their age. The information below can assist clinicians and patients in using steps as a way to understand what those age-related fitness goals can be and guide them through stages of fair, good, and excellent fitness levels.

LONG-TERM FITNESS GOALS FOR HEALTHY ADULTS BY AGE

Fair physical activity

15–30 years:	7,500–10,000 steps per day
31–60 years:	5,000–10,000 steps per day
61–80 years:	3,000–6,000 steps per day

Good physical activity

15–30 years:	15,000–20,000 steps per day
31–60 years:	13,000–15,000 steps per day
61–80 years:	8,000–13,000 steps per day

Excellent physical activity

15–80 years:	20,000+ steps per day

To begin your steps program, calculate your baseline, or the number of steps you're taking per day before you begin the program, and set your walking goals. It is important to gradually increase your activity level weekly to add steps to your baseline. If you have pain or a condition (eg, heart disease) that may interfere with your activity tolerance, consult with a health professional to ensure that your steps program will safely improve your health.

To calculate your baseline:
A. Wear your pedometer every day for 1 week (7 days). Record your number of daily steps:

    Day 1 _____ Day 5 _____

    Day 2 _____ Day 6 _____

    Day 3 _____ Day 7 _____

    Day 4 _____

B. Total steps for the week: _____

C. Divide the total by 7: _____ = Baseline average steps per day

To calculate your daily goal:
Look at the number of steps you took each day for your first week. What was the highest number of steps you took in one day? Circle it, and use this number as your benchmark to set your daily goal. Try to keep your steps up to that number each day for the next week. Continue to record your steps in a daily log (see below for a suggested format for your daily log).

To upgrade your walking program:
When you have met your goal for 1 week, add 200 to 500 steps to your daily goal. Continue adding 200 to 500 steps to your goal each week, if you have met your previous week's goals, until you meet the recommended long-term goal for people of your age and health status. Your physical therapist can help you determine your long-term goal for a healthy lifestyle.

DAILY STEPS LOG

Monthly goal: _____		Write in your weekly goal below at the start of each week:
Date	No. of steps	Comments
Weekly average =		Weekly goal:

Resource
1. Tudor-Locke C. Taking steps toward increased physical activity: Using pedometers to measure and motivate. *Res Digest*. 2002;3(17):1-8.

Prevention of Further Injury by Increasing Strength and Muscle Mass

Life demands frequent bursts of intense physical effort, such as carrying grocery bags, lifting children into car seats, carrying laundry baskets up and down stairs, lifting gallons of milk or cases of wine, pushing lawn mowers or snow shovels, and raking leaves. Human beings were designed to lift heavy things. The biochemical signals triggered by brief but intense muscle contractions prompt improvements and adaptations in muscle tone, size, and power.[129] The benefits are an increase in strength and a decrease in risk of injury. A strength-training program featuring natural, total-body movements such as squats, lunges, push-ups and pull-ups, rowing, and overhead lifting helps develop and maintain lean muscle mass, increase metabolism to maintain low levels of body fat, increase bone density, improve balance, prevent injuries, and balance hormone and blood glucose levels.[129] Workouts of short duration (10–20 minutes), high intensity, and fairly regular frequency (two to three times per week) can produce these results.[117] Workouts that are too long and too frequent, that include exercises that are too similar, and that do not recognize naturally occurring heavy lifting during the course of everyday life may result in overtraining.

To ready a patient for everyday life, a workout routine should focus on exercises that engage a variety of muscles in real-life movement patterns. Squats, lunges, pull-ups, push-ups, waist-to-shoulder reaches, waist-to-overhead reaches, and asymmetrical one-hand carries are common functional exercises involving movements that occur in everyday life activities. A strength-training session should start with a brief warm-up of 2 minutes of, for example, push-ups, jumping jacks, jumping rope, or squatting to increase blood flow to the muscles and prepare for the intended activities. Movements are repeated with quality form at a comfortable pace through the full motion for the number of repetitions intended. Strength training recruits as many muscle fibers as possible to fully load the muscle and reach fatigue, triggering biochemical signals to grow stronger by recruiting new fibers.[129]

The clinician should recommend that patients work with weight equipment and focus on the large muscles of the body, chest, back, shoulders, buttocks, thighs, and calves working together to get the best metabolic value. Patients should lift comfortable weights for 12 repetitions each, two to three times per week. When patients can lift the weight 14 times, they are ready to safely increase the weight by 5% to 10%. Starting with 5% increases ensures a pace that minimizes delayed exercise effects but results in changes. Patients can decide themselves whether functional or isolated strengthening is the best type of strength training for them.

Intermittent Brief Periods of Fast Activity to Restore Immune System Health

Progression of exercise is an important aspect of active care. As patients achieve recommended guidelines for low-intensity exercise and strength training, they can progress to brief, high-intensity activity. Maximum-effort activity fine-tunes patients' bodies and helps increase energy levels, improve athletic performance, improve immune and metabolic system health, and minimize the effects of aging by promoting the release of testosterone and human growth hormone in both women and men.[129] Modern research confirms that, as with our ancestors, occasional series of short, intense bursts can have a more profound impact on overall fitness and weight loss than a medium-paced jog lasting several times as long.[129] High-intensity interval training (HIIT), which increases metabolic rate, decreases appetite, develops more calorie-burning lean muscle tissue, and improves insulin sensitivity, leads to effective weight loss.

Sprinting in any form is a physically stressful activity that requires time to progress to maximal effort and activate benefits. The preparatory activity can be as simple as light walking, progressing to fast walking, jogging, running, and then sprinting; but if less impact is desired, the patient can swim or use a stationary bike, elliptical, or rower. Maximal sprints occur every 72 hours for athletes in training; patients, however, need to start HIIT gradually, perhaps once every other week, and allow plenty of recovery time after the first sessions. Recovery time from all-out effort is necessary to allow the repair that follows training and to enable strength gains. When patients do not allow sufficient recovery time from an HIIT or strength training workout, repair fails to occur, and cumulative stress on the tissues can lead to chronic inflammation, tissue failure, and injury. As patients' fitness level improves, recovery time between sessions and sprints can be shortened.

Novices should start with three to four sprints, short of full speed, with long rest periods. For example, a novice may begin with 1- to 2-minute exertion intervals to get his or her heart rate up above 75% to 90%, followed by 3- to 5-minute recovery intervals to get the heart rate back down below 75% (the lower, the better). As the body adapts, the patient can increase to six to eight sprints of 8 to 60 seconds each (finishing under 20 minutes) followed by shorter recovery periods (1–2 minutes) as the heart rate indicates. The clinician should never advocate pushing the body through intense exercise if the patient shows signs of fatigue, soreness, sickness, or a compromised immune system. These illness signals warrant more extended periods of rest and recovery.

The time to exercise and achieve maximum benefit is when the body feels refreshed. An important message regarding HIIT is that it is not about speed, but about effort. As long as the patient perceives the activity as heavy exertion, the effort is sufficient to gain the benefits. Clinicians should remind their more disabled patients of this guidance.

Diet

It is not common in physical therapy practice to inform patients about how their diet affects their pain. When pain mechanisms are dominated by the CNS, however, the foods patients select to fuel themselves may have an influence on their pain; this is especially true for those who have comorbidities such as hypertension, Alzheimer's disease, endometriosis, osteoporosis, chronic obstructive pulmonary disease, menopause, obesity, arthritis, heart disease, diabetes, and certain diet-related cancers.[132-135]

Rates of obesity, arthritis, heart disease, diabetes, and cancer have shown alarming increases, and many point to food industry practices as the cause of inflammatory problems, including chronic pain.[136,137] Human-made products that are foreign to our genes and disturb the normal, healthy function of the body when ingested are increasingly present in the food supply.[136] The modern diet is based largely on grains, refined starches, sugar and carbonated beverages, and engineered foods such as heavily processed, packaged, fried, and preserved foods. These foods contain substances that may promote inflammation and perpetuate chronic pain. Anti-inflammatory foods include the following[136]:

- Fruits and vegetables (especially potatoes)
- Nuts
- Fresh fish, wild game, and grass- or pasture-fed meat
- Omega 3 eggs
- Organic extra virgin olive oil, organic coconut oil
- Organic butter
- Dark chocolate
- Stout beer, red wine
- Balsamic vinegar
- Spices such as ginger, turmeric, garlic, oregano, marjoram, and cumin

Proinflammatory foods include the following[136]:

- Refined grains, whole grains
- Grain and flour products
- Grain-fed meat and eggs
- Most packaged and processed foods
- Deep-fried foods
- Trans fat (eg, some margarine, processed foods)
- Corn, safflower, sunflower, soybean oil
- Most commercial salad dressings

Processed grains in particular, including wheat, rice, and corn flour products such as bread, pasta, crackers, snack foods, baked goods, and boxed cereals, promote inflammatory responses.[135,137] Conventional knowledge presented in commercials, diet plans, and even government health commission recommendations is that grains should be the primary source of calories. However, humans are genetically adapted to eat a diet that consists largely of vegetation (fruits, vegetables, and nuts) and animals that eat vegetation, commonly referred to as a Paleolithic (hunter–gatherer) or low-inflammation diet.[135-138] Human genes and digestive systems have not had time to adapt to the unfamiliar protein structure and excessive carbohydrate load of all forms of cultivated grains, even whole grains.[135,137] The repeated insulin response from these foods drives our cellular DNA to inflammatory responses throughout the body.

Inflammatory responses are a cumulative problem over time. Rarely do patients think their symptoms could be coming from the foods they select. In patients with chronic pain, diets high in carbohydrates contribute to a spike in insulin in the bloodstream, signaling their body to store fat and produce inflammatory by-products. Clinicians should investigate patients' diets to identify any inflammatory culprits; for example, a flare-up may follow a weekend of heavy inflammatory food consumption. In addition to weight gain, overstressing insulin response systems over years and decades can lead to general system failure in the form of type 2 diabetes, obesity, cardiovascular disease, diet-related cancers, and chronic musculoskeletal pain.[123,125]

Clinicians should recommend to their patients simple principles for healthy eating to reduce inflammatory reactivity, consistent with the patients' readiness to make dietary changes. A desirable ratio of muscle mass to body fat is only 20% related to activities; 80% is related to dietary choices. Recommendations should focus on quality sources of animal protein (organic, free-range, or wild sources of meat, fowl, and fish), an assortment of colorful vegetables and fresh fruits, and healthy sources of fat (eg, nuts and seeds, their derivative butters, certain oils, avocados).[135,137] Humans thrive on eating an ever-changing variety of natural foods that satisfy and nourish, at times and in amounts that fluctuate according to mood, environmental circumstances, activity level, and many other factors.[129] Clinicians should recommend avoidance of preservative-containing, packaged, and high-glycemic and high-carbohydrate foods; encourage a low inflammatory diet; and discover patients' individual reactivity to specific foods.[136] Although clinicians can identify potential sources of threat to patients' bodies, immune systems, and pain control systems by screening their diets, a consultation with a certified clinical nutritionist or dietitian is always appropriate when patients have poor dietary habits. **Table 7.3** summarizes interventions for patients with the affective pain mechanism. **Appendix 7.G** provides a comparison among all three central pain mechanisms for intervention strategies.

TABLE 7.3 Interventions for the Affective Pain Mechanism

Category	Interventions
Education on central nervous system pain mechanisms	Explanation of the nondamaging nature of pain: Hurt vs harm, interpretation of inputs
	Pain mechanism education
	Discussion of the role of negative emotions, harmful and damaging thoughts, and beliefs regarding pain: Pain journal
	Training in coping strategies for loneliness, depression, anxiety, negative repressed emotions, fear of motion or activity: Relaxation, diaphragmatic breathing
	Explanation of the Activity Pyramid: Green, yellow, and red lights, flare-up management for graded exposure to meaningful function
	Identification of the activity baseline and explanation of the no-worse concept: Goal is to return control to the patient
Education on conscious factors	Stages of readiness to change
	Contribution of negative emotions to pain, depression, anxiety, anger, fear
	Individualized treatment based on screening tool results
	Interdisciplinary cognitive–behavioral therapy program if indicated as best use of patient resources
Education on unconscious factors	Progression and treatment of tension myositis syndrome
	Mechanism of unconscious factors in chronic pain—the brain triggers ischemia to protect the person from repressed negative emotions, causing pain related to current life pressures, childhood experiences and relationships, and perfectionism trait
	Referral to a psychologist for a thorough evaluation
	Recommended reading of John E. Sarno's: *The Mindbody Prescription: Healing the Body, Healing the Pain*[139]; *Healing Back Pain: The Mind-Body Connection*[140]; and *The Divided Mind: The Epidemic of Mindbody Disorders*.[14]
Activity	Pacing and graded exposure to activity: Build low aerobic activity, HR 55%–75% of maximum, 2–5 hours per week; Use Figure 7.5 step program to assist with building low-intensity aerobic activity.
	Weight training to build upper and lower extremity strength: Start with isolated movements, progress to function, HR 55%–75% of maximum, two times a week
	Deep muscle training for spine postural stabilization: Progression to function, HR 55%–75% of maximum, two times a week
	High-intensity interval training (HIIT): Progress to 10-20 min, HR >75% of maximum, one to two times a week
	Mechanical examination

Abbreviation: HR = heart rate.

Conclusion

Psychosocial factors are important and treatable correlates of disabling musculoskeletal pain. Biomedical treatments (eg, surgery, injection, medication, exercises) are only one aspect of the care of such pain; they are best reserved for discrete, objective, verifiable pathological processes, and their use should be supported by strong scientific evidence. The best targets for treatment of the affective pain mechanism are improving patients' coping with depression and anxiety, addressing the tendency to misinterpret or overinterpret pain, and discovering unconscious repressed negative emotions. Comprehensive biopsychosocial treatment is more effective than traditional biomedical treatment alone for patients with dominating affective pain mechanism. The pain mechanism classification system can lead to better use of resources, decreased disability and health care utilization, and increased comfort and quality of life for these patients.

KEY MESSAGES

- Pain is more likely to cause an emotional disturbance than to result from it; however, current or past psychological trauma and states can initiate the pain response and may be the underlying reason that patients with the affective pain mechanism have not achieved pain control.

- In patients with the affective pain mechanism, pain is influenced by characteristics of the conscious mind (ie, depression, anxiety, insomnia, anger, illness behavior, and social and cultural factors) and of the unconscious mind (ie, repressed negative emotions related to current life pressures, residual anger from childhood relationships and experiences, and the type A personality and perfectionism).

- The psychology of the health care provider may be as important as the psychology of the patient in the management of disabling musculoskeletal pain. Patients are better served by clinicians who use the biopsychosocial model of illness and who provide them with current, detailed descriptions of the neurophysiology of pain.

- The three components in the evaluation of patients with the affective pain mechanism are (1) readiness to change education and assessment, (2) use of psychosocial screening tools, and (3) assessment of coping strategies.

- The three key elements of intervention for patients with the affective pain mechanism are (1) the biopsychosocial approach, (2) motivational interviewing, and (3) nonpharmacy approaches to pain.

- For patients with the affective pain mechanism, the cognitive and behavioral dimensions of pain are in need of change. Patients' motivation to change their pain-related behaviors must come from within themselves. The clinician's recommendations are effective only when the patient recognizes the value of the recommendations and acts on them.

- Management of chronic affective pain should include the nonpharmacy approaches of sleep restoration, relaxation training, active exercise, and diet.

References

1. Finnerup NB, Sindrup SH, Jensen TS. Chronic neuropathic pain: Mechanisms, drug targets and measurement. *Fundam Clin Pharmacol.* 2007;21:129-136.
2. Schweinhardt P, Sauro KM, Bushnell MC. Fibromyalgia: A disorder of the brain? *Neuroscientist.* 2008;14:415-421.
3. Hoffman BM, Papas RK, Chatkoff DK, Kerns RD. Meta-analysis of psychological interventions for chronic low back pain. *Health Psychol.* 2007;26:1-9.

4. Nicholas MK, Linton SJ, Watson PJ, Main CJ. Early identification and management of psychological risk factors ("yellow flags") in patients with low back pain: A reappraisal. *Phys Ther.* 2011;91:737-753.
5. Spence SH. Cognitive–behaviour therapy in the treatment of chronic, occupational pain of the upper limbs: A 2 yr follow-up. *Behav Res Ther.* 1991;29:503-509.
6. Richardson GM, McGrath PJ. Cognitive–behavioral therapy for migraine headaches: A minimal-therapist-contact approach versus a clinic-based approach. *Headache.* 2005;29:352-357.
7. Vlaeyen JW, Teeken-Gruben NJ, Goossens ME, et al. Cognitive–educational treatment of fibromyalgia: A randomized clinical trial: I. Clinical effects. *J Rheumatol.* 1996;23:1237-1245.
8. Bradley LA. Pathophysiological mechanisms of fibromyalgia and related disorders. *J Clin Psychiatry.* 2008;69(2):6-13.
9. Mannion AF, Junge A, Taimela S, et al. Active therapy for chronic low back pain: Part 3. Factors influencing self rated disability and its change following therapy. *Spine.* 2001;26:920-929.
10. Hoogendoorn WE, van Poppel MN, Bongers PM, et al. Systematic review of psychosocial factors at work and private life as risk factors for back pain. *Spine.* 2000;25:2114-2125.
11. Linton SJ. A review of psychological risk factors in back and neck pain. *Spine.* 2000;9:1148-1156.
12. Pincus T, Burton A, Vogel S, Field AP. A systematic review of psychological factors as predictors of chronicity/disability in prospective cohorts of low back pain. *Spine.* 2002;27:E109-E120.
13. Gallagher RM, Verma S. Mood and anxiety disorders in chronic pain. In: Dworkin RH, Breitbart WS, eds. *Psychological Aspects of Pain: A Handbook for Healthcare Providers.* Seattle, WA: IASP Press; 2004:139-178.
14. Sarno JE. *The Divided Mind: The Epidemic of Mindbody Disorders.* New York: HarperCollins; 2007.
15. Bloodworth D, Calvillo O, Smith K, et al. Chronic pain syndromes: Evaluation and treatment. In: Braddom RL, ed. *Physical Medicine and Rehabilitation.* 2nd ed. Philadelphia, PA: Saunders, 2001:913-933.
16. Kendall NA, Linton SJ, Main CJ. *Guide to Assessing Psychosocial Yellow Flags in Acute Low Back Pain: Risk Factors for Long-Term Disability and Work Loss.* Wellington, New Zealand: Accident Rehabilitation and Compensation Insurance Corporation of New Zealand and the National Health Committee; 1997.
17. Grol R, Buchan H. Clinical guidelines: What can we do to increase their use? *Med J Aust.* 2006;185:301-302.
18. Blyth FM, Macfarlane GJ, Nicholas MK. The contribution of psychosocial factors to the development of chronic pain: The key to better outcomes for patients? *Pain.* 2007;129:8 11.
19. Hudson JI, Mangweth B, Pope HG Jr, et al. Family study of affective spectrum disorder. *Arch Gen Psychiatry.* 2003;60:170-177.
20. Apkarian AV, Sosa Y, Sonty S, et al. Chronic back pain is associated with decreased prefrontal and thalamic gray matter density. *J Neurosci.* 2004;24:10410-10415.
21. DeGood DE, Tait RC. Assessment of pain beliefs and pain coping. In: Turk DC, Melzack R, eds. *Handbook of Pain Assessment.* 2nd ed. New York: Guilford Press; 2001:320-345.
22. Jensen MP, Turner JA, Romano JM, Karoly P. Coping with chronic pain: A critical review of the literature. *Pain.* 1991;47:249-283.
23. Smith TW, Aberger EW, Follick MJ, Ahern DK. Cognitive distortions and psychological distress in chronic low back pain. *J Consult Clin Psychol.* 1986;54:573-575.
24. Smith TW, Peck JR, Ward JR. Helplessness and depression in rheumatoid arthritis. *Health Psychol.* 1990;9:377-389.
25. Tota-Faucette ME, Gil KM, Williams DA, Keefe FJ, Goli V. Predictors of response to pain management treatment: The role of family environment and changes in cognitive processes. *Clin J Pain.* 1993;9:115-123.
26. Dolce JJ, Crocker MF, Moletteire C, Doleys DM. Exercise quotas, anticipatory concern and self-efficacy expectancies in chronic pain: A preliminary report. *Pain.* 1986;24:365-372.
27. Lorig K, Chastain RL, Ung E, Shoor R, Holman HR. Development and evaluation of a scale to measure perceived self-efficacy in people with arthritis. *Arthritis Rheum.* 1989;32:37-44.
28. Lefebvre JC, Keefe FJ, Affleck G, et al. The relationship of arthritis self efficacy to daily pain, daily mood, and daily pain coping in rheumatoid arthritis patients. *Pain.* 1999;80:425-435.
29. Ring D, Kadzielski J, Fabian L, Zurakowski D, Malhotra LR, Jupiter JB. Self-reported upper extremity health status correlated with depression. *J Bone Joint Surg Am.* 2006;88:1983-1988.
30. Lawson K, Reesor KA, Keefe FJ, Turner JA. Dimensions of pain-related cognitive coping: Cross-validation of the factor structure of the Coping Strategy Questionnaire. *Pain.* 1990;43:195-204.
31. Tunks ER, Crook J, Weir R. Epidemiology of chronic pain with psychological comorbidity: Prevalence, risk, course, and prognosis. *Can J Psychiatry.* 2008;53:224-234.

32. Parsons S, Breen A, Foster NE, et al. Prevalence and comparative troublesomeness by age of musculoskeletal pain in different body locations. *Fam Pract.* 2007;24:308-316.
33. Chiechanowski P, Sullivan M, Jensen M, Romano J, Summers H. The relationship of attachment style to depression, catastrophizing and health care utilizations in patients with chronic pain. *Pain.* 2003;104:627-637.
34. Bair MJ, Robinson RL, Eckert GJ, Stang PE, Croghan TW, Kroenke K. Impact of pain on depression treatment response in primary care. *Psychosom Med.* 2004;66:17-22.
35. Richardson C, Glenn S, Horgan M, Nurmikko T. A prospective study of factors associated with the presence of phantom limb pain six months after major lower limb amputation in patients with peripheral vascular disease [published correction appears in *J Pain.* 2007;8:998]. *J Pain.* 2007;8:793-801.
36. Ring D, Kadzielski J, Malhotra L, Lee SG, Jupiter JB. Psychological factors associated with idiopathic arm pain. *J Bone Joint Surg Am.* 2005;87:374-380.
37. Hill JC, Lewis M, Sim J, Hay EM, Dziedzic K. Predictors of poor outcome in patients with neck pain treated in physical therapy. *Clin J Pain.* 2007;23:683-690.
38. Sternberg B. Insomnia, depression, and anxiety [course handouts]. Concord, CA: Institute for Natural Resources; March 2009.
39. Wakefield J, Horwitz A. *The Loss of Sadness: How Psychiatry Transformed Normal Sorrow Into Depressive Disorder.* Oxford, England: Oxford University Press; 2007.
40. Moussavi S, Chatterji S, Verdes E, Tandon A, Patel V, Ustun B. Depression, chronic diseases, and decrements in health: Results from the World Health Surveys. *Lancet.* 2003;370:851-858.
41. Bair MJ, Robinson RL, Katon W, Kroenke K. Depression and pain comorbidity: A literature review. *Arch Intern Med.* 2003;163:2433-2445.
42. Gureje O, Simon GE, Von Korff M. A cross-national study of the course of persistent pain in primary care. *Pain.* 2001;92:195-200.
43. van den Berg B, Grievink L, Stellato RK, Yzermans CJ, Lebret E. Symptoms and related functioning in a traumatized community. *Arch Inter Med.* 2005;165:2402-2407.
44. Mariano AJ. Chronic pain and spinal cord injury. *Clin J Pain.* 1992;8:87-92.
45. Cairns DM, Adkins RH, Scott MD. Pain and depression in acute traumatic spinal cord injury: Origins of chronic problematic pain? *Arch Phys Med Rehabil.* 1996;77:329-335.
46. Gormsen L, Rosenberg R, Bach FW, Jensen TS. Depression, anxiety, health-related quality of life and pain in patients with chronic fibromyalgia and neuropathic pain. *Eur J Pain.* 2009;14:127.
47. Otto M, Bach FW, Jensen TS, Sindrup SH. Health related quality of life and its predictive role for analgesic effect in patients with painful polyneuropathy. *Eur J Pain.* 2007;11:572-578.
48. Gustorff B, Dorner T, Likar R, et al. Prevalence of self-reported neuropathic pain and impact on quality of life: A prospective representative survey. *Acta Anaesthesiol Scand.* 2008;52:132-136.
49. Svendsen KB, Jensen TS, Hansen HJ, Bach FW. Sensory function and quality of life in patients with multiple sclerosis and pain. *Pain.* 2005;114:175-181.
50. Poleshuck EL, Green CR. Socioeconomic disadvantage and pain. *Pain.* 2008;136:235-238.
51. Edwards RR, Smith MT, Kudel I, Haythornthwaite J. Pain related catastrophizing as a risk factor for suicidal ideation in chronic pain. *Pain.* 2006;126:272-279.
52. Fishbain DA, Goldberg M, Meagher BR, Steele R, Rosomoff H. Male and female chronic pain patients categorized by DSM-III psychiatric diagnostic criteria. *Pain.* 1986;26:181-197.
53. Williams LS, Jones WJ, Shen J, Robinson RL, Weinberger M, Kroenke K. Prevalence and impact of pain and depression in neurology outpatients. *J Neurol Neurosurg Psychiatry.* 2003;74:1587-1589.
54. Bair MJ, Wu J, Damush TM, Sutherland JM, Kroenke K. Association of depression and anxiety alone and in combination with chronic musculoskeletal pain in primary care. *Psychosom Med.* 2008;70:890-897.
55. Conrad PJ. The role of anxiety sensitivity in subjective and physiological responses to social and physical stressors. *Cogn Behav Ther.* 2006;35:216-225.
56. Barsky AJ, Ahern DK. Cognitive behavior therapy for hypochondriasis: A randomized controlled trial. *JAMA.* 2004;291:1464-1470.
57. Hadjistavropoulos HD, Hadjistavropoulos T. The relevance of health anxiety to chronic pain: Research findings and recommendations for assessment and treatment. *Curr Pain Headache Rep.* 2003;7:98-104.
58. Tofler I. "Free-floating" somatoform disorder. *Psychosomatics.* 2003;44:435-436.
59. Poleshuck EL, Bair MJ, Kroenke K, et al. Psychosocial stress and anxiety in musculoskeletal pain patients with and without depression. *Gen Hosp Psychiatry.* 2009;31:116-122.
60. Asmundson GJ, Norton PJ, Vlaeyen JW. Fear-avoidance models of chronic pain: An overview. In: Amundson GJ, Vlaeyen JW, Crombez G, eds. *Understanding and Treating Fear of Pain.* Oxford, England: Oxford University Press; 2004:3-24.

61. Asmundson GJG, Taylor S. PTSD and chronic pain: Cognitive behavioral perspective and practical implications. In: Young G, Kane AW, Nicholson K, eds. *Causality: Psychological Knowledge and Evidence in Court*. New York: Springer; 2006:225-241.
62. Barlow DH. *Anxiety and Its Disorders*. 2nd ed. New York: Guilford Press; 2002.
63. Barlow DH. Unraveling the mysteries of anxiety and its disorders from the perspective of emotion theory. *Am Psychol*. 2000;55:1247-1263.
64. Asmundson GJG, Vlaeyen JWS, Crombez G, eds. *Understanding and Treating Fear of Pain*. New York: Oxford University Press; 2004.
65. Asmundson GJG, Carleton RN. Fear of pain is elevated in adults with co-occurring trauma-related stress and social anxiety symptoms. *Cogn Behav Ther*. 2005;34:248-255.
66. Schmidt NB, Richey JA, Fitzpatrick KK. Discomfort intolerance: Development of a construct and measure relevant to panic disorder. *J Anxiety Disord*. 2006;20:263-280.
67. Antony MM. Why we worry: Understanding and treating anxiety disorders [course handouts]. Haddonfield, NJ: Institute for Brain Potential; 2009.
68. Reiss S. Theoretical perspectives on the fear of anxiety. *Clin Psychol Rev*. 1987;7:585-596.
69. Keogh E, Asmundson GJG. Negative affectivity, catastrophizing, and anxiety sensitivity. In: Amundson GJG, Vlaeyen JW, Crombez G, eds. *Understanding and Treating Fear of Pain*. Oxford, England: Oxford University Press; 2004:91-115.
70. Keogh E, Cochrane M. Anxiety sensitivity, cognitive bias and the experience of pain. *J Pain*. 2002;3:320-329.
71. Zvolensky MJ, Goodie JL, McNeil DW, Sperry JA, Sorrell JT. Anxiety sensitivity in the prediction of pain-related fear and anxiety in a heterogeneous chronic pain population. *Behav Res Ther*. 2001;39:683-696.
72. Stewart SH, Asmundson GJG. Anxiety sensitivity and its impact on pain experiences and conditions: A state of the art. *Cogn Behav Ther*. 2006;35:185-188.
73. McCracken LM, Keogh E. Acceptance, mindfulness, and values-based action may counteract fear and avoidance of emotions in chronic pain: An analysis of anxiety sensitivity. *J Pain*. 2009;10:408-415.
74. Sareen J, Cox BJ, Clara I, Asmundson GJ. The relationship between anxiety disorders and physical disorders in the US National Comorbidity Survey. *Depress Anxiety*. 2005;21:193-202.
75. McCracken LM, Dhingra L. A short version of the Pain Anxiety Symptoms Scale (PASS-20). Preliminary development and validity. *Pain Res Manage*. 2002;7(1):45-50.
76. Watt MC, Stewart SH, Lefaivre MJ, Ulman LS. A brief cognitive behavioral approach to reducing anxiety sensitivity decreases pain related anxiety. *Cogn Behav Ther*. 2006;35:248-256.
77. Neckelmann D. Insomnia, depression and anxiety [course handout]. Bergen, Norway: Haukeland University Hospital Department of Psychiatry; 2007.
78. National Sleep Foundation. *2003 Sleep in America Poll*. Washington, DC: National Sleep Foundation;; 2003.
79. Wilcox S, Brenes GA, Levine D, Sevick MA, Shumaker SA, Craven T. Factors related to sleep disturbance in older adults experiencing knee pain or knee pain with radiographic evidence of knee osteoarthritis. *J Am Geriatric Soc*. 2000;48:1241-1251.
80. Turk DC, Gatchel RJ, eds. *Psychological Approaches to Pain Management: A Practitioner's Handbook*. New York: Guilford Press; 1999.
81. Potter-Efron R. Understanding angry people: Recognizing, managing and healing anger [course notes]. Santa Rosa, CA: R. Cassidy Seminars; 2010.
82. Volavka J. *Neurobiology of Violence*. 2nd ed. Washington, DC: American Psychiatric Publishing; 2002.
83. Vlaeyen JW, Kole-Snijders AM, Boeren RG, van Eek H. Fear of movement/(re)injury in chronic low back pain and its relation to behavioral performance. *Pain*. 1995;62:363-372.
84. Fordyce WE. *Behavioral Methods for Chronic Pain and Illness*. St. Louis, MO: Mosby; 1976.
85. Vlaeyen JW, Seelen HA, Peters M, et al. Fear of movement/reinjury and muscular reactivity in chronic low back pain patients: An experimental investigation. *Pain*. 1999;82:297-304.
86. McCracken LM, ed. *Contextual Cognitive Behavioral Therapy for Chronic Pain*. Seattle, WA: IASP Press; 2005.
87. Liptom JA, Marbach JJ. Ethnicity and the pain experience. *Soc Sci Med*. 1984;19:1279-1298.
88. Unruh AM. Gender variations in clinical pain experience. *Pain*. 1996;65:123-167.
89. Zborowski M. *People in Pain*. San Francisco, CA: Jossey-Bass; 1969.
90. Turk DC, Monarch ES. *Biopsychological Approaches to Pain Management: A Practitioner's Handbook*. New York: Guilford Press; 1999.
91. Bachanas PJ, Roberts MC. Factors affecting children's attitudes toward healthcare and responses to stressful medical procedures. *J Pediatr Psychol*. 1995;20:261-275.
92. Bhandari M, Tornetta P 3rd. Evidence-based orthopaedics: A paradigm shift. *Clin Orthop Relat Res*. 2003;413:117-132.

93. Schünemann HJ, Bone L. Evidence-based orthopedics: A primer. *Clin Orthop Relat Res.* 2003; 413:117-132.
94. Doornberg JN, Ring D, Fabian LM, Malhotra L, Zurakowski D, Jupiter JB. Pain dominates measurements of elbow function and health status. *J Bone Joint Surg Am.* 2005;87:1725-1731.
95. Fernandez E, Turk DC. Sensory and affective components of pain: Separation and synthesis. *Psychol Bull.* 1992;112:205-217.
96. Moseley L. Unraveling the barriers to reconceptualization of the problem in chronic pain: The actual and perceived ability of patients and health professionals to understand the neurophysiology. *J Pain.* 2003;4:184-189.
97. Hahn SR, Thompson KS, Wills TA, Stern V, Budner NS. The difficult doctor–patient relationship: Somatization, personality and psychopathology. *J Clin Epidemiol.* 1994;47:647-657.
98. Schwenk TL, Marquez JT, Lefever RD, Cohen M. Physician and patient determinants of difficult physician–patient relationships. *J Fam Pract.* 1989;28:59-63.
99. Lowe B, Kroenke K, Herzog W, Gräfe K. Measuring depression outcome with a brief self-report instrument: Sensitivity to change of the Patient Health Questionnaire (PHQ-9). *J Affect Disord.* 2004;81:61-66.
100. Martin A, Rief W, Klaiberg A, Brachler E. Validity of the brief Patient Health Questionnaire Mood Scale (PHQ-9) in the general population. *Gen Hosp Psychiatry.* 2006;28:71-77
101. Waddel G, Newton M, et al. A Fear-Avoidance Beliefs Questionnaire (FABQ) and the role of fear avoidance beliefs in chronic low back pain and disability. *Pain.* 1993;52:157-168.
102. Linton SJ. A review of psychological risk factors in back and neck pain. *Spine.* 2000;9:1148-1156.
103. Linton SJ, Hallden BH. Can we screen for problematic back pain? A screening questionnaire for predicting outcome in acute and subacute back pain. *Clin J Pain.* 1998;14:1-7.
104. Linton SJ, Hallden K. Risk factors and the natural course of acute and recurrent musculoskeletal pain: Developing a screening instrument. In: Jensen TS, Turner JA, Wiesenfeld-Hallin Z, eds. *Proceedings of the 8th World Congress on Pain: Progress in Pain, Research, and Management.* Vol 8. Seattle, WA: IASP Press; 1997.
105. Abrams MP, Carleton RN, Asmundson GJG. An exploration of the psychometric properties of the PASS-20 with a nonclinical sample. *J Pain.* 2007;8:879-886.
106. Asmundson GJG, Collimore KC, Bernstein A, Zvolensky MJ, Hadjistavropoulos HD. Is the latent structure of fear of pain continuous or discontinuous among pain patients? Taxometric analysis of the Pain Anxiety Symptoms Scale. *J Pain.* 2007;8:387-395.
107. McCracken LM, Gross RT, Aikens J, Carnrike CL. The assessment of anxiety and fear in persons with chronic pain: A comparison of instruments. *Behav Res Ther.* 1996;34:927-933.
108. Larsen DK, Taylor S, Asmundson G. Exploratory factor analysis of the Pain Anxiety Symptoms Scale in patients with chronic pain complaints. *Pain.* 1997;69:27-34.
109. Feldner M, Hekmat H. Perceived control over anxiety-related events as a predictor of pain behaviors in a cold pressor tank. *J Behav Ther Exper Psychiatry.* 2001;32(4):191-202.
110. Ring DR, Kadzielski J. Malhotra L, Lee SG, Jupiter JB. Psychological factors associated with idiopathic arm pain. *J Bone Joint Surg.* 2005;87:374-380.
111. Kroenke K, Spitzer L, Williams J. The PHQ-9 validity of a brief depression severity measure. *J Gen Intern Med.* 2001;16(9):606-613.
112. Linton SJ. *New Avenues for the Prevention of Chronic Musculoskeletal Pain and Disability.* Amsterdam, The Netherlands: Elsevier; 2002.
113. Fairbank J, Couper J, Davies J, et al. The Oswestry Low Back Pain questionnaire. *Physiotherapy.* 1980;66:271-273.
114. Vernon H, Mior S. The Neck Disability Index: A study of reliability and validity. *J Manip Physiol Ther.* 1991;14(7):409-415.
115. Hudak P, Amadio PC, Bombadier C; Upper Extremity Collaborative Group. Development of an upper extremity outcome measure: The DASH (Disabilities of the Arm, Shoulder and Hand). *Am J Indust Med.* 1996;29:602-608.
116. Binkley J, Stratford P, Lott S, Riddle D. The Lower Extremity Functional Scale (LEFS): Scale development, measurement properties, and clinical application. *Phys Ther.* 1999;79:371-383.
117. Loeser JD. Introduction. In: G. M. Aronoff, ed. *Evaluation and Treatment of Chronic Pain.* 3rd ed. Baltimore, MD: Williams & Wilkins; 1999: xxiii-xxiv.
118. Waddell G. *The Back Pain Revolution.* 2nd ed. Edinburgh, Scotland: Elsevier; 2004.
119. Nachemson AL. Newest knowledge of low back pain: A critical look. *Clin Orthop.* 1992;279:8-20.
120. Jones SL, Jones PK, Katz J. Compliance for low-back pain patients in the emergency department: A randomized trial. *Spine.* 1988;13:553-556.

121. Moseley GL. Physiotherapy is effective for chronic low back pain: A randomised controlled trial. *Aust J Physiother.* 2002;48:43-49.
122. Symonds TL, Burton AK, Tillotson KM, Main CJ. Absence resulting from low back trouble can be reduced by psychosocial intervention at the work place. *Spine.* 1995;20:2738-2745.
123. Burton AK, Waddell G, Tillotson KM, Summerton N. Information and advice to patients with back pain can have a positive effect: A randomized controlled trial of a novel educational booklet in primary care. *Spine.* 1999;24:2484-2491.
124. Buchbinder R, Jolley D, Wyatt M. Population based intervention to change back pain beliefs and disability: Three part evaluation. *BMJ.* 2001;322:1516-1520.
125. Rollnick S, Miller W. What is motivational interviewing? *Behav Cog Psychother.* 1995;23:325-334.
126. Miller W, Rollnick S. *Motivational Interviewing: Preparing People to Change Addictive Behaviors.* New York: Guilford Press; 1991.
127. Emmons KM, Rollnick S. Motivational interviewing in health care settings: Opportunities and limitations. *Am J Prev Med.* 2001;20:68-74.
128. Prochaska JO, DiClemente CC, Norcross JC. In search of how people change: Applications to addictive behaviors. *Am Psychol.* 1992;47:1102-1114.
129. Sisson M. *The Primal Blueprint.* Malibu, CA: Primal Nutrition.
130. Hanson RW. Using relaxation and self-hypnosis for pain. In: *Self-Management of Chronic Pain: Patient Handbook.* New York: Guilford Press; 2000.
131. Tudor-Locke C. Taking steps toward increased physical activity: Using pedometers to measure and motivate. *Res Digest.* 2002;3(17):1-8.
132. Balkwill F, Mantovani A. Inflammation and cancer: Back to Virchow? *Lancet.* 2001;357:539-545.
133. Ban WQ, Man SF, Senthilselvan A, Sin DD. Association between chronic obstructive pulmonary disease and systemic inflammation: A systematic review and meta-analysis. *Thorax.* 2004;59:574-580.
134. Grimble RF. Inflammatory status and insulin resistance. *Curr Opin Clin Nutr Metab Care.* 2002;5:551-559.
135. Pfeilschifter J, Köditz R, Pfohl M, Schatz H. Changes in proinflammatory cytokine activity after menopause. *Endocr Rev.* 2002;23:90-119.
136. Recitas, LG. *The Plan: Eliminate the Surprising "Healthy" Foods That Are Making You Fat—and Lose Weight Fast.* New York: Hachette Book Group.
137. Seaman DR. Nutritional considerations for inflammation and pain. In: Liebenson C, ed. *Rehabilitation of Spine: A Practitioner's Manual.* 2nd ed. Baltimore, MD: Lippincott Williams & Wilkins; 2007:730-731.
138. O'Keefe JH Jr, Cordain L. Cardiovascular disease resulting from a diet and lifestyle at odds with our Paleolithic genome: How to become a 21st century hunter–gatherer. *Mayo Clin Proc.* 2004;79:101-108.
139. Sarno JE. *The Mindbody Prescription: Healing the Body, Healing the Pain.* New York: Warner Books; 1998.
140. Sarno JE. *Healing Back Pain: The Mind-Body Connection.* New York: Warner Books; 1991.

APPENDIX 7.A Orthopedic Outpatient, 38-Year-Old Female

Physical Therapy/Occupational Therapy Initial Evaluation

SUBJECTIVE FINDINGS

Chief complaint:	Right-sided head, neck, shoulder, arm, forearm, and hand pain, spreading to trunk on right side
Descriptors:	Sharp, dull, burning, pinching, numbness, tingling, choking, stabbing
Onset:	Patient stabbed in throat by mugger 3 yr ago when leaving work after night shift; couldn't scream; almost died
Frequency:	Constant
24-hr behavior:	No pattern in time of day; after activity always worse; each day starts the same
Subjective pain:	(Likert) / Faces scale: 9/10
Aggravating factors:	Speaking; swallowing; turning neck; raising arm; going out, especially to loud and crowded places; touching neck and arm
Relieving factors:	Quiet room, narcotic medication, meditation and prayer, being alone with husband who cares for her

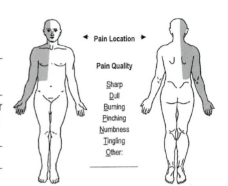

◀ Pain Location ▶

Pain Quality
Sharp
Dull
Burning
Pinching
Numbness
Tingling
Other:

PATIENT EDUCATION CONSIDERATIONS

Readiness to learn:	Ready and self-motivated (Extrinsically motivated) (Limitations (see below))
Limitations to learning:	(Cognitive) Physical Language Financial Cultural (Other:) Comprehension and concentration
Teaching method preferred:	(Handout) Verbal (Demonstration) (Practice) (Other:) Practice at home alone
Explain:	Fear of therapy, pain, massage, and "neck cracking"

MEDICAL HISTORY

Past medical history:	Irritable bowel syndrome, temporal mandibular disorder, and fibromyalgia diagnosed since onset of problem
Family history:	No significant medical history
Surgery and invasive procedures:	Trigger point injections at 2 different pain clinics: not helpful, worsened symptoms
Medications:	Narcotics, antidepressants, muscle relaxants—help patient tolerate pain to function Allergies: Penicillin
Previous treatments:	3 courses of physical therapy (MDT, stabilization and general strengthening, manual therapy and manipulations), without significant relief
Diagnostic tests:	X-ray: Negative MRI: Negative CT scan: EMG: Negative Other: Negative bone scan

PSYCHOSOCIAL FACTORS

Living situation:	Lives with husband, no children. Husband works full time and cares for her. She stays alone during day but sees a work counselor. See checklist of observed yellow flags.
Behavior:	Patient is frustrated, cooperative, and quiet. Husband is overprotective of patient and angry that health care system cannot get rid of his wife's pain.
Occupation:	Pediatric ICU nurse, off work since attack; does not want to return to night shift hours because location is too dangerous; would consider day shift once pain is relieved
Recreation and leisure:	Meditation and prayer, attends church 2x/wk; walks 3 blocks
Functional disability:	Cares for herself independently. Husband performs all household duties, including shopping, laundry, and outdoor chores, and drives her to appointments.
Concerns:	Patient is fearful regarding returning to work, safety, driving, lifting children, and working at the fast pace of the ICU. Pain is worsening, and patient fears not being able to communicate or swallow again. Pain is spreading to other areas of her right side. Patient has been unable to have children since the pain started.
Unhealthy coping forms:	Defensiveness, depression, with obsessions and compulsions

PROVISIONAL PAIN CLASSIFICATION (in order of dominance)

1. **Affective pain mechanism:** Posttraumatic stress disorder, depression
2. **Central sensitization**
3. **Peripheral neurogenic pain mechanism**—ischemia, remodeling phase

(continues on next page)

APPENDIX 7.A Orthopedic Outpatient, 38-Year-Old Female *(continued from previous page)*

PAIN EDUCATION TOPICS

1. Good vs bad pain, pain–brain connection, multidimensional (emotional, social, mechanical) nature of pain, description of dominating dimension and triggers to pain for treatment
2. Strategies to activate brain's pain control center, including deep breathing, time-out relaxation, and imagery, when performing safe activities at home
3. Strategies to improve meaningful and pleasurable function to improve limitation from pain and allow function to change pain
4. Effects of severe trauma and life-changing events on pain, pain psychology, coping
5. Interdisciplinary chronic pain management program, interdisciplinary cognitive–behavioral medicine, team approach
6. Ischemic musculoskeletal pain mechanism and the need for increased blood flow using movement and prolonged low-level heat
7. Connective tissue healing and remodeling guidelines, need for regular progressive movement, and no-worse concept and motion check for harm as indicators of safe progression
8. Musculoskeletal nerve pain and need for regular movement, green and red light movements and activities (eg, no-worse concept)
9. Posture, body mechanics, and pacing strategies for home activities, including shopping, laundry, and driving (eg, add 1-5 min per day)

Provisional classification supporting information:
- Onset, past intervention results, coping forms, concerns, and behaviors: affective pain mechanism
- Aggravating and alleviating factors, location, description: central sensitization, peripheral neurogenic pain mechanism

PSYCHOSOCIAL YELLOW FLAGS

Check all that apply.

Attitudes and beliefs about pain	✔	Belief that pain is harmful or disabling, resulting in avoidance behaviors (eg, guarding, fear of movement)
	✔	Belief that all pain must be abolished before attempting to return to work or normal activity
	✔	Expectation of increased pain with activity or work; lack of ability to predict capability
	✔	Catastrophizing, thinking the worst, misinterpreting bodily symptoms
		Belief that pain is uncontrollable
		Passive attitude toward rehabilitation
Behaviors	✔	Use of extended rest, disproportionate downtime
		Reduced activity level, with significant withdrawal from activities; boom-bust cycle of activity
	✔	Avoidance of normal activity, progressive substitution of lifestyle away from productive activity
		Report of extremely high intensity of pain (eg, "above 10" on a 0-10 scale)
		Excessive reliance on use of aids or appliances
	✔	Reduction in sleep quality since onset of pain
		High intake of alcohol or other substances (possibly as self-medication), with an increase since onset of pain
		Smoking

Compensation issues		Lack of financial incentive to return to work
		Delay in accessing income support and treatment cost, disputes over eligibility
		History of claims due to other injuries or pain problems
		History of extended time off work due to injury or other pain problems (eg, >12 weeks)
		Previous experience of ineffective case management (eg, absence of interest, perception of being treated punitively)
Diagnosis and treatment	✔	Experience with a health professional who sanctioned disability or did not provide interventions to improve function
	✔	Experience of conflicting diagnoses or explanations for pain, resulting in confusion
		Catastrophizing and fear (eg, of "ending up in a wheelchair") caused by diagnostic language
		Dramatization of pain by a health professional resulting in dependency on treatments and continuation of passive treatment
	✔	Frequent visits to a health professional in the past year (excluding the present episode of pain)
		Expectation of a "techno-fix" (eg, view of body as a machine)
	✔	Lack of satisfaction with previous treatment for pain
	✔	Acceptance of advice to withdraw from job
Emotions	✔	Fear of increased pain with activity or work
	✔	Depression, especially long-term low mood, loss of sense of enjoyment
	✔	Increased irritability
	✔	Anxiety about heightened awareness of body sensations, including sympathetic nervous system arousal
	✔	Feeling of being under stress and unable to maintain a sense of control
	✔	Presence of social anxiety or disinterest in social activity
	✔	Feeling of being useless and not needed
Family	✔	Overprotective partner or spouse (usually well intentioned) who emphasizes fear of harm or catastrophizes
	✔	Solicitous behaviors from spouse (eg, taking over tasks)
		Socially punitive responses from spouse (eg, ignoring, expressing frustration)
		Lack of support by family members for an attempt to return to work
		Lack of available support person with whom to talk about problems
Work	✔	History of manual work in industries such as fishing, forestry, farming, construction, nursing, trucking, migrant or contract labor
		Pattern of frequent job changes, experience of stress at work, job dissatisfaction, poor relationships with peers or supervisors, lack of vocational direction
	✔	Belief that work is harmful, will do damage, or is dangerous
		Unsupportive current work environment
		Low educational background, low socioeconomic status
	✔	Job that involves significant biomechanical demands such as lifting; manual handling of heavy items; extended sitting, standing, driving, or vibration; maintenance of sustained postures or movements; inflexible work schedule without breaks
		Minimal availability of selected duties and graduated return-to-work pathways with poor implementation
		Absence of interest of supervisor, peers, employer

(continues on next page)

APPENDIX 7.A Orthopedic Outpatient, 38-Year-Old Female *(continued from previous page)*

Physical Therapy/Occupational Therapy
Objective Evaluation

OBJECTIVE FINDINGS

Visits 1 and 2:	No mechanical evaluation performed • Allodynia with light touch in areas of pain and nonsymptomatic areas • FABQ Physical Activity 20; FABQ Work 42 • PHQ-9 20 (severe depression) • NDI 30 (severe disability) • Prochaska readiness stage: contemplation • Begin pain education, set movement guidelines based on NDI and PSFS
Visit 3:	Mechanical evaluation performed
Posture:	Forward head; entire body slouched to right side, cradling arm; correct posture—no effect on pain
Active range of motion:	Cervical protrusion nil loss; retraction moderate loss; flexion minimal loss; extension moderate loss; right lateral flexion, rotation nil loss; left lateral flexion, rotation moderate loss. Right upper extremity elevation flexion, abduction, external rotation, and internal rotation all minimal loss. All directions increase pain in neck and upper extremity. Left shoulder range of motion unremarkable, no effect on pain. Patient required rest breaks.
Repeated test movements:	Cervical retraction, extension, flexion, right lateral flexion, left lateral flexion sitting and lying, 5-6x each—increased pain but no worse as a result, no effect on mechanical exam or median nerve test. Patient required rest breaks.
Neurological exam:	Normal motor C3-T1; hypersensitivity right anterior lateral neck, shoulder, chest on right improves moving distally in arm.
Neurodynamic test:	Right MNT, moderate loss compared to left at shoulder, neck, elbow, wrist; repeated elbow extension, increased pain and worse as a result. Entrapment scalene right, scar from stab wound; indirect myofascial release to scar and scalene 5 min; repeated MNT, improved range of motion at all links, decrease in pain.

PROVISIONAL MECHANICAL CLASSIFICATION

Other chronic pain syndrome—cognitive–behavioral, psychological screen for posttraumatic stress disorder and depression

Peripheral neurogenic pain mechanism—ischemic, container dependent; scalene right, stab wound scar

PROVISIONAL PAIN CLASSIFICATION (in order of dominance)

1. **Affective pain mechanism**—depression and posttraumatic stress disorder
2. **Central sensitization**—fear of movement and work
3. **Peripheral neurogenic pain mechanism**—ischemic, container dependent; scalene right, stab wound scar

Intervention, Visits 1-3:

- Contact physician for referral to pain management program and interdisciplinary cognitive–behavioral program
- Refer to pain management program's outpatient psychology evaluation
- Begin pain education, take baseline measurements using NDI, PSFS, PHQ-9, FABQ
- Issue patient education handouts on active sleep restoration, Baseline Activity Tool, central nervous system, nerve pain education, relaxation, breathing
- Initiate Activity Pyramid baseline finding and charting for activities of daily living and low-level aerobic exercise

Resource Utilization Summary:

- Initial evaluation plus 2 outpatient visits before entering program
- Participation in full-day 4-wk program
- After completion of program, gradual return to part-time duty, day shift, ICU pediatric nursing
- Post program outpatient therapy for specific functions such as household and job-specific lifting and carrying activities 1x/wk for 4 wk, starting 2nd wk after completion of program

TREATMENT

Treatment:
- Provide posture strategies for computer and driving to encourage use of lordosis and decrease forward head; lumbar roll for desk and thoracic roll for car
- Review body mechanics strategies of "hip hinge" and lead with "heart not head" for work-related child care and household chores; reinforce get-up-and-move sitting strategies or neurodynamic movements during day for mechanical ischemic nerve pain and symptoms, median nerve bias
- Reinforce breathing and relaxation; redirect interpretation of emotional vs mechanical pain triggers
- Prescribe continuous low-level heat therapy for pain when patient cannot get up and stretch (eg, during extended computer use, driving, or nursing activity without breaks)
- Progress and pace full restoration of cervical ROM and strength, including UE neurological tissues; focus on scalene and median nerve
- Progress and pace full restoration of household chores, grocery shopping, and laundry
- Provide upgraded gym program: improve postural awareness of lordosis and forward head; use physio ball and alternating arm movements and resisted push, pull, waist-to-overhead UE functional patterns

Treatment summary: **Preprogram 3 outpatient visits; full-day 4-wk interdisciplinary cognitive–behavioral program; postprogram 4 outpatient visits; entire treatment 14 wk.** Progress desensitization of central and mechanical ischemic pain mechanisms, with progressive movement directed at UE neurodynamic tissues and spine and emphasis on alignment to meet function load and ROM demands; education on the meaning of and expectations for symptoms

(continues on next page)

APPENDIX 7.A Orthopedic Outpatient, 38-Year-Old Female *(continued from previous page)*

Outcome tool summary:		Initial	Discharge
PSFS:	Sit and work at computer, 1-2 hr	0	9
	Perform regular household tasks and weekly grocery shopping	0	7
	Lift 25 lb and carry 10 ft (job related)	0	7
	Pain limitation to function	3	10
	Pain intensity rating	9 (3 pain medications)	3 (1 pain medication)
		Visit 2	Visit 4
PHQ-9		20 (severe depression)	7 (mild depression)
FABQ		Activity 20; Work 53	Activity 2; Work 12
NDI		30 (severe disability)	12 (mild disability)

Abbreviations: CT = computed tomography; EMG = electromyography; FABQ = Fear-Avoidance Beliefs Questionnaire; ICU = intensive care unit; MNT = median nerve test; MRI = magnetic resonance imaging; NDI = Neck Disability Index; PHQ-9 = Patient Health Questionnaire; PSFS = Patient-Specific Functional Scale; ROM = range of motion; UE = upper extremity.

APPENDIX 7.B Orthopedic Outpatient, 62-Year-Old Male

Physical Therapy/Occupational Therapy Initial Evaluation

SUBJECTIVE FINDINGS

Chief complaint:	Recent: left cervical, shoulder, posterior arm, forearm, hand pain
	Chronic: left low back pain, sacroiliac region to left buttock
Descriptors:	UE: weakness, hand and triceps; pain, numbness, or tingling, entire arm; dull ache, neck and shoulder; occipital headaches
	Back: sharp, stabbing, dull, ache, exploding, fireworks
Onset:	UE: no apparent reason, progressive, starting at neck before heart procedure 12 wk ago, then radiating to hand after procedure
	Back: lumbar surgery 1 yr ago, problems before but worse after surgery, status unchanged for last 6 months with other problems. Was scheduled for lumbar fusion when pretesting found heart problem requiring heart surgery; "heart is bad." No further lumbar surgery planned at this time.
Frequency:	UE: intermittent
	Back: constant
24-hr behavior:	UE: AM worse, PM worse, better as day progresses; Back: same, no change based on time of day
Subjective pain:	(Likert) Faces scale: UE 0-6/10; back 5/10
Aggravating factors:	UE: reaching, drumming, typing, lying in bed with 2 pillows, any form of housework, cardiac rehab exercises
	Back: movement in all directions, exercise, family and job stress
Relieving factors:	Medication, heat, relaxation

Pain Location

Pain Quality
Sharp
Dull
Burning
Pinching
Numbness
Tingling
Other:

PATIENT EDUCATION CONSIDERATIONS

Readiness to learn:	(Ready and self-motivated) Extrinsically motivated (Limitations (see below))
Limitations to learning:	Cognitive Physical Language Financial Cultural
	(Other:) Fear avoidance related to activity and job
Teaching method preferred:	(Handout) (Verbal) (Demonstration) (Practice) Other: Likes to write out own instructions
Explain:	Anxiety related to heart health, son, and job; possible job opportunity; need for further lumbar surgery; inability to exercise because of pain

(continues on next page)

> **APPENDIX 7.B Orthopedic Outpatient, 62-Year-Old Male** *(continued from previous page)*

MEDICAL HISTORY

Past medical history:	General anxiety disorder, high blood pressure, chronic back pain, thyroid disorder, heart disease
Family history:	Heart disease, anxiety, depression, cancer
Surgery and invasive procedures:	Single lumbar fusion >10 yr ago, lumbar discectomy 1 yr ago, heart surgery 12 wk ago
Medications:	Oxycodone, hydrocodone/acetaminophen, acetaminophen, duloxetine, gabapentin, thyroid and heart medication, muscle relaxants (12 other medications listed) Allergies: Sulfa, latex
Previous treatments:	Physical therapy for back, several episodes pre- and postsurgery; mechanical therapy for back; acupuncture; no therapy for neck; currently in cardiac rehab 3x/wk

	X-ray:	MRI:	CT scan:	EMG:	Other:
Diagnostic tests, neck:	Degenerative changes	Degenerative changes, HNP C6-7		Lower cervical radiculopathy	
Diagnostic tests, back:	Degenerative changes	Degenerative changes, old fusion, significant scarring nerve root left L3	Normal	Normal	Normal bone scan

PSYCHOSOCIAL FACTORS

Living situation:	Lives with wife. Has 2 grown children and 4 grandchildren <6 yr old; often babysits. Insomnia for years, worse since heart procedure and neck problem. See checklist of observed yellow flags.
Behavior:	Patient is fearful and anxious regarding worsening weakness in UE. He is overwhelmed by additional comorbidities recently identified with heart problems and is unsure about the future, a third back surgery, and his ability to pursue a job opportunity. He is anxious about mortality and "doesn't want to die, yet."
Occupation:	Retired as police officer for many years; retired as community college professor since last year. Is interested in applying for a curriculum director job with the police department, which would combine both his interests and be his "dream job"; unsure if he can handle the position because of pain. Cares for 2 grandchildren (infant and 4-yr-old) 2 days/wk. Does light household chores (eg, takes garbage out).
Recreation and leisure:	Currently does cardiac rehab 3x/wk, light UE weights 3x/wk. Running was a form of stress release and very important to him in the past, but he has not run in over 5 yr and has unrealistic expectations about his ability to return to running.
Functional disability:	Cares for self independently. Wants to take on more chores related to outdoor and remodeling home but is afraid of hurting himself.
Concerns:	Declining ability to work, exercise, and sleep; doubt whether strength, endurance, and health are sufficient to pursue job opportunity; family-related stress regarding son; concern about relationship with police department; stress regarding declining health
Unhealthy coping forms:	Anxious coping, internalization and stress-related symptoms, obsessions and compulsions regarding high-level exercise (running, heavy weightlifting)

PROVISIONAL PAIN CLASSIFICATION (in order of dominance)

1. **Affective pain mechanism**—generalized anxiety disorder
2. **Central sensitization**—fear avoidance
3. **Peripheral neurogenic pain mechanism, ischemic**—remodeling phase, both cervical and lumbar

PAIN EDUCATION TOPICS

1. Mechanical, emotional, and social pain inputs, journaling to identify dominant culprits and achieve best control
2. Strategies to activate the brain's pain and emotion control center, including deep breathing, imagery, and time-out relaxation
3. Meaningful and pleasurable function to improve limitation from pain, graded exposure
4. Pain psychology, coping with anxiety
5. Ischemic musculoskeletal pain mechanism and need for increased blood flow using movement and prolonged low-level heat
6. Connective tissue healing and remodeling guidelines, need for regular progressive movement, and no-worse concept and motion checks as indicators of safe progression and no harm
7. Peripheral neurogenic pain mechanism and need for evaluation of cervical spine and reevaluation of lumbar spine for direct mechanical therapy

Provisional classification supporting information:

- Onset, past medical history, behavior, functional disability, coping forms—affective pain mechanism
- Location of symptoms, aggravating and alleviating factors, 24-hour behavior—peripheral neurogenic pain mechanism, ischemia

PSYCHOSOCIAL YELLOW FLAGS

Check all that apply.

Attitudes and beliefs about pain	✔	Belief that pain is harmful or disabling, resulting in avoidance behaviors (eg, guarding, fear of movement)
	✔	Belief that all pain must be abolished before attempting to return to work or normal activity
	✔	Expectation of increased pain with activity or work; lack of ability to predict capability
	✔	Catastrophizing, thinking the worst, misinterpreting bodily symptoms
		Belief that pain is uncontrollable
		Passive attitude toward rehabilitation
Behaviors	✔	Use of extended rest, disproportionate downtime
	✔	Reduced activity level, with significant withdrawal from activities; boom-bust cycle of activity
	✔	Avoidance of normal activity, progressive substitution of lifestyle away from productive activity
		Report of extremely high intensity of pain (eg, "above 10" on a 0-10 scale)
		Excessive reliance on use of aids or appliances
	✔	Reduction in sleep quality since onset of pain
	✔	High intake of alcohol or other substances (possibly as self-medication), with an increase since onset of pain
		Smoking

(continues on next page)

APPENDIX 7.B Orthopedic Outpatient, 62-Year-Old Male *(continued from previous page)*

Compensation issues	Lack of financial incentive to return to work
	Delay in accessing income support and treatment cost, disputes over eligibility
	✔ History of claims due to other injuries or pain problems
	✔ History of extended time off work due to injury or other pain problems (eg, >12 weeks)
	Previous experience of ineffective case management (eg, absence of interest, perception of being treated punitively)
Diagnosis and treatment	Experience with a health professional who sanctioned disability or did not provide interventions to improve function
	✔ Experience of conflicting diagnoses or explanations for pain, resulting in confusion
	Catastrophizing and fear (eg, of "ending up in a wheelchair") caused by diagnostic language
	Dramatization of pain by a health professional resulting in dependency on treatments and continuation of passive treatment
	✔ Frequent visits to a health professional in the past year (excluding the present episode of pain)
	✔ Expectation of a "techno-fix" (eg, view of body as a machine)
	✔ Lack of satisfaction with previous treatment for pain
	✔ Acceptance of advice to withdraw from job
Emotions	✔ Fear of increased pain with activity or work
	✔ Depression, especially long-term low mood, loss of sense of enjoyment
	✔ Increased irritability
	✔ Anxiety about heightened awareness of body sensations, including sympathetic nervous system arousal
	✔ Feeling of being under stress and unable to maintain a sense of control
	✔ Presence of social anxiety or disinterest in social activity
	✔ Feeling of being useless and not needed
Family	Overprotective partner or spouse (usually well intentioned) who emphasizes fear of harm or catastrophizes
	Solicitous behaviors from spouse (eg, taking over tasks)
	Socially punitive responses from spouse (eg, ignoring, expressing frustration)
	Lack of support by family members for an attempt to return to work
	✔ Lack of available support person with whom to talk about problems
Work	✔ History of manual work in industries such as fishing, forestry, farming, construction, nursing, trucking, migrant or contract labor
	Pattern of frequent job changes, experience of stress at work, job dissatisfaction, poor relationships with peers or supervisors, lack of vocational direction
	✔ Belief that work is harmful, will do damage, or is dangerous
	Unsupportive current work environment
	Low educational background, low socioeconomic status
	Job that involves significant biomechanical demands such as lifting; manual handling of heavy items; extended sitting, standing, driving, or vibration; maintenance of sustained postures or movements; inflexible work schedule without breaks
	Minimal availability of selected duties and graduated return-to-work pathways with poor implementation
	Absence of interest of supervisor, peers, employer

Physical Therapy/Occupational Therapy Objective Evaluation

OBJECTIVE FINDINGS

Visit 1:	• Partial cervical mechanical evaluation performed, no back evaluation performed • Education regarding pain journal to help identify mechanical, emotional, and social inputs • FABQ Physical Activity Neck 25, Back 25; FABQ Work Neck 33, Back 40 • PASS 61/100 (high level of pain-related anxiety) • Yellow Flag Risk Form 65 (moderate risk of chronic disability) • ODI 45 (severe disability) • NDI 24 (moderate disability) • Prochaska readiness stage—preparation • Movement goals based on NDI, ODI, and PSFS results
Posture:	Forward head, correct posture—decreased hand tingling and numbness sustained 5 min, abolished hand symptoms, increased triceps strength 3-/5 to 3+/5
Active range of motion:	Cervical protrusion nil loss, retraction moderate loss, flexion nil loss, extension moderate loss, cervical rotation right nil loss and left moderate loss, lateral flexion right nil loss and left moderate loss; pain during and at end of motion in all directions, sharp pain present in rotation, lateral flexion left end of all directions. Retraction least painful direction.
Repeated test movements:	Protrusion: Produces, increases, peripheralizes hand symptoms; weaker triceps 2/5; no change in motion; more painful in rotation and lateral flexion left as a result
	Retraction: Active progressed to patient overpressure; decreased or abolished all below-elbow symptoms; decreased upper arm symptoms, increased triceps strength to 3+/5, improved left rotation and lateral flexion range and pain during range; improved range of motion for neurodynamic median and ulnar nerve tests
Neurological and neurodynamic exam:	Decreased light touch to C7, C8 dermatome left. Weakness in lumbricals left 2/5; left 5th digit abduction 3-/5; triceps, wrist extensor 4/5; wrist flexor 4/5. Weaker triceps reflex on left. Positive ulnar nerve and median nerve neurodynamic tests, moderate loss in range for both, increased pain and worse as a result for repeated movement screen at elbow.

Visit 1: PROVISIONAL MECHANICAL CLASSIFICATION

Cervical derangement—unilateral, asymmetrical, below elbow, with motor loss; partial centralization

Other chronic pain—behavioral/psychological screen for health-related anxiety

Visit 1: PROVISIONAL PAIN CLASSIFICATION (in order of dominance)

1. **Affective pain mechanism**—pain-related anxiety
2. **Central sensitization**—fear of movement and work
3. **Peripheral neurogenic pain mechanism, container related**—cervical spine disc
4. **Peripheral neurogenic pain mechanism**—lumbar spine
5. **Ischemia pain mechanism**—remodeling phase, cervical and lumbar spine

(continues on next page)

APPENDIX 7.B Orthopedic Outpatient, 62-Year-Old Male *(continued from previous page)*

Intervention Visit 1-3:
- Contact physician for referral to outpatient psychology evaluation and anxiety management
- Begin pain journal education and active sleep restoration
- Take baseline measurements—ODI, PSFS, PASS, FABQ, Yellow Flag Risk Form
- Education posture—prevent forward head and apply to activities of daily living
- Active retraction with patient overpressure 10x for 10 sec each, every hour; check strength and range of motion and signs of centralization

Visit 4:	Evaluation of low back complaints—lumbar mechanical evaluation; pretest symptoms 6/10 left low back, 4/10 left sacroiliac joint and buttock
Posture:	Normal lordosis
Active range of motion:	Flexion: Nil loss, decreased pain
	Extension: Nil loss, increased pain (worst direction)
	Left side glide: Pain limits range, increased pain
	Right side glide: Nil loss, decreased pain
Repeated test movements:	Flexion: Sitting, decreased pain, no effect; lying, decreased pain, no effect
	Extension: Standing, increased pain, no effect; prone, increased pain, no effect
	Left side glide: Standing increased pain, no effect
	Right side glide: Decreased pain, no effect
	Repeated left pelvic posterior rotation and anterior rotation: Increased pain, no effect
Neurological exam:	Normal motor and sensory L1-S1; negative straight leg raise, slump bilateral. Two-point discrimination test: Left low back quadrant, 8 cm; right low back quadrant, 4 cm
MMT trunk/ special tests:	4/5 abdominals, side plank endurance 40 sec bilateral, plank 30 sec, 3/5 erector spinae; all tests increase pain, no worse as a result; positive provocation quadrant test left immediate increase. No effect with any sacroiliac joint provocation test.

Visit 4: PROVISIONAL MECHANICAL CLASSIFICATION

Other function—mechanically inconclusive, chronic pain return to function, consider sensory-motor approach
Other chronic pain—psychological screen for health-related anxiety

Visit 4: PROVISIONAL PAIN CLASSIFICATION (in order of dominance)

1. **Affective pain mechanism**—pain-related anxiety
2. **Central sensitization**—fear of movement and work
3. **Peripheral neurogenic pain mechanism, container related**—cervical spine derangement
4. **Motor/autonomic, lumbar spine**—mechanically inconclusive; lateral foramina stenosis left, primary sensory motor dysfunction

Intervention Visits 4-20:
- Follow up on psychology referral for anxiety management strategies
- Review pain journal for inputs and strategize on emotion–anxiety–pain connection and mechanical pain connections
- Deep breathing and time-out relaxation practice
- Progress full centralization of cervical derangement with extension and lateral flexion procedures and posture education
- Sensory–motor–cortical remodeling for low back pain consisting of 4 stages[1]:
  - Stage 1: Sensory localization retraining to determine site of stimulus; motor retraining in laterality recognition using Recognise software (Neuro Orthopaedic Institute, Adelaide City, Australia)
  - Stage 2: Sensory localization and stimulus type retraining to determine site and size of probe; motor retraining in imagined movements using videotape of model performing movements small to full range
  - Stage 3: Graphesthesia training to determine letters and numbers of varying size and orientation; motor retraining in local muscle stabilization, diaphragm breathing with pelvic floor and postural bracing, plank, side plank, birddog
  - Stage 4: Graphesthesia training to determine 3-letter words of varying size and orientation, overlapping letters; motor retraining for full range movements forward and backward, side glide left and right, integration with upper and lower body, 3 plane core
- Education regarding tissue remodeling, pain behavior for effective remodeling using the no-worse concept, traffic light guide, and *Explain Pain* book[2]

Resource Utilization Summary:
- Initial evaluation plus 19 visits; 1x/wk for total of 20 visits in 20 wk
- Initial evaluation from psychology, ongoing treatment 1x/wk

TREATMENT

Treatment:
- Provide posture strategies for computer use and driving; lifting and sustained postures for child care, computer use, and drumming to encourage neutral spine and decrease forward head; small lumbar roll for desk and thoracic roll for car
- Review body mechanics strategies of "hip hinge" and lead with "heart not head" for work-related and household chores; reinforce get-up-and-move sitting strategies or stretching during day for mechanical pain
- Reinforce use of deep breathing, imagery, and relaxation; redirect interpretation of emotional vs mechanical pain triggers
- Prescribe continuous low-level heat therapy for pain when patient cannot get up and stretch (eg, during extended computer use, driving, or child care activity without breaks)
- Progress and pace full restoration of cervical ROM and strength
- Progress and pace full restoration of household chores (eg, grocery shopping, laundry) and outdoor lawn and home maintenance
- Provide upgraded gym program to strengthen upper body, improve postural awareness of neutral spine, and prevent forward head using weightlifting for neck and upper extremities and push, pull, and waist-to-overhead UE functional patterns
- Progress core stability exercise and cardiovascular, high-intensity interval training after completion of sensory–motor–cortical training program detailed above

(continues on next page)

APPENDIX 7.B Orthopedic Outpatient, 62-Year-Old Male *(continued from previous page)*

Treatment summary: **20 total visits over 20 wk.** Progress desensitization of central and mechanical ischemic pain mechanisms with progressive movement directed at cervical spine and emphasis on alignment to meet function load and ROM demands; provide education on the meaning of and expectations for symptoms and anxiety control and relaxation for stress management. The more acute problem related to the cervical spine showed mechanical pain mechanisms dominating, whereas chronic low back complaints require central sensitization pain mechanism management program for best results. Managing and identifying the dominating mechanism guided results for two distinct problems.

Outcome tool summary:

PSFS:

	Initial	Discharge
Do prolonged typing or drumming, 2 hr (neck)	0	9
Perform regular outdoor household tasks such as weekly lawn care and garbage removal (back)	3	7
Lift 30 lb (grandkid) and carry 10 ft (neck and back)	0	7
Pain limitation to function	3	10
Pain intensity rating	Neck 6, back 5 with medications	Neck 0, back 3; oxycodone and hydrocodone/ acetaminophen discontinued; only acetaminophen for pain

	Visit 1	Visit 20
PASS	61/100	15/100
FABQ	Neck Activity 25, Work 33	Neck Activity 5, Work 1
	Back Activity 25, Work 40	Back Activity 8, Work 3
Yellow Flag Risk Form	65 (moderate risk of chronic disability)	35 (low risk of chronic disability)
ODI	45 (severe disability)	20 (moderate disability)
NDI	24 (moderate disability)	5 (mild disability)

Abbreviations: CT = computed tomography; EMG = electromyography; FABQ = Fear-Avoidance Beliefs Questionnaire; HNP = herniated nucleus pulposus; MRI = magnetic resonance imaging; NDI = Neck Disability Index; ODI = Oswestry Disability Index; PASS = Pain Anxiety Symptom Scale; PSFS = Patient-Specific Functional Scale; ROM = range of motion; UE = upper extremity.

Resources
1. Wand BM, O'Connell NE, Di Pietro F, Bulsara M. Managing chronic nonspecific low back pain with a sensorimotor retraining approach: Exploratory multiple-baseline study of 3 participants. *Phys Ther.* 2011;91:535-546.
2. Butler D, Moseley L. *Explain Pain.* Adelaide, Australia: Noigroup Publications; 2003.

APPENDIX 7.C Orthopedic Outpatient, 55-Year-Old Male

Physical Therapy/Occupational Therapy Initial Evaluation

SUBJECTIVE FINDINGS

Chief complaint:	Bilateral posterolateral cervical spine, radiates to suboccipital in form of headaches
Descriptors:	Dull headache, pinching, tingling, sharp in neck
Onset:	Motor vehicle accident 2 yr ago, broadsided by driver running red light; no insurance coverage; progressively worsening last 8 mo
Frequency:	Constant symptoms, sharper with movement
24-hr behavior:	No pattern in time of day; after activity always worse; each day starts the same
Subjective pain:	(Likert) / Faces scale: 7/10
Aggravating factors:	Any motion causes sharp neck pain, prolonged activity causes headache, stress increases all symptoms
Relieving factors:	Medication, heat, relaxation

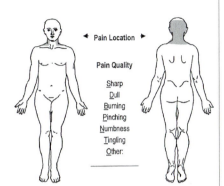

PATIENT EDUCATION CONSIDERATIONS

Readiness to learn:	Ready and self-motivated (Extrinsically motivated) (Limitations (see below))
Limitations to learning:	Cognitive Physical Language Financial Cultural (Other:) Anger
Teaching method preferred:	Handout Verbal (Demonstration) (Practice) Other:
Explain:	Anger and blame directed at driver and lack of insurance

(continues on next page)

> **APPENDIX 7.C** Orthopedic Outpatient, 55-Year-Old Male *(continued from previous page)*

MEDICAL HISTORY

Past medical history:	High blood pressure
Family history:	Depression
Surgery and invasive procedures:	Trigger point injections—temporarily helpful but too expensive to continue
Medications:	Narcotics, muscle relaxants—help patient tolerate pain to function Allergies: None
Previous treatments:	Physical therapy, massage and exercise, chiropractor manipulations and modalities did not help; last treatments >6 mo ago; did not follow exercise recommendations

Diagnostic tests: X-ray: Degenerative changes   MRI: Degenerative changes   CT scan: EMG: Other:

PSYCHOSOCIAL FACTORS

Living situation:	Lives with wife, 3 children ages 17, 14, and 12; works full-time as electrician; see checklist of observed yellow flags.
Behavior:	Patient is hostile but cooperative, is angry at driver and health care system for not getting rid of his pain, and engages in repeated front desk altercations regarding availability of appointments.
Occupation:	Electrician; works full-time; missed a lot of work over last 8 mo due to pain
Recreation and leisure:	Does not exercise; watches kids' sports; was a seasonal hunter but because of pain has been unable since accident
Functional disability:	Cares for self independently. Limits work to what needs to be done; tries to get others to do the work, causing stress on job and with coworkers. Wife and kids perform all household duties including shopping, laundry, outdoor chores, driving to kids' events. His focus is on continuing to work; "need money." Job is unsupportive for his situation.
Concerns:	Declining ability to work; safety on job site; lack of medical insurance; litigation regarding lack of insurance coverage and continued need for treatment; excessive use of medications, alcohol
Unhealthy coping forms:	Defensiveness, depression, internalization and stress-related symptoms, escape through substance use

PROVISIONAL PAIN CLASSIFICATION (order of dominance)

1. **Affective pain mechanism**: Anger
2. **Central sensitization**
3. **Ischemia**, remodeling phase

PAIN EDUCATION TOPICS

1. Mechanical, emotional, and social dimensions of pain; journaling to identify dominant dimension and direction of care
2. Strategies to activate brain's pain and emotion control center (eg, deep breathing, time-out relaxation)
3. Meaningful and pleasurable function to improve limitation from pain, no need for direct exercise, gradual exposure to fun
4. Pain psychology—coping with anger
5. Ischemic musculoskeletal pain—need for increased blood flow using movement and prolonged low-level heat
6. Connective tissue healing and remodeling guidelines; need for regular progressive movement; no-worse concept and motion checks as indicators of safe progression and no harm

Provisional classification supporting information:
- Onset, past interventions, behavior, functional disability, coping forms—affective pain mechanism
- Location of symptoms, behavior, aggravating and alleviating factors—central sensitization, ischemia

PSYCHOSOCIAL YELLOW FLAGS

Check all that apply.

Attitudes and beliefs about pain	✔ Belief that pain is harmful or disabling, resulting in avoidance behaviors (eg, guarding, fear of movement)
	✔ Belief that all pain must be abolished before attempting to return to work or normal activity
	✔ Expectation of increased pain with activity or work; lack of ability to predict capability
	✔ Catastrophizing, thinking the worst, misinterpreting bodily symptoms
	✔ Belief that pain is uncontrollable
	✔ Passive attitude toward rehabilitation
Behaviors	Use of extended rest, disproportionate downtime
	✔ Reduced activity level, with significant withdrawal from activities; boom-bust cycle of activity
	✔ Avoidance of normal activity, progressive substitution of lifestyle away from productive activity
	Report of extremely high intensity of pain (eg, "above 10" on a 0-10 scale)
	Excessive reliance on use of aids or appliances
	✔ Reduction in sleep quality since onset of pain
	✔ High intake of alcohol or other substances (possibly as self-medication), with an increase since onset of pain
	Smoking
Compensation issues	Lack of financial incentive to return to work
	✔ Delay in accessing income support and treatment cost, disputes over eligibility
	History of claims due to other injuries or pain problems
	History of extended time off work due to injury or other pain problems (eg, >12 weeks)
	Previous experience of ineffective case management (eg, absence of interest, perception of being treated punitively)

(continues on next page)

APPENDIX 7.C Orthopedic Outpatient, 55-Year-Old Male *(continued from previous page)*

Diagnosis and treatment	✔ Experience with a health professional who sanctioned disability or did not provide interventions to improve function
	✔ Experience of conflicting diagnoses or explanations for pain, resulting in confusion
	Catastrophizing and fear (eg, of "ending up in a wheelchair") caused by diagnostic language
	Dramatization of pain by a health professional resulting in dependency on treatments and continuation of passive treatment
	✔ Frequent visits to a health professional in the past year (excluding the present episode of pain)
	✔ Expectation of a "techno-fix" (eg, view of body as a machine)
	✔ Lack of satisfaction with previous treatment for pain
	Acceptance of advice to withdraw from job
Emotions	✔ Fear of increased pain with activity or work
	✔ Depression, especially long-term low mood, loss of sense of enjoyment
	✔ Increased irritability
	Anxiety about heightened awareness of body sensations, including sympathetic nervous system arousal
	✔ Feeling of being under stress and unable to maintain a sense of control
	✔ Presence of social anxiety or disinterest in social activity
	✔ Feeling of being useless and not needed
Family	Overprotective partner or spouse (usually well intentioned) who emphasizes fear of harm or catastrophizes
	Solicitous behaviors from spouse (eg, taking over tasks)
	Socially punitive responses from spouse (eg, ignoring, expressing frustration)
	Lack of support by family members for an attempt to return to work
	✔ Lack of available support person with whom to talk about problems
Work	✔ History of manual work in industries such as fishing, forestry, farming, construction, nursing, trucking, migrant or contract labor
	✔ Pattern of frequent job changes, experience of stress at work, job dissatisfaction, poor relationships with peers or supervisors, lack of vocational direction
	✔ Belief that work is harmful, will do damage, or is dangerous
	✔ Unsupportive current work environment
	Low educational background, low socioeconomic status
	✔ Job that involves significant biomechanical demands such as lifting; manual handling of heavy items; extended sitting, standing, driving, or vibration; maintenance of sustained postures or movements; inflexible work schedule without breaks
	Minimal availability of selected duties and graduated return-to-work pathways with poor implementation
	Absence of interest of supervisor, peers, employer

Physical Therapy/Occupational Therapy
Objective Evaluation

OBJECTIVE FINDINGS

Visit 1:	• Partial mechanical evaluation performed • Education on use of pain journal to help identify mechanical, emotional, and social triggers to pain intensity • FABQ Physical Activity 24, Work 48 • PHQ-9 15 (moderate to severe depression) • Yellow Flag Risk Form 60 (moderate risk of chronic disability) • NDI 24 (moderate disability) • Prochaska readiness stage: contemplation • Begin pain journal, set movement goals based on NDI and PSFS scores
Posture:	Forward head, correct posture—no effect on pain
Active range of motion:	Cervical protrusion nil loss, retraction moderate loss, flexion moderate loss, extension moderate loss, cervical rotation right and left moderate loss, lateral flexion right and left moderate loss; pain during and at end of motion in all directions, sharp pain present in rotation right and left at end of motions; lateral flexion least painful direction
Repeated test movements:	Screen of all motions, 10 reps each, increased pain but no worse from baseline, no effect mechanically on any motion
Neurological and neurodynamic exam:	Normal motor, sensory C3-T1, negative neurodynamic passive neck flexion test

PROVISIONAL MECHANICAL CLASSIFICATION

Dysfunction—articular, multiple directions

Other chronic pain—behavioral, psychological screen for depression and anger, risk for chronic disability

PROVISIONAL PAIN CLASSIFICATION (in order of dominance)

1. **Affective pain mechanism**—depression and anger, moderate risk for chronic disability
2. **Central sensitization**—fear of movement and work
3. **Ischemia**—cervical articular dysfunction, multiple directions

Intervention Visit 1:

- Contact physician for referral to outpatient psychology evaluation for depression and chronic disability risk
- Begin pain journal education, active sleep restoration, ischemic pain education
- Take baseline measurements: NDI, PSFS, PHQ-9, FABQ, Yellow Flag Risk Form
- Issue handouts on active sleep restoration, practical pain journal

Intervention Visits 2-8:

- Follow-up on psychology referral for anger management strategies
- Review pain journal for inputs and strategize on reducing connection between emotion (anger) and pain and between mechanics and pain
- Instruct in deep breathing and imagery identification and use, progress to time-out relaxation practice
- Begin movement remodeling in lateral planes, progress to sagittal and transverse planes
- Educate on tissue remodeling and pain behavior for effective remodeling using Activity Pyramid and traffic light guide

(continues on next page)

APPENDIX 7.C Orthopedic Outpatient, 55-Year-Old Male *(continued from previous page)*

Resource Utilization Summary:
- Initial evaluation plus 7 visits; 1x every 2 wk; total 8 visits over 16 wk
- Initial evaluation from psychology and recommended anger management course

TREATMENT

Treatment:	• Instruct in posture strategies for computer use, driving, lifting, and sustained postures for work to encourage use of lordosis and decrease forward head; provide lumbar roll for desk and thoracic roll for car
	• Review body mechanics strategies of "hip hinge" and lead with "heart not head" for work-related and household chores; reinforce get-up-and-move sitting strategies or stretching during day for mechanical pain
	• Reinforce deep breathing, imagery, and relaxation to redirect interpretation of emotional vs mechanical pain triggers
	• Continuous low-level heat therapy for pain when patient cannot get up and stretch (eg, during extended computer use, driving, or long periods of work activity without a break)
	• Progress and pace full restoration of cervical ROM and strength; progress to full restoration of household chores, including grocery shopping, laundry, outdoor chores, and home maintenance
	• Provide gym program to improve postural awareness of lordosis and decrease forward head with weightlifting for upper extremities and push, pull, waist-to-overhead UE functional patterns
	• Progress and pace return to shooting range to prepare for hunting season
Treatment summary:	**OP 8 visits over 16 wk.** Progress desensitization of central and mechanical ischemic pain mechanisms with progressive movement directed at spine with emphasis on alignment to meet functional load and ROM demands; provide education on the meaning of and expectations for symptoms and control of anger and other emotions

Outcome tool summary:		Initial	Discharge
PSFS:	Engage in prolonged above-head work for 2 hr	3	9
	Perform regular outdoor household tasks weekly (eg, lawn care, garbage removal)	0	7
	Lift 30 lb and carry 10 ft (job related)	0	7
	Pain limitation to function	3	10
	Pain intensity rating	7 (2 pain medications)	2 (no pain medications
		Visit 1	Visit 8
PHQ-9		15 (moderate to severe depression)	2 (no depression)
FABQ		Activity 24, Work 48	Activity 0, Work 0
Yellow Flag Risk Form		60 (moderate risk)	25 (low risk)
NDI		24 (moderate disability)	5 (mild disability)

Abbreviations: CT = computed tomography; EMG = electromyography; FABQ = Fear-Avoidance Beliefs Questionnaire; MRI = magnetic resonance imaging; NDI = Neck Disability Index; PHQ-9 = Patient Health Questionnaire; PSFS = Patient-Specific Functional Scale; ROM = range of motion; UE = upper extremity.

APPENDIX 7.D Orthopedic Outpatient: 48-Year-Old Male

Physical Therapy/Occupational Therapy Initial Evaluation

SUBJECTIVE FINDINGS

Chief complaint:	Central low back pain
Descriptors:	Dull, tightness
Onset:	Progressive since college; acute episodes for no apparent reason, most recent 3 yr ago, unchanged. Very active in exercise, fitness, and sports.
Frequency:	Intermittent
24-hr behavior:	No pattern in time of day, but stiffness in AM. Sleep disturbance, job and family stress.
Subjective pain:	(Likert) / Faces scale: 3/10 at worst, no pain at best
Aggravating factors:	Unsure activity, stress (job, family)
Relieving factors:	Yoga class, sometimes. On 2 occasions patient traveled with college friends and had no back pain, but symptoms returned within 1 day of return home; he found this unusual and thought he should mention.

Pain Location

Pain Quality
Sharp
Dull
Burning
Pinching
Numbness
Tingling
Other:

PATIENT EDUCATION CONSIDERATIONS

Readiness to learn:	(Ready and self-motivated) Extrinsically motivated Limitations (see below)
Limitations to learning:	Cognitive Physical Language Financial Cultural (Other:) None
Teaching method preferred:	(Handout) Verbal (Demonstration) (Practice) Other:
Explain:	

MEDICAL HISTORY

Past medical history:	Very healthy
Family history:	
Surgery and invasive procedures:	Trigger point injections at 2 different pain clinics—not helpful, worsened symptoms
Medications:	None Allergies: Penicillin
Previous treatments:	Physical therapy, massage and exercise, chiropractor manipulations and modalities, work hardening, McKenzie Method
Diagnostic tests:	X-ray: DDD L5-S1 MRI: DDD, DJD, herniated L5-S1 CT scan: EMG: Negative Other: Negative bone scan

PSYCHOSOCIAL FACTORS

Living situation:	Lives with wife and 3 sons (ages 12, 15, 17); very active family; coaches and referees boys' teams. Patient is oldest of 5 children, all living locally; parents are living; father has medical complications, and mother needs frequent help. Siblings are not in agreement about how to deal with changes in parents' medical status and living situation, causing stress.
Behavior:	Patient is cooperative and questioning whether stress is cause of pain; nothing has helped, and pain has steadily increased since college.
Occupation:	Patient owns a business; the past several years have been stressful financially, and he has had a hard time keeping employees.
Recreation and leisure:	Bikes, plays basketball, runs, swims, does yoga and cross-fit exercise, travels, takes active family trips (eg, kayaking, rock climbing)
Functional disability:	None—performs all daily living, household, occupation, and recreation activities, regardless of pain
Concerns:	Unsure about parents' situation, relationship with siblings, keeping employees, back pain related to stress
Unhealthy coping forms:	Defensiveness, depression, obsessions and compulsions

PROVISIONAL PAIN CLASSIFICATION

Affective pain mechanism—tension myositis syndrome, perfectionism trait

PAIN EDUCATION TOPICS

1. Good vs bad pain, pain–brain connection (ie, brain uses pain in body to distract from negative emotions in subconscious mind by causing ischemia in tissues ["victim"], but "culprit" is negative emotions in unconscious mind, so treat culprit, not victim)
2. Strategies to activate brain's pain control center, including deep breathing and time-out relaxation; identification of what could be looming in unconscious mind by journaling
3. Mechanical pain vs emotional pain—both cause ischemic response at tissue level, but source of ischemia is different (ie, tissue vs negative repressed emotion)
4. Tension myositis syndrome—definition, cause, and treatment

Provisional classification supporting information:

- Location, past interventions, psychosocial characteristics, concerns, coping forms—affective pain mechanism

(continues on next page)

APPENDIX 7.D Orthopedic Outpatient: 48-Year-Old Male

Physical Therapy/Occupational Therapy
Objective Evaluation

OBJECTIVE FINDINGS

Visit 1:	• Mechanical evaluation performed • PHQ-9 score 4 (none) • Yellow Flag Risk Form 21 (low risk of chronic disability) • ODI 8 (mild disability) • Prochaska readiness stage—action • Begin pain education, pain journaling
Posture:	Decrease lordosis, correct posture—no effect on pain
Active range of motion and repeated test movements:	No loss of lumbar ROM, flexion, extension, side glide right, side glide left No pain produced during exam, 20 reps each direction in standing Prone press up and knee to chest
Core endurance:	Plank 45/45 sec, side plank right 45/45 sec, side plank left 45/45 sec, bridge right 45/45 sec, bridge left 45/45 sec No pain during testing, patient has excellent awareness of posture Diaphragm breath analysis—good, intact
Neurological exam:	Negative slump, straight leg raise test bilaterally, repeated testing no effect, unable to reproduce pain
Special test:	Negative quadrant exam bilaterally, held test for 1 min
Palpation:	Upper trapezius, lumbar paraspinal, posterior and lateral glutei bilaterally—all positive for tenderness compared with other muscles

PROVISIONAL MECHANICAL CLASSIFICATION

Other—chronic pain, mechanically inconclusive

PROVISIONAL PAIN CLASSIFICATION

Affective pain mechanism—tension myositis syndrome

Intervention Visit 1:

- Contact physician for referral to psychology for investigative approach addressing repressed unconscious negative emotions
- Begin pain education, take baseline measurements (ODI, PHQ-9, Yellow Flag Risk Form)
- Issue information document on diagnosis, definition, and treatment of tension myositis syndrome and referral information for self-diagnosis and care planning

Resource Utilization Summary:

- Initial evaluation plus follow-up phone call, 6 wk
- Patient opted for psychology evaluation

TREATMENT

Treatment:
- Education regarding brain–pain connection, affective unconscious mind, perfectionism trait, and connection to back pain
- Differentiation of mechanical from emotional pain mechanisms and evaluation; history results

Treatment summary: Patient was referred for investigative psychology regarding unconscious repressed emotions and their connection to pain. At 6-wk follow-up call, patient had no pain and was very grateful for the thorough examination, explanation, and referral. No further treatment was necessary; he understood why he was in pain and why past treatments did not work.

Abbreviations: CT = computed tomography; DDD = degenerative disc disease; DJD = degenerative joint disease; EMG = electromyography; MRI = magnetic resonance imaging; ODI = Oswestry Disability Index; PHQ-9 = Patient Health Questionnaire; PSFS = Patient-Specific Functional Scale; ROM = range of motion.

APPENDIX 7.E Clinical Reasoning for Subjective CNS Pain Characteristics

Central Nervous System
Pain Mechanisms: Subjective Characteristics

Central Sensitization	Affective Pain Mechanism Conscious (C) vs Unconscious (U)	Autonomic/Motor Pain Mechanism
Location: Widespread, nonanatomical distribution of pain	**Location:** (C) Widespread, nonanatomical distribution; (U) axial low back pain, neck pain, headaches, knee pain (specific location)	**Location:** Widespread, nonanatomical distribution of pain to upper and/or lower extremity may include the spine, typically affects more than one nerve field
Frequency: Constant, unremitting, spontaneous, latent, paroxysmal pain; easily provoked pain with all activity	**Descriptors:** (C) Catastrophic emotional language; (U) dull, tight, weak, sharp with movement	**Frequency:** Constant unremitting, spontaneous, latent, paroxysmal pain
Descriptors: Catastrophic terms related to harm and unhealed tissue; pain threat high	**Frequency:** (C) Constant, spontaneous, latent, paroxysmal pain; (U) intermittent	**Descriptors:** Deep, dull, burning, aching, pulsating, stabbing, cold intolerance
Intensity: High severity, irritability	**Intensity:** (C) High severity, irritability; (U) low-grade irritant	**Intensity:** High severity, irritability
Onset: Chronic >3 months; past expected tissue healing & pathology recovery times; pain disproportionate to the nature and extent of injury or pathology	**Onset:** Chronic >3 months; past expected tissue healing/pathology recovery times; pain disproportionate to the nature and extent of injury or pathology	**Onset:** Chronic >3 months; past expected tissue healing/pathology recovery times; pain disproportionate to the nature and extent of injury or pathology; initial trauma managed poorly.
History: Failed interventions (medical, surgical, therapeutic)	**History:** Failed interventions (medical, surgical, therapeutic); (C) preexisting anxiety, depression, psychological trauma (ie, abuse, accident, work-related injury), CNS disorder (ie, SCI, MS, etc); (U) increased stress/repressed negative emotions regarding current life pressures, past childhood relationships with parents & siblings, characteristic of perfectionism	**History:** Immune, GI, endocrine, parasympathetic, and sympathetic systems symptoms and/or complications
24-hour behavior: Erratic, inconsistent, night pain, disturbed sleep	**24-hour behavior:** Inconsistent pain, night pain, disturbed sleep	**24-hour behavior:** Erratic, inconsistent, night pain, disturbed sleep
Psychosocial screen: Positive for pain behaviors (maladaptive and harmful beliefs/poor self-efficacy), high functional disability	**Psychosocial screen:** (C) Positive for negative emotions, altered family, work, social life, medical conflict, high functional disability; (U) appear negative on conscious level	**Psychosocial screen:** Positive for pain behaviors (maladaptive beliefs/poor self-efficacy), high functional disability
Aggravating or alleviating factors: Disproportionate, nonmechanical, unpredictable pattern in response to multiple nonspecific factors; heat helps; antiepileptic/antidepressant medications help		**Other clinical signs:** Swelling indicating lymphedema, spasticity, tone, discoloration of skin, skin and hair sensitivities, trophic changes, excessive sweating

APPENDIX 7.F Clinical Reasoning for Objective CNS Pain Characteristics

Central Nervous System
Pain Mechanisms: Objective Characteristics

Central Sensitization *Spinal Cord Facilitation*	Affective Pain Mechanism Conscious (C) vs Unconscious (U) *Emotional/Social Dysfunction*	Autonomic/Motor Pain Mechanism *Cortical Disinhibition*
Objective findings: Spinal cord facilitation signs; pain evoked easily **Movement testing:** Disproportionate inconsistent nonmechanical/anatomical pattern of pain provocation; no relationship between stimulus and response; common latency effect; result is worse; absence of tissue injury/pathology **Palpation:** Diffuse nonanatomic areas of pain or tenderness; light touch elicits noxious response (allodynia) in area of symptoms. **Posture:** Antalgic postures or movements; disuse atrophy of muscles **Neurological testing:** Positive for hyperalgesia, allodynia, hyperpathia **Proprioceptive screen:** Spine and extremity tests are negative **Breath assessment:** Sitting diaphragm breathing test: upper respiratory pattern **Yellow flag assessment:** Positive identification of catastrophization, fear-avoidance behavior, harmful thoughts, distress. **Readiness stage:** Precontemplation, contemplation, preparation **Fear Avoidance Beliefs Questionnaire (FABQ) score:** Physical activity ≥14 **Yellow flag risk score:** Over 55 indicates moderate risk of chronic disability **Outcome measures:** Disabilities of the Arm, Shoulder and Head, Oswestry Disability Index, Neck Disability Index, Lower Extremity Function Scale, with moderate disabilities (may choose others)	**Objective findings:** (C) Similar to central sensitivity with greater emotional component; (U) similar to ischemia; treatment ineffective. Tender points: upper trapezius, lumbar paraspinals, posterior lateral aspects of the gluteus maximus, bilaterally **Yellow flag assessment:** (C) Positive for distress, negative emotions, depression, anxiety, anger, altered family/work/social life, medical conflict, reduced coping skills with life-changing events (ie, SCI, loss, amputation, neurological impairment, etc); (U) appear negative on a conscious level but positive toward increased stress & repressed negative emotions regarding current life stressors, past childhood relationships with parents & siblings, characteristic of perfectionism at the unconscious level. **Psychometric tools:** Assist referral to (C) cognitive–behavioral therapy program and/or (U) investigative psychology • Yellow Flag Risk Form: Chronic disability risk assessment (>55 points) • Anger/depression: Patient Health Questionnaire (PHQ-9) (score >10) • Anxiety: Pain Anxiety Symptom Scale (higher score) • (U) Tension myositis syndrome information document (>3 yes answers)	**Objective findings:** Same as central sensitivity; in addition signs of: • Cortical dysfunction (spasticity, tone) • Autonomic nervous system dysfunction (skin discoloration, excessive sweating, trophic changes, hair excitability, lymph edema) • Involvement of sympathetic and parasympathetic systems **General illness** may be present from immune and GI system involvement. **Proprioceptive screen:** All spine and extremity tests are positive **Palpation:** Diffuse nonanatomic areas of pain/tenderness; light touch elicits noxious response in areas with/without symptoms often within the space around the skin **2-point discrimination:** Positive findings within area of symptoms; primary sensory cortex findings **Neurological testing:** Positive findings related to loss of graphesthesia (recognition of symbols drawn on skin), incomplete drawing of body outline for area of symptoms, signs of neglect present in left–right discrimination testing; positive findings in localization and precision sensory testing

APPENDIX 7.G Clinical Reasoning for CNS Pain Intervention

Central Nervous System Pain Mechanisms: Intervention		
Central Sensitization	**Affective Pain Mechanism Conscious (C) vs Unconscious (U)**	**Autonomic/Motor Pain Mechanism**
Education: • Explanation of the nondamaging nature of pain: hurt vs harm; interpretation of inputs • Pain mechanism education • Discussion of the role of negative emotions, thoughts, and beliefs; review pain journal • Training in coping strategies for fear of motion or activity; use relaxation, diaphragm breathing training • Explanation of the Activity Pyramid: Green, yellow, and red lights, flare-up management • Identification of the activity baseline and explanation of the no-worse concept; return control to patient **Activity:** • Graded exposure to patient-identified fearful/harmful activity; build low aerobic activity, HR at 55%-75% max, for 2-5 hr/wk • Weight training to build upper and lower extremity strength; start with isolated movements and progress to function at HR 55%-75% of maximum, 2x/wk • Deep muscle training for spine postural stabilization; progress to function, 2x/wk • High-intensity interval training (HIIT); progress to 10-20 min intervals, HR >75% of max, 1-2x/wk • Mechanical exam	Same as central sensitization **(C) Education:** • Regarding readiness stage • Negative emotions' contribution to pain • Focused discussion based on psychometric tools (PHQ-9, PASS, Yellow Flag Risk Form) • Interdisciplinary cognitive–behavioral therapy program, if Yellow Flag Risk Form score >55 **(U) Education:** Tension myositis syndrome; discuss treatment progression: • Understand mechanism; brain's efforts to protect are causing tissue ischemia • Acknowledge activation of mechanism related to unconscious repressed, negative emotions • Refer to investigative psychologist if unable to self-treat with John Sarno's books (*The Mindbody Prescription: Healing the Body, Healing the Pain; Healing Back Pain: The Mind-Body Connection; The Divided Mind: The Epidemic of Mindbody Disorders*) Patients must have **psychological evaluation**, if this mechanism is classified as dominating.	Education and activity same as central sensitization **Treatment for output systems with symptoms:** Lymphedema: Lymph massage, compression stockings Tone and spasticity: Facilitatory and inhibitory techniques Immune system and metabolic disorders: Build low aerobic activity, HR 55%-75% of maximum, 2-5 hr/wk; progress to 10-20 min HIIT, HR >75% of maximum, 1-2x/wk **Treatment for cortical disinhibition:** Sensorimotor retraining approach: 5 stages to progress, 3x/day *Sensory retraining:* (1) localization training, (2) localization and precision stimulus type, (3) graphesthesia with letters & numbers, (4) graphesthesia with 3-letter words, (5) graphesthesia with simple calculations • Progress visualization, size, orientation, speed, overlapping • Progress to next stage when accuracy is 80% *Motor retraining:* (1) left–right discrimination, (2) imagined movements, (3) reflective movements, (4) local isometric bracing, (5) small-range movements with feedback, (6) full-range movements with feedback (mirrors, palpation, elastic tape, watching, imagining) • Progress therapy as patient masters exercise

CHAPTER 8

Motor/Autonomic Pain Mechanism

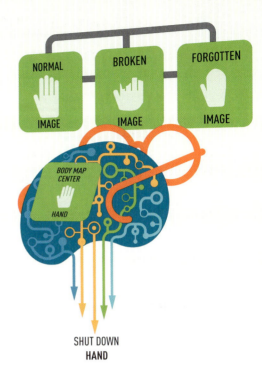

Readiness to change precedes all education and intervention.
—G. Lorimer Moseley

POINTS TO DISCUSS

- Complex regional pain syndrome and the physiological processes involved in the motor/autonomic pain mechanism
- Contributions of inflammatory mechanisms, vasomotor or autonomic dysfunctions, and cortical or neuroplastic changes in the central nervous system
- Principles of neural plasticity and cortical reorganization, including cortical representation, mirror neurons, facilitation and disinhibition, the body matrix, and their use in clinical pain practice
- Subjective and objective components of evaluation for the motor/autonomic pain mechanism
- Sensory screening tools (two-point touch discrimination, localization and precision testing, dermatographia, and stereognosis) and motor screening tools (gross motor proprioception screen, limb position sense screen, left–right discrimination testing)
- Treatment interventions, including patient education, training from the brain to periphery (graded motor imagery), and sensorimotor retraining from the periphery to the brain (stress loading, desensitization)

The motor/autonomic musculoskeletal pain mechanism is a complex multisystemic pain mechanism that manifests pain through an integration of all the body's systems (ie, neurological, cardiovascular, gastrointestinal, skeletal, endocrine, and immune). Patients with pain dominated by the motor/autonomic pain mechanism typically have visible signs or physical manifestations of the disorder that are not expressed in many of the other pain mechanisms. For example, patients may have trophic changes throughout the

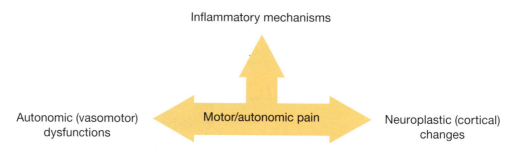

FIGURE 8.1 Processes in the motor/autonomic pain mechanism.

body or swelling and visual redness in their affected and unaffected extremities. Patients can also present with alterations in both peripheral and central modes of pain reception. Characteristically, patients in whom this mechanism is dominant present with the diagnosis of complex regional pain syndrome (CRPS).

The most important changes in the motor/autonomic pain mechanism are categorized as (1) facilitated inflammatory mechanisms, (2) autonomic or vasomotor dysfunctions, and (3) neuroplastic or cortical changes in the central nervous system (CNS) (see **Figure 8.1**).[1,2] Thus, this mechanism has inflammatory, sympathetic, and neuroplastic pathogeneses. Excitation of sensitized nociceptors and disinhibition of central descending inhibitory neurons may also be present.[3] Patients with the motor/autonomic pain mechanism can have central sensitization findings combined with cortical smudging or alterations in the discrete organization of the motor and sensory cortex resulting in changes in the ability to localize symptoms. Some top-down processing takes place, but local inflammatory mechanisms are occurring simultaneously. Research on changes in the immune context in the brain found increased permeability through the spinal cord into the brain after peripheral nerve injury,[4] demonstrating how quickly these changes can occur to sensitize central systems.

Neurogenic inflammation can be facilitated through inflammatory and autoimmune mechanisms via cytokines and nerve growth factor in patients with CRPS.[5] Cytokines can be thought of as linking the immune and nervous systems with items such as IL-6, IL-1β, and tumor necrosis factor-α, produced by the body's white blood cells and other cells of the nervous system.[6] In animal models, blockage of proinflammatory cytokines and anti-inflammatory cytokines reduced neuropathic hyperalgesias.[7] These cytokine changes with aberrant inflammatory processes can present with a mechanical hyperalgesia. Further sensitization of secondary nociceptive neurons in the spinal cord can also result.

Complex Regional Pain Syndrome

CRPS is a pain condition with characteristic symptoms of sensory, motor, or autonomic problems.[8,9] In 46% of cases, CRPS follows a traumatic event; other cases (5%–10%) can be spontaneous, and in many cases the cause is unknown.[1] Whether the mechanism of onset is spontaneous or traumatic, some evidence has been found for genetic susceptibility to CRPS. van de Beek et al[10] identified two distinct genetic location sites in people with CRPS and a genetic predisposition to dystonia associated with trauma. In addition to the mechanisms of genetics, trauma, and insidious onset, Geertzen et al[11] found that stressful life events were present more frequently in patients with CRPS; 79% of diagnosed patients had experienced a stressful life event compared with 21% of the control group. To date, no association has been found between CRPS type 1 and psychological factors, contrary to many popular beliefs.[12]

CRPS type 1 was formerly known as reflex sympathetic dystrophy (RSD) and results from damage to the nerves by illness or injury that is unidentifiable as opposed to CRPS type II, known as causalgia, with a documented nerve injury.[13]

CRPS often presents with edematous, trophic, and sweating changes, with discoloration or alterations in blood flow and vascularity. No specific test or diagnostic procedure is available to confirm this condition; diagnosis relies on history and physical examination. Tests such as two-point touch discrimination or body image drawings may aid clinicians in discerning whether premotor and sensorimotor parts of the brain have cortical versus just peripheral system involvement. Proposed clinical diagnostic criteria for CRPS (the Budapest criteria) were published in 2007[14] and validated in 2010 (see **Figure 8.2**).[15] Diagnosis can be aided by signs and symptoms in the categories of sensory, vasomotor, sudomotor/edema, and motor/trophic changes.[15]

FIGURE 8.2 Clinical Diagnostic Criteria ("Budapest Criteria") and Severity Score for Chronic Regional Pain Syndrome

Chronic regional pain syndrome (CRPS) includes an array of painful conditions that are characterized by a continuing (spontaneous and/or evoked) regional pain that is seemingly disproportionate in time or degree to the usual course of any known trauma or other lesion. The pain is regional (not in a specific nerve territory or dermatome) and usually has a distal predominance of abnormal sensory, motor, sudomotor, vasomotor, and/or trophic findings. The syndrome shows variable progression over time.

BUDAPEST CRITERIA FOR CLINICAL DIAGNOSIS

To make the clinical diagnosis, the following criteria must be met[1,2]:

1. Continuing pain, which is disproportionate to any inciting event

2. Must report at least one symptom in *three of the four* following categories:
   - **Sensory.** Reports of hyperesthesia and/or allodynia
   - **Vasomotor.** Reports of temperature asymmetry and/or skin color changes and/or skin color asymmetry
   - **Sudomotor/edema.** Reports of edema and/or sweating changes and/or sweating asymmetry
   - **Motor/trophic.** Reports of decreased range of motion and/or motor dysfunction (weakness, tremor, dystonia) and/or trophic changes (hair, nail, skin)

3. Must display at least one sign *at time of evaluation* in two or more of the following categories:
   - **Sensory.** Evidence of hyperalgesia (to pin prick) and/or allodynia (to light touch and/or temperature sensation and/or deep somatic pressure and/or joint movement)
   - **Vasomotor.** Evidence of temperature asymmetry (>1°C) and/or skin color changes and/or asymmetry

(continues on next page)

> **FIGURE 8.2** Clinical Diagnostic Criteria ("Budapest Criteria") and Severity Score for Chronic Regional Pain Syndrome
>
> *(continued from previous page)*
>
> - **Sudomotor/edema.** Evidence of edema and/or sweating changes and/or sweating asymmetry
> - **Motor/trophic.** Evidence of decreased range of motion and/or motor dysfunction (weakness, tremor, dystonia) and/or trophic changes (hair, nail, skin)
>
> 4. There is no other diagnosis that better explains the signs and symptoms.
>
> For research purposes, the diagnostic decision rule should be at least one symptom in all four symptom categories and at least one sign (observed at evaluation) in two or more sign categories.
>
> ## CRPS SEVERITY SCORE
>
> The CRPS severity score takes into account 17 features of the clinical history and physical examination to facilitate uniform communication regarding patients' clinical status for clinical or research purposes.[3] Presence of a symptom is scored 1; absence is scored 0.
>
> The following symptoms are self-reported by patients:
>
> 1. Allodynia/hyperpathia
> 2. Asymmetry in temperature
> 3. Asymmetry in skin color
> 4. Asymmetry in sweating
> 5. Asymmetry in edema
> 6. Trophic changes
> 7. Motor changes
> 8. Decreased active range of motion
>
> The following objective signs are found on examination:
>
> 9. Hyperpathia to pin prick
> 10. Allodynia
> 11. Temperature asymmetry by palpation
> 12. Asymmetry in skin color
> 13. Asymmetry in sweating
> 14. Asymmetry in edema
> 15. Trophic changes
> 16. Motor changes
> 17. Decreased active range of motion
>
> The number of positive findings is totaled; higher scores indicate greater severity.
>
> **Resources**
> 1. Harden RN, Bruehl S, Stanton-Hicks M, Wilson PR. Proposed new diagnostic criteria for complex regional pain syndrome. *Pain Med.* 2007;8:326-331.
> 2. Harden RN, Bruehl S, Perez RS, et al. Validation of proposed diagnostic criteria (the "Budapest criteria") for complex regional pain syndrome. *Pain.* 2010;150:268-274.
> 3. Harden RN, Bruehl S, Perez RS, et al. Development of a severity score for CRPS. *Pain.* 2010;151:870-876.

Traumatic events such as wrist and ankle fractures have been linked to progression of CRPS type 1. In rats with either immobilization and fracture or immobilization without coordinate fracture, the immobilization and fracture group experienced warmth, edema, and allodynia that diminished over 20 weeks. In rats that were only immobilized, however, these symptoms resolved within 2 weeks. In this study,

> A neurokinin receptor agonist partially reversed spontaneous extravasation, warmth, and edema in the hindpaw in both models, suggesting neurogenic inflammatory responses contribute to the development and maintenance of limb warmth and edema observed after fracture or immobilization. Mechanical allodynia was inhibited by the intrathecal administration of a neurokinin receptor antagonist, indicating that substance P signaling in the spinal cord contributes to nociceptive sensitization after fracture or immobilization.[16(p105)]

Many people have fractures, however, and do not develop CRPS. When they are damaged, local tissue cells can produce neurokinins. These neurokinins vary among individuals, and when tissues are injured, unique abnormalities may exist. Neuromodulators may play a role in sensitizing the CNS structures of patients with a propensity for the disorder.

As discussed throughout this text, classification of dominating pain mechanisms aids in clinical treatment and investigation of improved outcomes. Future research is needed to identify whether stages or subtypes of CRPS exist that may dictate differences in treatment. For now, one clinical sign in this patient population is the finding of temperature subtypes referred to as "hot CPRS," in which the skin is warm or red, and "cold CRPS," in which the skin is cold or blue. There has been much discussion about these subtypes; however, more research is needed to determine chronicity and treatment outcomes.[17] Bruehl et al[18] proposed that three possible subtypes of CRPS may exist (but did not find evidence that they follow a sequential order): (1) a subtype with vasomotor signs predominating, (2) a subtype with neuropathic pain and sensory abnormalities predominating, and (3) a classic RSD subtype with motor and trophic signs predominating. This research supports the presence in patients with the motor/autonomic pain mechanism of an additional ischemic pain mechanism or inflammatory neuropathic pain mechanism that may not initially be labeled as such.

The clinician must first be able to recognize the dominant pain mechanism in patients who present with multiple mechanisms. Then, the clinician must educate the patients accordingly, create treatment plans for all mechanisms, and give priority to the dominant mechanism. For example, a patient with the autonomic/motor pain mechanism has progressed with function and ambulation and activities of daily living performance, but in a later visit reports experiencing anger about the fracture or trauma that caused the symptoms and a pain flare-up. The clinician must acknowledge the affective components of this patient's pain (ie, the links between negative emotions, coping, and symptoms) and address the temporary change in dominating mechanism that has worsened the patient's symptoms. If the clinician uses methods directed only at the motor/autonomic mechanism (eg, a graded motor imagery program and sensorimotor training) and does nothing to address the anger, the treatment session may be futile. Vasomotor signs can coincide with inflammatory mechanisms in such patients and contribute to symptoms associated with CRPS such as a "functional inhibition of sympathetic vasoconstrictor neurons and consecutive vasodilation."[1(p652)]

Maladaptive neuroplasticity can also play a role in the motor/autonomic pain mechanism. The pain component of CRPS is often influenced by the sympathetic innervations of deep somatic structures.[19] Acerra and Moseley[20] showed that some patients with CRPS type 1 feel pain or paresthesia in the affected limb after watching reflected images of the unaffected limb. The clinician may also observe bony changes (eg, periarticular osteopenia) present in individuals with CRPS, possibly because of disuse.

Maihofner et al[21,22] demonstrated cortical representation changes in the brain on magnetoencephalography contralateral to the affected arm. In addition to changes in central processing, the presence of mechanical hyperalgesia has been linked to mislocalizations during sensory stimulation[22]; healthy nervous systems typically do not mislocalize symptoms. This finding demonstrates the central component on the central–peripheral continuum that manifests as a mislocalization of sensory stimulation and motor/autonomic physical characteristics. Mislocalization of sensory stimuli may be accompanied by a distorted sense of the size of the affected limb because of changes in the patient's primary sensory cortex.[23]

Geha et al[24] demonstrated a reorganization of white matter connectivity in certain regions of the brain in patients with chronic CRPS compared with healthy control subjects. These patients showed alterations in branching patterns, with increased branching in the ventromedial prefrontal cortex to the insula and decreased branching in the basal ganglion (the basal ganglion aids in action selection and motor control). Brain studies have demonstrated alterations in lateral or medial prefrontal cortex depending on the condition.[24] Areas of involvement in patients with chronic pain may be related to regions that involve emotions, decision making, and perception of pain. These findings provide evidence supporting the idea that the anatomical abnormalities contribute to the affective and symptomatic presentation in patients with motor/autonomic pain and that these patients present with significant processing and emotional brain changes that dominate their experience of pain.

It has been demonstrated that attention to or anticipation of pain at a specific location of the body prioritizes tactile stimuli at that location in normal individuals.[25] The healthy brain prioritizes tactile information from threatened body parts. In other words, when someone is fearful of injury at a particular body part, attention is biased toward that body part. When patients with chronic unilateral back pain judged which of a pair of identical stimuli occurred first, they were slower to recognize the stimulus nearer the involved side of the back. This finding supports the idea that there is a spatial disruption of sensory input with chronic pain states and that this disruption may cause symptoms.[26]

Moseley[23] found that interventions in an appropriate sequence can activate cortical motor networks and improve pain and disability in patients with CRPS originating with wrist fracture. He found that graded motor imagery, a program of training in left–right discrimination, followed by imagined movements and then mirror movements, was helpful in remodeling motor areas of the brain in these patients. It may be necessary to remodel the brain by activating neurons that prepare the limb for movement versus neurons that execute the movement.[23] Multiple systems may be in play with the motor/autonomic pain mechanism, and cortical representations or neurosignatures may trigger pain responses in multiple dimensions. An examination of all threats to the physiological system and their interplay guides clinicians in remodeling and restoring the cortex. Active, nonthreatening brain-down movement training may help reverse the effects of motor/autonomic pain, but if the patient is fearful of movement, the emotional or cognitive context involving fear avoidance may limit success and should be addressed first.

Principles of Neuroplasticity and Cortical Reorganization

Many approaches under a medical model involve erroneous attempts to treat patients with central pain mechanisms at a local tissue level via surgery, injections, or medications. Patients with sympathetic mediated pain may or may not respond to sympathetic blocks. In a study of children with CRPS,[27] patients were given either intravenous (IV) lidocaine and lumbar sympathetic saline or lumbar sympathetic lidocaine and IV saline. Children who had the lumbar sympathetic blockade as opposed to the IV route had significant reductions in pain intensity of allodynia to brush, pinprick, and pinprick temporal summation and verbal pain scores. The authors concluded that some components of pain may be mediated by abnormal sympathetic efferent activity.[27] Although there may be abnormalities in efferent activity, local injections are not always efficacious in all patients with central pain mechanisms or CRPS, perhaps because of the cortical or neuroplastic changes that may also occur in the CNS. A systematic review of the role of local anesthetic sympathetic blockade in CRPS concluded that questions remain about the effectiveness of local blockade as a treatment modality; fewer than one-third of patients obtained full relief.[28] This indicates the need to subgroup CNS mechanisms more effectively to identify the best intervention.

Because it is unclear what mechanisms are dominant in CRPS, it is difficult to standardize treatment or compare studies based on study design without identifying the CNS pain mechanisms involved. In addition, some patients present with the motor/autonomic pain mechanism but do not have CRPS. Ongoing pain states can have multiple mechanisms of action that all need clinical consideration, but typically with the motor/autonomic pain mechanism, the sympathetic nervous system is overemphasized. Evidence suggests that if a disorder has a component of sympathetic maintained pain, it is not the abnormal sympathetic nervous system itself that causes the discomfort, but rather abnormal sensitivity to normal sympathetic secretions in injured nerves and peripheral nociceptor terminals.[29] This evidence suggests that the discomfort stems from how the patient interprets those signals and whether a cognitive, emotional, or cortical component is dominating. If the clinician can target the trigger to increased sensitivity or perceived threat to the system, then pain or suffering may be quicker to change.

In CNS pain mechanisms, it is important to think neurobiologically and reflect on ways to affect the mind without inadvertently stimulating the nervous system and creating more pain. Sometimes there are ways to creatively tap into the brain without moving any external structures. The principles of cortical representation, mirror neurons, facilitation and disinhibition, and the body matrix can aid the clinician in remodeling the CNS system from the brain down.

Cortical Representation

Pain is an output of the brain. In the somatosensory cortex, the human brain has a somatotopic map representing the body present from birth. The density of the skin's receptors is different in various areas of the body (eg, the hand has more receptors on the skin than the back). Receptor density allows for different representations of the skin's sensory surfaces in the brain. This brain map can alter based on the individual's level of activity or function. For example, people who use their hands more, such as pianists or artists, have a greater receptor density in the hand somatotopic map represented in their brain than people who do not use their hands for a fine-motor craft. Increased cortical representation occurs in people whose function, use, and activity dictate a greater need for a body part, such as performing artists or professional athletes.[30]

This concept is evident in patients who have had a limb amputated. Phantom limb pain demonstrates that the system is more complex than a simple feedback loop. Alterations in somatotopic maps of limbs found in the brain shortly after amputation are thought to be due to the removal of inhibitory mechanisms of existing neurons. In addition, it is thought that deafferentation causes central neural changes because this inhibitory control is removed.[31] This phenomenon demonstrates alterations in plasticity of the neural projections and loss of sensory input in the somatosensory cortex. Interestingly, if phantom limb pain is treated with opioids, the cortical reorganization is altered, and less potential reorganization occurs.[32]

In addition to phantom limb experiences, reorganization of the representation in the primary somatosensory cortex has been shown to occur with CRPS. The cortical hand representation in patients with symptomatic CRPS was smaller on the affected limb side, and representation shifted toward the lips.[21] Flor et al[33] also demonstrated a medial shift indicating cortical reorganization in patients with chronic lower back pain compared with healthy controls.

Cortical disinhibition has also been shown to occur in pain patients. When cortical disinhibition dominates, two-point touch discrimination and acuity of touch diminish, and a brain-down remodeling approach to sensory and motor function (ie, treatment first of the CNS and brain) is necessary to successfully treat pain in other areas of the body. This remodeling can occur via cortical mechanisms, such as refinement of tactile acuity and discrimination of touch by promoting recognition of the type (eg, pen cap vs pen tip) and location (eg, right or left hand, points 1–6) of sensation.[34] It appears that stimulating patients' attention to the task of acuity, and possibly cortical representation, can be helpful in treatment of the motor/autonomic pain mechanism.[34]

Mirror Neurons

Another way to tap into the cortex is through mirror neurons. Mirror neurons are a class of neurons that discharge when a task is performed, observed, heard, or even smelled.[20,35] Mirror neurons are organized into two major networks located in the parietal lobe and premotor cortex and are also found in the anterior insula and anterior midcingulate cortex.[36,37] They were first discovered in the premotor cortex of monkeys and have become clinically relevant as a way to facilitate rehabilitation techniques,[38] especially for clinicians who work with individuals with the dominant motor/autonomic pain mechanism. Just as Acerra and Moseley[20] demonstrated that patients may present with pain in the absence of sensory inputs, activation of a potential mirror neuron response is a powerful tool the clinician can use in tapping into treatment options.

Emotionally, mirror neurons help bridge first- and third-person experiences, for example, they help improve one person's understanding of common elements of another person's experience in complex philosophical realms such as pain or emotions. Observation of another person in an emotional state can activate a representation of that state in the observer.[39] Because the patient's mood can influence the clinician's mood and vice versa, communication and motivational interviewing are important skills enabling the clinician to treat depressed or anxious and agitated patients. Pain-related empathy involves attention to the pain aspect of the observed stimuli; it requires the top-down attention of the person observing the painful situation and does not occur automatically.[40]

The context or meaning of a painful situation also influences a person's perception of pain. For instance, patients who experienced an uncomfortable stimulus while observing a red (ie, signifying harmful) or a blue (ie, signifying less harmful) visual cue interpreted the stimulus as more painful and intense when they observed the red visual cue.[41] If a patient associates an image or a task with greater threat or harm, he or she may have a greater negative reaction or interpretation, and potentially vice versa. The clinician's understanding of each patient's fear hierarchy of movement, activities, places, people, and emotions can aid him or her in individualizing the desensitization and remodeling program to target the movements, images, or interactions that have the highest priority for the patient.

In addition to emotions and empathy, the observation of an action leads to the activation of parts of the same neural network and parts of its execution.[37,42] Motor memories can be created through performance and observation to affect the plasticity of the motor cortex.[43] Interestingly, patients who have had a limb amputated who watch the intact limb of another person being touched can experience sensation in their phantom limb. Ramachandran and Brang[44] hypothesized that people with an intact hand do not experience the phenomenon because the intact hand sends a signal in the motor neuron system that does not allow conscious awareness to occur. This research supports the use of observation of movement or of tactile stimulation and mirror therapy in the rehabilitation of patients who have experienced a stroke, motor/autonomic pain mechanism, or phantom pain.

Different mirror neurons fire with different intentions for a task. These neurons are organized by intention or motor plan.[45] For example, when a patient with arm pain is asked to reach for an object and bring it into his or her mouth, certain mirror neurons will fire. If the patient is asked to put that object into a container, however, the intention is different, and different mirror neurons are stimulated. Hearing the sounds of the task can also stimulate the mirror mechanism.[45] Mirror neurons thus provide a method of remodeling or desensitizing the cortical representation of patients with chronic pain by allowing them to think about or watch a movement before actually executing it.

Facilitation and Disinhibition

Many people maintain a system of motor control in which one upper or lower limb is dominant. Neurologically, humans have an innate or built-in neglect of the nondominant limb[46] that may be based on the brain's somatotopic representation. With pathology, changes favor a similar mechanism by which the brain slightly loses interest in the nondominant side or slightly favors the side of dominance. With pain, two fundamental concepts are facilitation and disinhibition. *Facilitation* can be thought of as a state of hypersensitivity or learning at a synaptic level. Facilitation functions in an overprotective way; with persistent pain, stimuli that normally would not be perceived as painful cause the patient to adapt in ways that limit his or her activity level or range of available pain-free motion. *Disinhibition* involves a neurological loss of precision or a loss of inhibition centrally that causes the pain reaction to be indistinct. Phantom limb pain could be associated with this cortical process. The patient becomes unable to discriminate areas of the body in pain or to describe pain with specificity. Instead of being able to identify the specific part of the forearm that hurts, for example, the patient perceives that the entire forearm hurts.[46] The presence of spreading symptoms and dystonias in CRPS demonstrates not only that a local inflammatory neuropathic sensitization is present, but also that supraspinal or neuroplasticity changes are responsible for the spontaneous spread of symptoms and dystonias.[47,48]

Body Matrix

Melzack[49] coined the term *neuromatrix* to describe a multidimensional experience produced by multiple areas of the brain that affects how the body perceives itself. Moseley et al[50] discussed a body matrix that can be represented cortically through the brain's somatotopic representations in the homunculus (a visual representation of the body's abstract anatomic representation in the cerebrum), peripersonal spatial representation, and the body's own spatial representations. Peripersonal spatial representation involves the idea of ownership of the body and the area surrounding the body. The ability to perceive this representation is centered around the specific body part and specific side of involvement.[51] Visual distortions and the illusion of ownership of the body part contribute to the perception of pain by the body and brain. A study of patients with CRPS showed that viewing the affected arm through a magnifying lens condition resulted in greater swelling and greater perception of chronic pain.[50]

Subjective Evaluation for the Motor/Autonomic Pain Mechanism

The central and sympathetic nervous systems are fully involved in the production of pain for patients presenting with the motor/autonomic pain mechanism. Once again, patient education and movement guidelines; pacing and graded exposure to activities perceived as being fearful, harmful, and meaningful; assessment and treatment of yellow flags; a thorough mechanical evaluation when appropriate; neuroplastic remodeling; and a potential referral to psychology based on negative emotions and coping abilities are the guidelines for treatment of this condition.

An important outcome of evaluation is to understand which pain mechanism is dominating. Is the patient coping well with the condition and not experiencing significant worries and concerns but needs to move more? Or does the patient need to focus on the affective component and better manage the psychological perspective before the physical aspects can be addressed? The subjective evaluation helps the clinician identify the pattern of the dominating mechanism. Typically, increased pain and hyperalgesia with notable sensory symptom changes are present in patients with CNS pain mechanisms. Patients with the motor/autonomic pain mechanism may complain of a deep, boring pain with only mild sensory symptoms and may have complaints consistent with sensory gain or sensory loss fueled by an aberrant inflammatory mechanism or neuroplastic changes. Identifying the dominant mechanism can ensure early and accurate intervention and may preclude the need to treat other identified operant mechanisms. The following sections describe characteristics that are identifiable in the subjective evaluation when the motor/autonomic mechanism is dominating.

Location

Typically, the clinical features of motor/autonomic pain involve an extremity; sometimes the entire extremity and sometimes just part of the extremity is affected. For example, just the patient's wrist and hand may be involved, or the pain may spread from the shoulder all the way to the fingers. Often, more than one nerve field is involved. A glove-like distribution in the extremity, as opposed to a dermatomal or sensory nerve distribution, is more typical. Because this mechanism involves the cortical representation of the patient's body part, however, it can manifest itself in any area of the body. Axial regions may be involved, and chronic pelvic pain may also be present in patients with the motor/autonomic pain mechanism.[52]

Frequency of Pain

Patients' pain is most likely constant; patients rarely report to clinicians that the pain ever shuts off or that any measure offers relief. Typically there is no identifiable movement or mechanical pattern to the pain.

Descriptors

Patients may use terms such as "deep," "dull," "burning," "aching," "pulsating," or "stabbing." Symptoms may be vague or difficult for patients to describe. Cold sensitivities are common. Patients may have difficulty describing awareness of the extremity or the precise location of the symptoms.

Onset

Onset may be cumulative over years and involve multiple episodes of benign events at a certain area or areas of the body. Occasionally the onset is traumatic; however, the symptoms typically persist for more than 3 to 4 months following the trauma. Although the course of the disorder is relatively unknown, sympathetic dysfunction is observed at onset and tends to level out as the disorder progresses.[52]

24-Hour Behavior

Often there is no consistency in time of day for pain complaints. However, many patients complain of pain at night.

Psychological and Social Status

Patients report that stress typically makes the pain worse. They may have symptoms related to the immune system, such as mirror joint pain on the other limb; gastrointestinal issues, such as intermittent complaints of vomiting, diarrhea, or irritable bowel syndrome; or endocrine system involvement with metabolic changes. They may often be affected by their emotions but fail to recognize it or have a complex history involving emotional or personality disorders.

Thoughts, Beliefs, and Culture

Worrisome thoughts and beliefs can create pain. Often patients have a distorted body image. Increased epinephrine and norepinephrine in venous plasma concentrations may come from the pain of CRPS, affective components, or both.[53] Deeply entrenched personality disorders, social phobias, anxiety disorders, or depression may be involved. The use of objective tests and measures can help the clinician distinguish which symptoms are related to what mechanism. **Table 8.1** lists the subjective clinical characteristics of the motor/autonomic pain mechanism. **Appendix 8.A** shows a comparison of all the subjective clinical characteristics of the central pain mechanisms.

TABLE 8.1 Subjective and Objective Characteristics of Motor/Autonomic Pain

Characteristic	Findings for Motor/Autonomic Pain
Subjective	
Location	Widespread, nonanatomical distribution of pain to upper and/or lower extremity; may include the spine, and typically affects more than one nerve field; may have mirror pains and involve one whole side of the body
Frequency	Constant, unremitting, spontaneous, latent, paroxysmal
Descriptors	Deep, dull, burning, aching, pulsating, stabbing, cold intolerance, warmth, hypersensitivity
Intensity	High severity, irritability
Onset	Chronic; >3 months past expected tissue healing or pathology recovery time; pain is disproportionate to nature and extent of injury or pathology; initial trauma may have been managed poorly

(continues on next page)

TABLE 8.1 Subjective and Objective Characteristics of Motor/Autonomic Pain

(continued from previous page)

Characteristic	Findings for Motor/Autonomic Pain
Subjective	
History	Immune, gastrointestinal, endocrine, parasympathetic, and sympathetic system symptoms and/or complications
24-hour behavior	Erratic, inconsistent; night pain, disturbed sleep
Psychosocial screen	Positive for pain behaviors (maladaptive beliefs, poor self-efficacy), high functional disability, negative emotions
Other clinical signs	Swelling indicating lymphedema, spasticity, tone, discoloration of skin, skin and hair sensitivities, trophic changes, excessive sweating
Objective findings for motor/autonomic pain	
	Same as for the central sensitization and affective pain mechanisms; in addition, signs of • Cortical dysfunction (spasticity, tone) • Autonomic nervous system dysfunction (skin discoloration, excessive sweating, trophic changes, hair excitability, lymphedema), skin hypersensitivities • Involvement of sympathetic and parasympathetic system, distorted body image
General illness	Present immune and gastrointestinal system involvement
Proprioception screen	Quadruped spinal flexion and extension difficulties, or limb difficulties depending on the presence of extremity dysfunction
Palpation	Diffuse nonanatomic areas of pain or tenderness; light touch elicits noxious response in areas with and without symptoms, often within the space around the skin
Two-point touch discrimination	Positive findings within area of symptoms; primary sensory cortex findings
Neurological testing	Positive findings: Loss of graphesthesia (recognition of symbols drawn on skin), incomplete drawing of body outline for area of symptoms, signs of neglect in left–right discrimination testing; loss of localization and precision

Objective Evaluation for the Motor/Autonomic Pain Mechanism

Clinical Examination

Patients with the motor/autonomic pain mechanism may complain of gross motor weakness and fine-motor issues involving tapping and grasping. Impairments such as lymphedema may be present. Patients may report sensations of warmth or swelling that may change but may not be clinically identifiable and do not present like chemical inflammation. On the uninvolved extremity, patients may display gross trophic changes as the body matches the changes in the involved extremity to the uninvolved side. Patients may demonstrate features such as spasticity, dystonia, discoloration, hypersensitivity, hyperalgesia, or allodynia.

Harden et al[54] developed a CRPS severity score that discriminates between patients with and without the condition and has validity as an index of severity. The 17 diagnostic criteria include yes/no self-reports of allodynia and hyperpathia, asymmetric temperature, skin color asymmetry, asymmetrical edema, trophic changes, motor changes, and decreased active range of motion (ROM). The signs observed on examination include hyperpathia to pin prick, temperature asymmetry by palpation, skin color asymmetry, sweating asymmetry, asymmetrical edema, trophic changes, motor changes, and decreased active ROM. **Figure 8.2** outlines the Budapest diagnostic criteria for CRPS and the application of Harden et al's[54] severity score.

Sensory Screening Tools

Patients with central sensitization pain mechanisms typically have intact two-point touch discrimination, localization and precision testing, and dermatographia and stereognosis. Those with the autonomic motor pain mechanism, however, show impaired performance on these tests. Tactile acuity can be difficult to interpret, so consistency in testing is important and may differentiate between the two CNS pain mechanisms.

Two-Point Touch Discrimination

Tactile discrimination allows us to identify distinct types of touch sensation based on various receptor sensitivities to mechanical, thermal, and chemical stimuli. The body's receptors can adapt in reaction to stimuli. Certain receptors are slow adapting and continue to signal the brain for a relatively long time once a stimulus is removed, whereas rapidly adapting receptors signal during the onset and sometimes at the removal of stimulation but do not continue firing. Different noxious stimuli can cause differences in perception of pain based on the level of the frequency applied (ie, fast or slow).[55] Recognition of sensory input occurs in the somatosensory cortex, where the sensory maps are located in the homunculus. When patients are in pain, this typical map can become smudged and distorted and can lose representation, as in stroke neglect. As a result, the receptor fields or density of the receptors can change. The individual's ability to detect two separate points can become distorted because there are no longer two different fields. When this lack of discrimination is combined with the patient's emotions, prior life experiences, and thoughts, worries, and concerns, the cortical map can be further altered.

Two-point touch discrimination relies on the primary sensory cortex and is associated with a greater threshold on the affected limb in patients with CRPS. Therefore, if the patient does not have any problems with two-point touch discrimination, there are no problems with the primary sensory cortex, and there is no reason to practice tactile or sensory retraining.[46] The two-point touch discrimination test comprises the following steps:

- Have the patient maintain a comfortable position with eyes closed.
- Gently but firmly apply a mechanical caliper to the patient's skin in the area to be tested on the unaffected limb or trunk. (When testing the foot, divide testing into four areas: hind foot, midfoot, forefoot, and great toe.) The caliper points should initially be placed close enough together so the patient recognizes the touch as one distinct point. Application of force should be light, about 10 g to 15 g, which corresponds to the very first small blanching around the prongs. Test pressure several times to make sure the ends are blunt enough to ensure touch without pain.
- Gradually separate the caliper points in 1-mm increments until the patient recognizes two separate points of contact on his or her skin. Both prongs need to touch simultaneously; the most common testing error is unintentionally placing the prongs on the skin at different times. Occasionally touch with one prong only to ensure that the patient

will not report two points of contact. Record the smallest distance between points at which the patient detects two separate points, called the *threshold*.
- Repeat the procedure, but record the number after decreasing the distance between the two points of the caliper in 1-mm increments until the patient perceives only one point of contact, and average the two threshold numbers. If the procedure is performed and the patient is unclear on the value two consecutive trials, record the perceived value of the threshold distance. Document the procedure thoroughly.
- Repeat the procedure on the identical area on the affected side of the patient's body. If on the trunk, cross the patient's midline.[56]

The threshold of pressure perception increases significantly with age.[57] For normative data for two-point touch discrimination thresholds, refer to **Table 8.2**.

TABLE 8.2 Two-Point Touch Discrimination Threshold Normative Values

Location	Norm
Arms[69]	
Upper lateral arm	42.4 mm
Lower lateral arm	37.8 mm
Mid medial arm	45.4 mm
Mid posterior arm	39.8 mm
Mid lateral forearm	35.9 mm
Mid medial forearm	31.5 mm
Mid posterior forearm	30.7 mm
1st dorsal interosseous muscle	21.0 mm
Palmar surface distal phalanx, thumb	2.6 mm
Palmar surface distal phalanx, long finger	2.6 mm
Palmar surface distal phalanx, little finger	2.5 mm
Trunk[a,70]	
Normal	40.0 mm
Over iliac crest	44.9 mm
Lateral to umbilicus	36.4 mm
Inferior angle of the scapula	52.2 mm
Face[70]	
Over eyebrow	14.9 mm
Cheek	11.9 mm
Lateral neck	35.2 mm
Legs[71]	
Proximal anterior thigh	40.0 mm
Distal anterior thigh	23.2 mm
Mid lateral thigh	42.5 mm

Location	Norm
Mid medial thigh	38.5 mm
Mid posterior thigh	42.2 mm
Proximal lateral leg	37.7 mm
Distal lateral leg	41.6 mm
Medial leg	4.4 mm
Lower leg	25.0 mm
Hind foot	18.0 mm
Mid foot	15.0 mm
Forefoot	13.0 mm
Big toe	5.0 mm
Tip	6.6 mm

[a]Sensitivity decreased from distal to proximal and correlated to the relative size of the cortical areas representing the body part.

It is important to restore accurate cortical representation for the patient's pain perception to improve. Two-point touch discrimination can be used not only to screen for the motor/autonomic pain mechanism, but also to promote accuracy of patients' cortical representation of the extremities. In addition, patients' observation of tactile stimulation can enhance the acuity of the limb and decrease pain.[34,58]

Localization and Precision Testing

These tests can be used in the extremity and spine. They test the tactile acuity to static points and stimulus discrimination between sharp and dull. The spinal cortical sensory test is used to screen for localization and precision in the cervical, lumbar, or thoracic spine (see **Figure 8.3**). This test is performed as follows:

- The patient is positioned in prone or the most comfortable position. Expose the area to be tested to allow skin contact.
- Place six small circles numbered 1 to 6 on the patient's back in two rows of three. Give the patient a reference diagram with circles numbered 1 to 6 in the same pattern as on the back.
- Touch a number on the patient's back with just enough uniform pressure to blanch the skin color. To test localization, ask the patient what number is being touched. To test precision, alternate between sharp and dull stimuli and ask the patient to identify where and which stimulus you are using. Record all responses.
- Perform a minimum of 20 trials.
- Indicate the number of correct trials, and calculate the percentage of correct answers. If 80% (16) of the trials are correct, progress testing to other locations and stimulus types. A positive test (below 80% correct) indicates a need for sensory retraining as part of the patient's rehabilitation program, especially if asymmetry exists in uninvolved areas or if there is bilateral involvement.

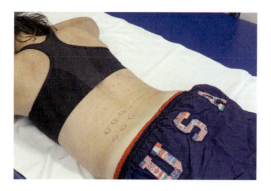 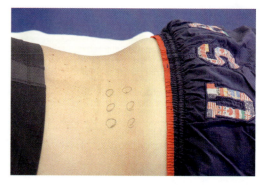

FIGURE 8.3 Prone lumbar localization and precision testing. The patient is positioned in prone or the most comfortable position. Expose the area to be tested to allow skin contact. Place six small circles numbered 1 to 6 on the patient's back in two rows of three. Give the patient a reference diagram with circles numbered 1 to 6 in the same pattern as on the back.

Dermatographia and Stereognosis

Patients with the motor/autonomic pain mechanism can present with dermatographia and poor stereognosis.[59] Dermatographia is raising and reddening of the skin in response to light scratching. Stereognosis is the ability to recognize forms or shapes with the sense of touch; the test can be externally applied to the skin, or the patient can be asked to grasp an object and identify it. With these tests, letters and numbers can be drawn on the skin in different orientations and sizes to test tactile acuity. The target baseline should be 80% accuracy, confirming the need for CNS sensory remodeling treatment.

Motor Screening Tools

Motor screening tools provide a general sense of how patients move and how aware they are of the position of their limbs or spinal posture in space. The tools allow the clinician to screen the general cortical wiring of the motor cortex and assess the patients' spatial perception. Patients may have just sensory or just motor deficits. The recommendation for practice is to screen both, as the intervention will have to be specific for the deficit.

Gross Motor Proprioception Screen

In patients with the motor/autonomic pain mechanism, a trial of the cat-and-camel exercise (see **Figure 8.4**) can reveal a decrease in the ability to perform with good motor control or proprioceptive awareness of the spine. Many patients with motor/autonomic pain struggle with segmental spinal movements and display either slouch or extended position, demonstrating a lack of awareness of the positions or inability to move in and out of positions. For affected extremities, distal areas such as the thumb or great toe can be used to assess proprioception with traditional sagittal plane testing. If this trial demonstrates an inability, a left–right discrimination test is needed.

Limb Position Sense Screen

Proprioception can be assessed through the extremities. A study showed that patients with CRPS were significantly less accurate in the positioning of both the affected and unaffected

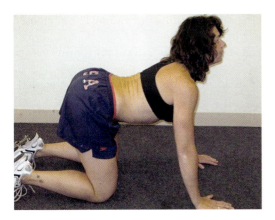 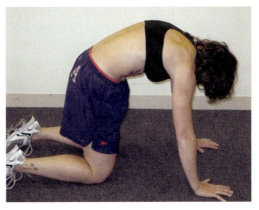

FIGURE 8.4 Patient performing the cat (left) and camel (right) exercise as a gross motor segmental spine proprioception screen.

limbs compared with healthy volunteers; their positioning improved when they were able to view the limb.[60] This altered proprioception could be explained by altered central processing within cortical centers that are responsible for limb representation.

For the limb position sense screen, the clinician can assess proprioception in several ways. If the pain is nonaxial, he or she can compare the limb position of the affected side to that of the unaffected side as a pass-fail scenario. Using one limb at a time, the clinician asks the patient to position the extremity in a series of horizontal or vertical positions corresponding to the hours of a clock, allowing a margin of error as long as the patient gets in close proximity to the clock number and symmetrical to the noninvolved limb. Another option is to place the patient's limb in space with the patient's eyes closed and ask him or her to report his or her clock hour position; the clinician has provided some tactile feedback in the process. The clinician could ask the patient to use the patient's nose as a reference point and turn the head in that direction on the horizontal (eg, "Turn your nose to 2:00, imagining that 12:00 is directly in front of you") or assess sagittal plan motion on the vertical using the head (eg, "Imagining that your nose is pointing to 3:00, point your nose toward 1:00 on the vertical"). The pelvis could be used as a reference point for the lumbar spine (eg, "Imagine your pelvic bones are pointed toward 12:00. Rotate your pelvic bones to point your belly button toward 2:00"). The cervical spine or extremities could be assessed in supine or standing as well.

Left–Right Image Discrimination Testing

Left–right image discrimination testing can help the clinician screen for signs of cortical representation. Flash cards, smart phone apps, or the Recognise program (Neuro Orthopedic Institute, Adelaide, Australia) can be helpful adjuncts to screen and treat patients for extremity or spine conditions presenting with loss of left–right discrimination. Left–right discrimination testing is conducted as follows (**Figure 8.5**):

- Compile 20 images of the body region affected in the patient. The images should portray either a direct view of the involved area or an orientation (90°, 180°, 270°) of the body part.
- Allow the patient to view each picture for approximately 5 to 30 seconds. When testing an extremity, ask the patient, "Is it an image of the left or right side?" When testing

the spine, ask the patient, "Is the person in the image turning or bending left or right?" Responses should be timed using a computer or timer.
- Record accuracy and speed. A positive screen is less than 80% accuracy for an average of 1.5-seconds assessment of 20 pictures.
- Review findings to identify any asymmetry in accuracy and speed between the unaffected and affected areas.

Appendix 8.B lists a comparison of all the objective clinical characteristics of the central pain mechanisms.

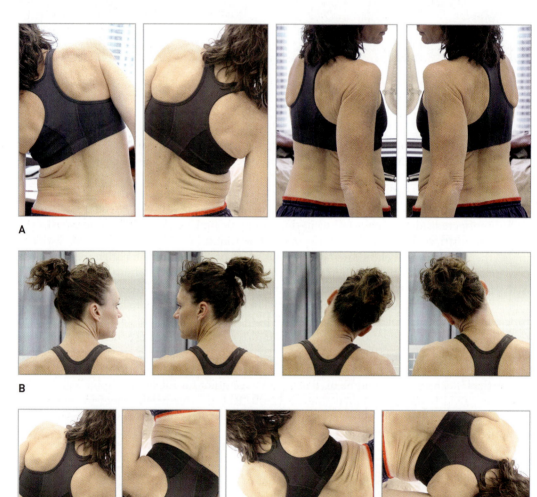

FIGURE 8.5 Images of the (**A**) lumbar spine and (**B**) cervical spine in sidebending and rotation. (**C**) Pictures would be rotated in different views (upright, image rotated 180° degrees, image rotated 270°, image rotated 90°) and to determine laterality (right/left side).

Intervention for the Motor/Autonomic Pain Mechanism

Treatment for patients with pain dominated by the motor/autonomic pain mechanism requires an approach that starts in the brain and progresses to the body, retraining both sensory and motor function in the primary somatomotor cortex of the brain. Patients with central deficits related to body image or movement beliefs have a difficult time with movement retraining from the periphery up. Addressing the movement from the cortical representation down can aid attempts to remodel function from the body up and can be effective when previous attempts at periphery-based exercise approaches have failed. The clinician must consider the context, physical movement limitations, and all potential stressors in all aspects of this remodeling restoring program. The following questions drive the specific intervention: (1) Is the patient in a state of readiness to begin a cortical-based remodeling program? (2) What contexts and movements are most painful, fearful, and meaningful to the patient? (3) Can the clinician train the brain representation to aid the body function?

The goals for treatment of the motor/autonomic pain mechanism focus on improving the understanding and awareness of this mechanism, strength, ROM, and function, as the body representation allows, through gradual exposure to a task or visual or sensory experience. Progression of exposure must be gradual enough that the image, stimulus, activity, context, or emotion does not stimulate an unwanted system response. As with any form of remodeling exercise, a "no-worse" response is an indication that symptom production is safe and necessary for progress; the goal is to excite below the activation threshold of the stimulus without provoking a protective response 24 hours later. In addition, to assist in restoration of movement, it is important to decrease catecholamine levels by reducing anxiety, fear, and frustration. Relaxation, motor imagery, and meditation have all been shown to be valuable additions to active treatment (see explanations in Chapters 6 and 7).

Patient Education

Patient education is the foundation of intervention for CNS pain mechanisms. Patients' readiness to become their own experts by understanding the problem, self-assessing behaviors, and participating in solution-based care is the premise of the education provided. Patients need to understand the pain mechanisms, improve their pain knowledge, and change their attitude and approach to pain. In addition, education should include information about the physiology of pain and neuroscience in general, which has been strongly linked to decreased pain ratings and disability and reductions in negative thinking.[61] Patient education includes use of journaling as self-assessment to uncover the relationship between negative thoughts about movement and their effect on symptoms. Patients may require cognitive–behavioral treatment strategies described in Chapters 6 and 7.

If patients continue to struggle with the management of their condition, a more comprehensive multidisciplinary approach to care may be the best use of resources. Determination of the patients' level of readiness to make behavior changes and selection of appropriate interventions will guide a successful rehabilitation program. Specific education areas could include aerobic conditioning, postural correction, pain mechanism education, visualization, and desensitization. The care plan may include detailed attention to the areas of flexibility, edema control, isometric and isotonic strengthening, stress loading, graded motor imagery, active movement, and ergonomics.

Training from the Brain to the Periphery

Through graded exposure to a task or image, patients are able to change the body part's representation in the brain. *Graded motor imagery* is a rehabilitation process consisting of left–right discrimination recognition tasks, imagined movements, and mirror therapy. Moseley[62,63] demonstrated that graded motor imagery resulted in significant improvements in neuropathic pain scores in patients with CRPS and pathological pain. A systematic review concluded that there is good level 2 evidence that graded motor imagery is effective in reducing pain in adults with CRPS type 1.[64] Progression is based on the amount of brain activity required to perform the task. Just like exercise from the periphery, intensity and specificity are needed for the best outcome. **Figure 8.6** is a patient education handout describing graded motor imagery.

Left–Right Discrimination

Left–right discrimination recognition tasks involve *implicit motor imagery*, or unconscious recognition by the brain, with speed and accuracy, of which upper or lower extremity, left or right, appears in a series of images. Images of the body parts in different positions, from different angles, and in different contexts may be used from a magazine, computer pictures, or Recognise flash cards or program. Patients can perform this task one to three times a day as a remodeling exercise. When the patient has improved to 80% accuracy, the images can be rotated clockwise 90°, 180°, and 270°, and the task repeated. The patient can change the environments, mood, and speed to identify the image. The goal is to improve speed and accuracy of recognition of the body part, thereby contributing to the brain's representation of the body part. Baseline data from testing can help the clinician assess metrics regarding the patient's progress (refer to **Figure 8.5**).

Imagined Movements

Once patients improve in left–right discrimination, they can progress to imagined movements of the body part, sometimes called *explicit motor imagery*. Simply envisioning or watching another person do functional and meaningful tasks using the body part that is affected in the patient activates areas in the patient's brain that correspond to that body part. Moseley[63] noted that limb left–right discrimination activates premotor but not primary motor cortices, whereas imagined movements activate both. The clinician can fine-tune the patient's imagined movement exercise to include certain contexts and functions that the patient perceives as fearful, harmful, and meaningful, which will assist the patient in progressing toward physical performance of the activities.

Patients look at an image of the extremity and spend 30 seconds to 1 minute imagining their body part in the position they are observing. Patients can imagine either viewing themselves from a distance or, for more of a challenge, moving their body part into position. When patients are able to do this without any irritating effects to their system, they can progress to imagining the body part in different contexts, under different scenarios, with different emotions (eg, with wind blowing around the arm in a reaching overhead position, while swimming in the ocean with leg kicking in plantarflexion, while sitting in a hot tub with the arm hanging dependently in supination). Clinically, we recommend a dosage of 30- to 60-second sets (up to 5 minutes) of three for three to four times a day.[65]

FIGURE 8.6 Graded Motor Imagery Patient Education Handout

Graded Motor Imagery

Graded motor imagery (GMI) is a sequential program consisting of three components: (1) left–right discrimination, (2) imagined movements, and (3) mirror therapy. The purpose of a GMI program is to change the way your brain thinks about pain and movement. Your occupational or physical therapist will help you develop a personal program to guide you through each of these stages.

HOW DOES THIS THERAPY WORK?
Research has shown that the brain is able to reorganize or adapt following injury or trauma. However, the ways in which the brain reorganizes or adapts can be helpful or not so helpful when the brain is deprived of the sensory stimulation it was designed to process.

HOW DOES GMI THERAPY REORGANIZE THE BRAIN?
A GMI program will gradually and systematically help you redevelop the nerve pathways in the brain that normally are activated before and during a movement. GMI is like exercise for neurons in the brain. Reactivation of these neurons in a gradual and purposeful way will help diminish pain and other disturbing sensations.

TO BEGIN: WATCHING THE MOVEMENTS OF OTHERS
Watching other people move prepares your brain for movement. You will be asked to watch or observe people moving the body part that is giving you pain to prepare your brain and body to move. Watching another person perform this movement provides the least amount of activation in the brain, so you need to start here. If you are able to watch other people move their body part without experiencing an increase in pain, you can move on to stage 1 of the sequence. If watching people move causes you to experience an increase in pain, focusing on the movement of a person or animal you love can activate your brain's pleasure centers (which are closely related to the pain centers in the brain), allowing you to better tolerate the pain. By focusing on an individual or animal you love, you activate the pleasure centers, and your pain levels may begin to diminish.

Stage 1: Left–Right Discrimination
Increasing your ability to differentiate left from right can help prepare your brain for movement. Studies have shown that people with chronic pain may be slower or unable to recognize whether pictures of their affected body part show the right or left side. You will be asked to view pictures of your affected body part in different positions to help your brain improve the ability to distinguish left from right, and you and your therapist will keep track of your accuracy and speed in naming left and right. Once you can exercise this skill without increasing your pain level, you can move on to stage 2.

Stage 2: Imagined Movements
Mirror neurons are activated when you think about performing an action. We do this all day long without even knowing it. Imagined movements involve the process of imagining

(continues on next page)

> **FIGURE 8.6** Graded Motor Imagery Patient Education Handout
>
> *(continued from previous page)*
>
> yourself moving, touching, and experiencing feelings associated with activities you do or want to do in your own mind without actually moving. Again, you are exercising your brain, with no motion required. It is important to visualize painless, coordinated actions and positions.
>
> **Stage 3: Mirror Therapy**
> The brain uses visual information in addition to information from tissues. In mirror therapy, you use a mirror box or standing mirror to trick your brain into seeing your affected body part functioning normally. The brain may give greater priority to what it sees than what it feels; observing the reflection of the unaffected side helps your brain believe your affected side is working well and appears normal. Mirror therapy helps builds endurance of the movement image in the brain, which is a preparatory step to actual movement of the involved area.
>
> **Resource**
> Moseley GL, Butler DS, Beames TB, Giles TJ. *The Graded Motor Imagery Handbook*. Adelaide, Australia: Noigroup Publications; 2012.
>
> Adapted from Elizabeth Gaffron, OTR/L

Mirror Therapy

In the final stage of graded motor imagery, mirror therapy, the patient moves the unaffected limb while viewing the movement in the mirror, which tricks the brain into perceiving that the painful limb is performing the motion. As with imagined movements, observation of a task in a mirror can neurologically represent the task in the brain's motor program. Mirrored movements should be pain free or no worse as a result. If symptoms are produced or increased, the movements are too advanced for the patient to benefit from this intervention. Clinicians can start unilaterally and progress to bilateral therapy as tolerated, eventually progressing to use of the involved extremity.

As active use of the involved limb becomes less painful, the patient can start to move it in whatever available ROM is comfortable. The patient can begin to initiate movement with the involved limb behind the mirror as he or she watches the uninvolved limb move. The patient can then slowly progress his or her ROM as tolerated. As use of the involved limb becomes less painful, the patient can progress to object manipulation, sliding, and tapping and then to isometrics and active ROM. Eventually the patient can progress to full motion with the involved limb using active punch and pull reaching patterns with the upper extremity or kicking and reaching tasks with the lower extremity.

Patients with axial symptoms begin by recognizing their own back by touching it or watching their hand touch it in the mirror, initiating right- and left-sided spinal motions while watching and touching the painful area. Patients can then progress to imagined movements of side bending and rotation, flexion, and extension of the spine. Research has demonstrated that viewing the back as it moves can result in less pain than moving the spine without visual feedback; not only was the pain intensity lower, but the average time to ease was shorter with visual feedback.[66] Patients can use this simple strategy as they progress from watching themselves move to watching themselves perform functional movement patterns.

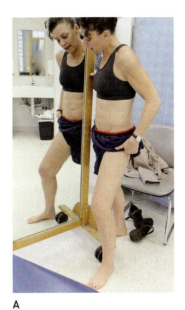
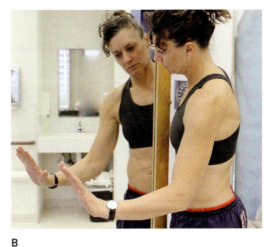

FIGURE 8.7 Mirror therapy training for the (**A**) lower extremity and (**B**) upper extremity.

Brain remodeling guidelines for the back are the same as for many other tissues (three to four times a day, with the patient remaining no worse as a result). **Appendix 8.C** describes a case demonstrating the use of mirror therapy as a treatment intervention. See **Figure 8.7** for pictures of mirror box or lower and upper extremity training in front of a mirror.

Training from the Periphery to the Brain

Stress Loading Protocols

Watson and Carlson[67] described an active stress loading program in the treatment of reflex sympathetic dystrophy of the hand. The use of active traction and exercise helps produce stressful use of the extremity without overly taxing the painful joints with large movements, allowing the body to adapt to the stresses placed on it. The premise is that the stressful exercise helps override the abnormal CNS processing; overload of the neural, vascular, sensorimotor, and musculoskeletal systems is required to achieve a training effect and break the pain cycle. Clinicians should avoid excessive joint mobilization, passive ROM, dynamic splinting, or the use of casting on the painful extremity.[53]

The concept of stress loading typically involves both scrubbing (compression) and carrying (traction). For traction, the patient might carry objects on the affected side and assume a normal arm swing during walking and then add weight to maximum tolerance. Scrubbing involves applying and approximating as much pressure as possible using a back-and-forth motion; ideally the patient uses weightbearing with maximal pressure and contraction of muscle groups. Typically patients begin with 1 to 5 pounds based on their individual tolerance. Compliance with stress loading is critical; treatment typically focuses on 3 minutes at a time for three times a day.[65] Patients then progress from 1 to 2 minutes per week to 15 minutes for five times a day. Other ways to progress scrubbing are to upgrade scrubbing styles and to use different positions or angles with a greater load. Although stress loading protocols have been included in some clinical guidelines, little direct evidence supports their effectiveness other than anecdotally. **Figure 8.8** is a patient education handout on stress loading.

> **FIGURE 8.8** Stress Loading Patient Education Handout
>
> ## Stress Loading
>
> *Stress loading* is use of active traction and compression exercises to produce stress in the extremity with minimal motion of the painful joints. Stress loading follows the basics of exercise physiology: Your body adapts in response to demands placed on it. Your response to pain has been changed, so now any stimulus is interpreted as a painful stimulus. Stressful exercise is needed to override what has become "abnormally normal" for that area. An overload is required to achieve a training effect and to break the pain cycle that you and your body are experiencing. This means you need to do something to overload your neural, vascular, sensorimotor, and musculoskeletal systems in order to break the existing pain patterns your body is feeling.
>
> Stress loading consists of two simple exercises:
>
> 1. *Scrubbing* is using a scrub brush with the affected extremity to apply as much pressure as possible using a back-and-forth motion. Ideally, you apply weight through the affected limb for maximum pressure and contraction of all your muscle groups. The clinician may make modifications to ensure that you are able to perform the scrubbing.
> 2. *Carrying* involves lifting and transporting a weighted backpack, suitcase, or purse in the hand on the affected side. You'll carry the weight throughout the day while you stand or walk. Your arm should hang down so it swings normally as you walk. The weight of the bag should be at maximum tolerance; most people start with 1 to 5 pounds and add weight as their tolerance increases. Sometimes the handle can be built up so the weight is comfortable in the hand.
>
> ### YOUR PERFORMANCE IS CRITICAL
>
> You must take an active role in this treatment to achieve good results. Stress loading won't work if you don't load the extremity to produce the stress. You need to do the scrubbing and carrying exercises consistently, both in the clinic and at home. Your therapist may give you a log sheet to record your scrubbing and carrying to help you perform these exercises regularly.

Desensitization

Desensitization can be used to decrease or normalize the body's response to particular sensations. The stimulus should be consistent for short periods and applied frequently throughout the day. Patients should start with the least painful stimulus and gradually progress to increasingly noxious stimuli. The process can begin with different textures or fabrics (eg, silk, wool, Velcro) and different levels of pressure. Vibration or heat and cold can be used. Sometimes the use of compression garments, beginning with a light elasticized sock or stocking, can aid the process of edema management. The patient can wear a watch or a piece of jewelry on the involved extremity to begin restoration of function and eventually allow tolerance of the tactile stimulation of accessories. **Figure 8.9** is a patient education handout on desensitization. The case described in **Appendix 8.D** included manual desensitization as part of a home exercise program for chronic radicular pain that presented as mechanically inconclusive.

FIGURE 8.9 Desensitization Patient Education Handout

Desensitization

Desensitization can be an effective way to treat hypersensitivity that causes pain, especially when used in combination with other medical and therapeutic interventions.

WHAT IS DESENSITIZATION?
Desensitization is a treatment technique used to make the painful area of your body less sensitive to particular stimuli. This technique is used to *normalize* your body's response to particular sensations.

HOW DOES DESENSITIZATION WORK?
A desensitization program provides consistent stimuli to the affected area for short periods of time, frequently throughout the day. These small bursts of therapeutic activity shower the brain with sensory input. The brain responds to this demand by becoming accustomed to the sensation, thereby gradually decreasing your body's pain response to the stimuli. In short, your body gets used to it. The stimuli become tolerable and no longer elicit the maximal pain response.

WHAT IS USED TO DESENSITIZE AN AREA?
Desensitization involves application of unpleasant stimuli to the hypersensitive area. These stimuli are sensations your body is routinely exposed to and that do not elicit a painful response in nonaffected areas of the body and thus are not harmful or damaging. The items used to produce stimuli for desensitization vary depending on what the affected area interprets as painful. Examples are different textures or fabrics, light or deep pressure, vibration, and heat or cold.

WHAT DOES A DESENSITIZATION PROGRAM CONSIST OF?
Your desensitization program will progress gradually from stimuli that produce the least painful response to stimuli that produce the most painful response. Once your affected area begins to tolerate a stimulus, the next stimulus is incorporated. For example, a desensitization program may progress from a very soft material stimulus (eg, silk) to a rougher material (eg, wool) or a textured fabric (eg, Velcro). This progression may take several days to several weeks, depending on your level of hypersensitivity and your daily effort.

WILL DESENSITIZATION GET RID OF MY PAIN?
Desensitization may minimize your body's painful response to various stimuli; however, the affected area may still feel uncomfortable when in contact with particular stimuli. The goal of desensitization is to inhibit or interrupt the body's interpretation of routine stimuli as painful. These stimuli may not become pleasant or enjoyable, but they will no longer provoke an extreme pain response.

Adapted from Melanie E. Swan, OTR/L

Sensorimotor Retraining Programs

Little research has examined the use of sensorimotor retraining programs in the spine or extremities, other than some work with phantom limb pain and CRPS, but remodeling of the cortical representation has been discussed in the literature and in this chapter. Wand et al[68] developed a sensorimotor retraining program that achieved positive outcomes in three patients; the need for a larger sample size is evident. Sensorimotor retraining programs retrain the sensory and motor systems both separately and simultaneously.

The initial goal of the sensory stage is to train the patient to localize a stimulus to the region under treatment. As described in the section "Localization and Precision Testing," the stimulus is applied to points on the affected limb or back, and the patient is asked to specify the location of the stimulus. Patients with great difficulty localizing can first visualize stimuli applied to the area by viewing their application in a mirror. Once the patient is at least 80% accurate, the visualization is removed. The next goal is to improve the patient's precision in discriminating sharp versus dull stimuli (see the "Localization and Precision Testing" section). The patient then progresses to graphesthesia training, which comprises tasks of progressive difficulty beginning with recognition of letters of varying sizes and orientations and increased speed of drawing; progressing to recognition of three-letter words of different sizes and orientations, increased speed of drawing words, and recognition of overlapping letters; and finally progressing to calculation of simple sums, drawing numbers of different sizes and orientations, increased speed of drawing numbers, and recognition of overlapping numbers.[68]

The motor stage of the retraining program begins with left–right discrimination, imagined movements, and then active muscle contraction. Isometric local recruitment involves methods of isolating deep stabilizers such as the transverse abdominal muscles and multifidus. Once this is mastered, co-contraction with the pelvic floor and diaphragm activation are stressed. Wand et al[68] advocated initial use of local muscle co-contraction for lumbar spine programs based on congruence with cortical representations. Patients progress to dissociation exercises and then to small movements using visual feedback from a mirror. Tactile feedback through segmental palpation and tape can aid in proprioceptive control. Patients can use repositioning training and then movements with an external reference, such as placing the body part in space according to a picture or verbal command. As patients are able to improve motor control in the cortex, they can progress to active isolated control with less pain, less threat, and greater awareness. Small movements progress to large, full-range movements in a similar order.

Appendix 8.E summarizes the case of a patient treated with sensorimotor retraining and a graded activity program. This case demonstrates the value of pain mechanism classification. CNS pain mechanism classification allowed the clinician to use clinical reasoning to identify the dominant mechanism and initiate a brain-down approach. Patient education regarding pain mechanisms, graded exposure to function, activation of psychology intervention, and cortical sensorimotor remodeling all were apparent in her success. Her case was finalized with a body-up approach and accurate mechanical diagnosis because persistent symptoms related to the lumbar spine were dominating at the end of her care. **Table 8.3** summarizes interventions for patients with the motor/autonomic pain mechanism. Refer to **Appendix 8.F** for a summary of CNS pain mechanism interventions.

TABLE 8.3 Interventions for the Motor/Autonomic Pain Mechanism

Category	Interventions
Education for central nervous system pain mechanisms	Explanation of the nondamaging nature of pain: Hurt vs harm, interpretation of inputs
	Pain mechanism education
	Discussion of the role of negative emotions, harmful and damaging thoughts, and beliefs regarding pain: Pain journal
	Training in coping strategies for loneliness, depression, anxiety, negative repressed emotions, fear of motion or activity: Relaxation, diaphragmatic breathing
	Explanation of the Activity Pyramid: Green, yellow, and red lights, flare-up management for graded exposure to meaningful function
	Identification of the activity baseline and explanation of the no-worse concept: Goal is to return control to the patient
Activity for central nervous system pain mechanisms	Pacing and graded exposure to activity: Build low aerobic activity, HR 55%–75% of maximum, 2 to 5 hours per week
	Weight training to build upper and lower extremity strength: Start with isolated movements, progress to function, HR 55%-75% of maximum, two times per week
	Deep muscle training for spine postural stabilization: Progression to function, HR 55%-75% of maximum, two times per week
	HIIT: Progress to 10 to 20 min, HR >75% of maximum, one to two times per week
	Mechanical examination
Activity for motor autonomic pain	Referral to interdisciplinary cognitive–behavioral program (Yellow Flag Risk Form score >55 points)
	Treatment for output systems with symptoms • Lymphedema: Lymph massage, compression stockings • Tone and spasticity: Facilitatory and inhibitory techniques (eg, dynamic neuromuscular stimulation) • Immune system and metabolic disorders: Build low aerobic activity, HR 55%–75% of maximum, 2–5 hours per week; progress to 10- to 20-min HIIT, HR >75% of maximum, one to two times per week
	Treatment for cortical disinhibition: Sensorimotor retraining, five stages to progress, three times per day *Sensory retraining:* (1) localization training, (2) localization and stimulus type, (3) graphesthesia with letters and numbers, (4) graphesthesia with three-letter words, (5) graphesthesia with simple calculations • Progress visualization, size, orientation, speed, overlapping • Progress to next stage when accuracy is 80% *Motor retraining:* (1) left–right discrimination, (2) imagined movements, (3) reflective movements, (4) local isometric bracing, (5) small-range movements with feedback, (6) full-range movements with feedback (mirrors, palpation, elastic tape, watching, imagining)
	Progress therapy as patient masters exercise

Abbreviation: HIIT = high-intensity interval training; HR = heart rate.

Conclusion

The complexities of the multisystemic pattern of the motor/autonomic musculoskeletal pain mechanism manifest pain through an integration of all body systems. Pathways in complex pain syndromes cause changes in sensory and cortical systems. Clinicians need to consider how to reorganize the brain from central and peripheral subsystems as the individual is remodeling and rehabilitating. This reorganization can occur in premotor and presensory regions of the brain, but the system must recognize and achieve each task-specific level before rehabilitation is progressed from intrinsic to extrinsic factors during sensory and motor tasks.

KEY MESSAGES

- The motor/autonomic musculoskeletal pain mechanism is a complex, multisystemic pattern that manifests pain through an integration of all body systems.
- Complex regional pain syndrome (CRPS) often presents with edematous, trophic, and sweating changes and discoloration or alterations in blood flow and vascularity. No specific test or diagnostic procedure is available to confirm this condition; diagnosis relies on history and examination.
- Patients with motor/autonomic pain may demonstrate features such as spasticity, tone, discoloration, hypersensitivity, hyperalgesia, or allodynia.
- Three pathways in CRPS cause the major changes that take place: (1) facilitated inflammatory mechanisms, (2) vasomotor or autonomic dysfunctions, and (3) cortical or neuroplastic changes.
- Mirror neurons are a class of neurons that discharge when a task is performed, observed, heard, or even smelled. They provide a powerful tool for treating motor/autonomic pain.
- With the motor/autonomic pain mechanism, the patient's ability to detect two separate points (ie, tactile discrimination) or two distinct fields of sensation can become distorted. The resultant cortical map can be altered by lack of discrimination combined with the patient's emotions and prior life experiences.
- Graded motor imagery, consisting of left-right discrimination, imagined movements, and mirror therapy, can be effective in reducing pain in patients with the motor/autonomic pain mechanism.
- Desensitization can be used to decrease an area's sensitivity to a particular stimulus. The application may feel unpleasant to hypersensitive areas but should be tolerable enough not to produce a pain response.
- Sensorimotor retraining programs in the spine or extremities may help prime the cortical system and allow the patient to participate in a restoration of function program. Sensory retraining occurs in conjunction with motor retraining, and therapy is not progressed until the patient has mastered the previous level.

References

1. Maihofner C, Seifert F, Markovic K. Complex regional pain syndromes: New pathophysiological concepts and therapies. *Eur J Neurol.* 2010;17:649-660.
2. Louw A, Puentedura, L. Complex regional pain syndrome. Paper presented at: Combined Sections Meeting of the American Physical Therapy Association; February 2012; Chicago, IL.
3. Drummond PD. Sensory disturbances in complex regional pain syndrome: Clinical observations, autonomic interactions, and possible mechanisms. *Pain Med.* 2010;11:1257-1266.
4. Beggs S, Liu XJ, Kwan C, Salter MW. Peripheral nerve injury and TRPV1-expressing primary afferent C-fibers cause opening of the blood-brain barrier. *Mol Pain.* 2010;6:74.

5. Huygen FJ, Ramdhani N, van Toorenenbergen A, Klein J, Zijlstra FJ. Mast cells are involved in inflammatory reactions during complex regional pain syndrome type 1. *Immunol Lett*. 2004;91:147-154.
6. Kohr D, Tschernatsch M, Schmitz K, et al. Autoantibodies in complex regional pain syndrome bind to a differentiation-dependent neuronal surface autoantigen. *Pain*. 2009;143:246-251.
7. Sommer C, Kress M. Recent findings on how proinflammatory cytokines cause pain: Peripheral mechanisms in inflammatory and neuropathic hyperalgesia. *Neurosci Lett*. 2004;361:184-187.
8. Hsu ES. Practical management of complex regional pain syndrome. *Am J Ther*. 2009;16:147-154.
9. Maihofner C, Neundorfer B, Birklein F, Handwerker HO. Mislocalization of tactile stimulation in patients with complex regional pain syndrome. *J Neurol*. 2006;253:772-779.
10. van de Beek WJ, Roep BO, van der Slik AR, Giphart MJ, van Hilten BJ. Susceptibility loci for complex regional pain syndrome. *Pain*. 2003;103:93-97.
11. Geertzen JH, de Bruijn-Kofman AT, de Bruijn HP, van de Wiel HB, Dijkstra PU. Stressful life events and psychological dysfunction in complex regional pain syndrome type I. *Clin J Pain*. 1998;14:143-147.
12. Beerthuizen A, Stronks DL, Huygen FJ, Passchier J, Klein J, Spijker AV. The association between psychological factors and the development of complex regional pain syndrome type 1 (CRPS1)—a prospective multicenter study. *Eur J Pain*. 2011;15:971-975.
13. Merskey HNB. *Classification of Chronic Pain: Description of Chronic Pain Syndromes and Definition of Pain Terms. Report by the International Association for the Study of Pain Task Force on Taxonomy*. 2nd ed. Seattle, WA: IASP Press; 1994.
14. Harden RN, Bruehl S, Stanton-Hicks M, Wilson PR. Proposed new diagnostic criteria for complex regional pain syndrome. *Pain Med*. 2007;8:326-331.
15. Harden RN, Bruehl S, Perez RS, et al. Validation of proposed diagnostic criteria (the "Budapest criteria") for complex regional pain syndrome. *Pain*. 2010;150:268-274.
16. Guo TZ, Offley SC, Boyd EA, Jacobs CR, Kingery WS. Substance P signaling contributes to the vascular and nociceptive abnormalities observed in a tibial fracture rat model of complex regional pain syndrome type I. *Pain*. 2004;108:95-107.
17. Bruehl S. Complex regional pain syndrome: Outcomes and subtypes. *Clin J Pain*. 2009;25:598-599.
18. Bruehl S, Harden RN, Galer BS, Saltz S, Backonja M, Stanton-Hicks M. Complex regional pain syndrome: Are there distinct subtypes and sequential stages of the syndrome? *Pain*. 2002;95:119-124.
19. Schattschneider J, Binder A, Siebrecht D, Wasner G, Baron R. Complex regional pain syndromes: The influence of cutaneous and deep somatic sympathetic innervation on pain. *Clin J Pain*. 2006;22:240-244.
20. Acerra NE, Moseley GL. Dysynchiria: Watching the mirror image of the unaffected limb elicits pain on the affected side. *Neurology*. 2005;65:751-753.
21. Maihofner C, Handwerker HO, Neundorfer B, Birklein F. Patterns of cortical reorganization in complex regional pain syndrome. *Neurology*. 2003;61:1707-1715.
22. Maihofner C, Handwerker HO, Neundorfer B, Birklein F. Cortical reorganization during recovery from complex regional pain syndrome. *Neurology*. 2004;63:693-701.
23. Moseley GL. Distorted body image in complex regional pain syndrome. *Neurology*. 2005;65:773.
24. Geha PY, Baliki MN, Harden RN, Bauer WR, Parrish TB, Apkarian AV. The brain in chronic CRPS pain: Abnormal gray-white matter interactions in emotional and autonomic regions. *Neuron*. 2008;60:570-581.
25. Vanden Bulcke C, Van Damme S, Durnez W, Crombez G. The anticipation of pain at a specific location of the body prioritizes tactile stimuli at that location. *Pain*. 2013;154:1464-1468.
26. Moseley GL, Gallagher L, Gallace A. Neglect-like tactile dysfunction in chronic back pain. *Neurology*. 2012;79:327-332.
27. Meier PM, Zurakowski D, Berde CB, Sethna NF. Lumbar sympathetic blockade in children with complex regional pain syndromes: A double blind placebo-controlled crossover trial. *Anesthesiology*. 2009;111:372-380.
28. Cepeda MS, Lau J, Carr DB. Defining the therapeutic role of local anesthetic sympathetic blockade in complex regional pain syndrome: A narrative and systematic review. *Clin J Pain*. 2002;18:216-233.
29. Janig W, Stanton-Hicks M. *Reflex Sympathetic Dystrophy*. Seattle, WA: IASP Press; 1996.
30. Elbert T, Pantev C, Wienbruch C, Rockstroh B, Taub E. Increased cortical representation of the fingers of the left hand in string players. *Science*. 1995;270:305-307.
31. Melzack R, Coderre TJ, Katz J, Vaccarino AL. Central neuroplasticity and pathological pain. *Ann N Y Acad Sci*. 2001;933:157-174.
32. Huse E, Larbig W, Flor H, Birbaumer N. The effect of opioids on phantom limb pain and cortical reorganization. *Pain*. 2001;90:47-55.
33. Flor H, Braun C, Elbert T, Birbaumer N. Extensive reorganization of primary somatosensory cortex in chronic back pain patients. *Neurosci Lett*. 1997;224:5-8.
34. Moseley GL, Zalucki NM, Wiech K. Tactile discrimination, but not tactile stimulation alone, reduces chronic limb pain. *Pain*. 2008;137:600-608.

35. Kohler E, Keysers C, Umilta MA, et al. Hearing sounds, understanding actions: Action representation in mirror neurons. *Science*. 2002;297:846-848.
36. Rizzolatti G, Fabbri-Destro M, Cattaneo L. Mirror neurons and their clinical relevance. *Nat Clin Pract Neurol*. 2009;5:24-34.
37. Danziger N, Faillenot I, Peyron R. Can we share a pain we never felt? Neural correlates of empathy in patients with congenital insensitivity to pain. *Neuron*. 2009;61:203-212.
38. Cattaneo L, Rizzolatti G. The mirror neuron system. *Arch Neurol*. 2009;66:557-560.
39. Singer T, Seymour B, O'Doherty J, et al. Empathy for pain involves the affective but not sensory components of pain. *Science*. 2004;303:1157-1162.
40. Gu X, Han S. Attention and reality constraints on the neural processes of empathy for pain. *Neuroimage*. 2007;36:256-267.
41. Moseley GL, Arntz A. The context of a noxious stimulus affects the pain it evokes. *Pain*. 2007;133:64-71.
42. Gallese V, Keysers C, Rizzolatti G. A unifying view of the basis of social cognition. *Trends Cogn Sci*. 2004;8:396-403.
43. Stefan K, Classen J, Celnik P, Cohen LG. Concurrent action observation modulates practice-induced motor memory formation. *Eur J Neurosci*. 2008;27:730-738.
44. Ramachandran VS, Brang D. Sensations evoked in patients with amputation from watching an individual whose corresponding intact limb is being touched. *Arch Neurol*. 2009;66:1281-1284.
45. Fogassi L, Ferrari PF, Gesierich B, Rozzi S, Chersi F, Rizzolatti G. Parietal lobe: From action organization to intention understanding. *Science*. 2005;308:662-667.
46. Moseley G. Neuroscience and chronic pain: Enhancing clinical application. Presented at: Annual Mike Hage Musculoskeletal Team Building Course, Rehabilitation Institute of Chicago; May 21-22, 2011; Chicago, IL.
47. van Rijn MA, Marinus J, Putter H, et al. Spreading of complex regional pain syndrome: Not a random process. *J Neural Transm*. 2011;118:1301-1309.
48. van Rijn MA, Marinus J, Putter H, van Hilten JJ. Onset and progression of dystonia in complex regional pain syndrome. *Pain*. 2007;130:287-293.
49. Melzack R. Phantom limbs and the concept of a neuromatrix. *Trends Neurosci*. 1990;13(3):88-92.
50. Moseley GL, Gallace A, Spence C. Bodily illusions in health and disease: Physiological and clinical perspectives and the concept of a cortical "body matrix." *Neurosci Biobehav Rev*. 2012;36:34-46.
51. Makin TR, Holmes NP, Ehrsson HH. On the other hand: Dummy hands and peripersonal space. *Behav Brain Res*. 2008;191:1-10.
52. Gradl G, Schurmann M. Sympathetic dysfunction as a temporary phenomenon in acute posttraumatic CRPS I. *Clin Auton Res*. 2005;15:29-34.
53. Harden RN, Rudin NJ, Bruehl S, et al. Increased systemic catecholamines in complex regional pain syndrome and relationship to psychological factors: A pilot study. *Anesth Analg*. 2004;99:1478-1485.
54. Harden RN, Bruehl S, Perez RS, et al. Development of a severity score for CRPS. *Pain*. 2010;151:870-876.
55. Defrin R, Pope G, Davis KD. Interactions between spatial summation, 2-point discrimination and habituation of heat pain. *Eur J Pain*. 2008;12:900-909.
56. Lundborg G, Rosen B. The two-point discrimination test — Time for a re-appraisal? *J Hand Surg (Edinburgh, Scotland)*. 2004;29:418-422.
57. Kaneko A, Asai N, Kanda T. The influence of age on pressure perception of static and moving two-point discrimination in normal subjects. *J Hand Ther*. 2005;18:421-424.
58. Moseley GL, Wiech K. The effect of tactile discrimination training is enhanced when patients watch the reflected image of their unaffected limb during training. *Pain*. 2009;144:314-319.
59. Kolar P. Dynamic neuromuscular stabilization: A developmental kinesiology approach. Presented at: Rehabilitation Institute of Chicago; June 15-17, 2009; Chicago, IL.
60. Lewis JS, Kersten P, McPherson KM, et al. Wherever is my arm? Impaired upper limb position accuracy in complex regional pain syndrome. *Pain*. 2010;149:463-469.
61. Moseley GL, Nicholas MK, Hodges PW. A randomized controlled trial of intensive neurophysiology education in chronic low back pain. *Clin J Pain*. 2004;20:324-330.
62. Moseley GL. Graded motor imagery is effective for long-standing complex regional pain syndrome: A randomised controlled trial. *Pain*. 2004;108:192-198.
63. Moseley GL. Graded motor imagery for pathologic pain: A randomized controlled trial. *Neurology*. 2006;67:2129-2134.
64. Daly AE, Bialocerkowski AE. Does evidence support physiotherapy management of adult complex regional pain syndrome type one? A systematic review. *Eur J Pain*. 2009;13:339-353.
65. Dickstein R, Deutsch JE. Motor imagery in physical therapist practice. *Phys Ther*. 2007;87(7):942-953.
66. Wand BM, Tulloch VM, George PJ, et al. Seeing it helps: Movement-related back pain is reduced by visualization of the back during movement. *Clin J Pain*. 2012;28:602-608.

67. Watson HK, Carlson L. Treatment of reflex sympathetic dystrophy of the hand with an active "stress loading" program. *J Hand Surg Am*. 1987;12:779-785.
68. Wand BM, O'Connell NE, Di Pietro F, Bulsara M. Managing chronic nonspecific low back pain with a sensorimotor retraining approach: Exploratory multiple-baseline study of 3 participants. *Phys Ther*. 2011;91:535-546.
69. Nolan, MF. Two-point discrimination assessment in the upper limb in young adult men and women. *Phys Ther*. 1982;62:965-969.
70. Nolan MF. Quantitative measure of cutaneous sensation: Two-point discrimination values for the face and trunk. *Phys Ther*. 1985;65:181-185.
71. Nolan MF. Limits of two-point discrimination ability in the lower limb in young adult men and women. *Phys Ther*. 1983;63:1424-1428.

APPENDIX 8.A Clinical Reasoning for Subjective CNS Pain Characteristics

	Central Nervous System Pain Mechanisms: Subjective Characteristics	
Central Sensitization	**Affective Pain Mechanism** Conscious (C) vs Unconscious (U)	**Autonomic/Motor Pain Mechanism**
Location: Widespread, nonanatomical distribution of pain **Frequency:** Constant, unremitting, spontaneous, latent, paroxysmal pain; easily provoked pain with all activity **Descriptors:** Catastrophic terms related to harm and unhealed tissue; pain threat high **Intensity:** High severity, irritability **Onset:** Chronic >3 months; past expected tissue healing & pathology recovery times; pain disproportionate to the nature and extent of injury or pathology **History:** Failed interventions (medical, surgical, therapeutic) **24-hour behavior:** Erratic, inconsistent, night pain, disturbed sleep **Psychosocial screen:** Positive for pain behaviors (maladaptive and harmful beliefs/poor self-efficacy), high functional disability **Aggravating or alleviating factors:** Disproportionate, nonmechanical, unpredictable pattern in response to multiple nonspecific factors; heat helps; antiepileptic/antidepressant medications help	**Location:** (C) Widespread, nonanatomical distribution; (U) axial low back pain, neck pain, headaches, knee pain (specific location) **Descriptors:** (C) Catastrophic emotional language; (U) dull, tight, weak, sharp with movement **Frequency:** (C) Constant, spontaneous, latent, paroxysmal pain; (U) intermittent **Intensity:** (C) High severity, irritability; (U) low-grade irritant **Onset:** Chronic >3 months; past expected tissue healing/pathology recovery times; pain disproportionate to the nature and extent of injury or pathology **History:** Failed interventions (medical, surgical, therapeutic); (C) preexisting anxiety, depression, psychological trauma (ie, abuse, accident, work-related injury), CNS disorder (ie, SCI, MS, etc); (U) increased stress/repressed negative emotions regarding current life pressures, past childhood relationships with parents & siblings, characteristic of perfectionism **24-hour behavior:** Inconsistent pain, night pain, disturbed sleep **Psychosocial screen:** (C) Positive for negative emotions, altered family, work, social life, medical conflict, high functional disability; (U) appear negative on conscious level	**Location:** Widespread, nonanatomical distribution of pain to upper and/or lower extremity may include the spine, typically affects more than one nerve field **Frequency:** Constant unremitting, spontaneous, latent, paroxysmal pain **Descriptors:** Deep, dull, burning, aching, pulsating, stabbing, cold intolerance **Intensity:** High severity, irritability **Onset:** Chronic >3 months; past expected tissue healing/pathology recovery times; pain disproportionate to the nature and extent of injury or pathology; initial trauma managed poorly. **History:** Immune, GI, endocrine, parasympathetic, and sympathetic systems symptoms and/or complications **24-hour behavior:** Erratic, inconsistent, night pain, disturbed sleep **Psychosocial screen:** Positive for pain behaviors (maladaptive beliefs/poor self-efficacy), high functional disability **Other clinical signs:** Swelling indicating lymphedema, spasticity, tone, discoloration of skin, skin and hair sensitivities, trophic changes, excessive sweating

APPENDIX 8.B Clinical Reasoning for Objective CNS Pain Characteristics

Central Nervous System Pain Mechanisms: Objective Characteristics		
Central Sensitization *Spinal Cord Facilitation*	**Affective Pain Mechanism** **Conscious (C) vs Unconscious (U)** *Emotional/Social Dysfunction*	**Autonomic/Motor Pain Mechanism** *Cortical Disinhibition*
Objective findings: Spinal cord facilitation signs; pain evoked easily **Movement testing:** Disproportionate inconsistent nonmechanical/anatomical pattern of pain provocation; no relationship between stimulus and response; common latency effect; result is worse; absence of tissue injury/pathology **Palpation:** Diffuse nonanatomic areas of pain or tenderness; light touch elicits noxious response (allodynia) in area of symptoms. **Posture:** Antalgic postures or movements; disuse atrophy of muscles **Neurological testing:** Positive for hyperalgesia, allodynia, hyperpathia **Proprioceptive screen:** Spine and extremity tests are negative **Breath assessment:** Sitting diaphragm breathing test: upper respiratory pattern **Yellow flag assessment:** Positive identification of catastrophization, fear-avoidance behavior, harmful thoughts, distress. **Readiness stage:** Precontemplation, contemplation, preparation **Fear Avoidance Beliefs Questionnaire (FABQ) score:** Physical activity ≥14 **Yellow flag risk score:** Over 55 indicates moderate risk of chronic disability **Outcome measures:** Disabilities of the Arm, Shoulder and Head, Oswestry Disability Index, Neck Disability Index, Lower Extremity Function Scale, with moderate disabilities (may choose others)	**Objective findings:** (C) Similar to central sensitivity with greater emotional component; (U) similar to ischemia; treatment ineffective. Tender points: upper trapezius, lumbar paraspinals, posterior lateral aspects of the gluteus maximus, bilaterally **Yellow flag assessment:** (C) Positive for distress, negative emotions, depression, anxiety, anger, altered family/work/social life, medical conflict, reduced coping skills with life-changing events (ie, SCI, loss, amputation, neurological impairment, etc); (U) appear negative on a conscious level but positive toward increased stress & repressed negative emotions regarding current life stressors, past childhood relationships with parents & siblings, characteristic of perfectionism at the unconscious level. **Psychometric tools:** Assist referral to (C) cognitive–behavioral therapy program and/or (U) investigative psychology • Yellow Flag Risk Form: Chronic disability risk assessment (>55 points) • Anger/depression: Patient Health Questionnaire (PHQ-9) (score >10) • Anxiety: Pain Anxiety Symptom Scale (higher score) • (U) Tension myositis syndrome information document (>3 yes answers)	**Objective findings:** Same as central sensitivity; in addition signs of: • Cortical dysfunction (spasticity, tone) • Autonomic nervous system dysfunction (skin discoloration, excessive sweating, trophic changes, hair excitability, lymph edema) • Involvement of sympathetic and parasympathetic systems **General illness** may be present from immune and GI system involvement. **Proprioceptive screen:** All spine and extremity tests are positive **Palpation:** Diffuse nonanatomic areas of pain/tenderness; light touch elicits noxious response in areas with/without symptoms often within the space around the skin **2-point discrimination:** Positive findings within area of symptoms; primary sensory cortex findings **Neurological testing:** Positive findings related to loss of graphesthesia (recognition of symbols drawn on skin), incomplete drawing of body outline for area of symptoms, signs of neglect present in left–right discrimination testing; positive findings in localization and precision sensory testing

APPENDIX 8.C Orthopedic Outpatient, 10-Yr-Old Male

Physical Therapy/Occupational Therapy Initial Evaluation

SUBJECTIVE FINDINGS

Chief complaint:	Constant R hand, forearm, arm, shoulder pain
Descriptors:	Dull, burning, sharp, cramping, swollen, discolored, spasms; "cannot touch arm"
Onset:	6 mo ago, car door was slammed on hand, resulting in fracture. Forearm and hand were casted above elbow for 12 wk and put in a sling. No follow-up was given; not known why patient was casted so long. Cast removed at ER when grandparents took him because it hurt so much.
Frequency:	Constant R arm pain
24-hr behavior:	Worse in PM and AM and with UE use
Subjective pain:	Likert / (Faces) scale: Severe pain
Aggravating factors:	Any activity with hand and UE causes spasticity and swelling
Relieving factors:	Putting arm in sling, use of antiseizure medications and muscle relaxants

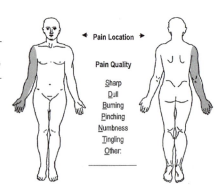

◄ Pain Location ►

Pain Quality
Sharp
Dull
Burning
Pinching
Numbness
Tingling
Other: _____

PATIENT EDUCATION CONSIDERATIONS

Readiness to learn:	Ready and self-motivated Extrinsically motivated (Limitations (see below))
Limitations to learning:	Cognitive Physical Language Financial Cultural (Other:) Grandparents speak no English
Teaching method preferred:	(Handout) Verbal (Demonstration) (Practice) (Other:) Interpreter; pictures
Explain:	Grandparents bring him to therapy (mom works full time), grandparents speak only German

MEDICAL HISTORY

Past medical history:	Healthy before fracture, now "cannot touch arm"
Family history:	No significant family history
Surgery and invasive procedures:	Cast was not removed for a prolonged period of time.
Medications:	Antiseizure medication, muscle relaxants, and ibuprofen all help in some way — Allergies: None
Previous treatments:	No prior treatment, other than immobilization
Diagnostic tests:	X-ray: Healed fracture MRI: Negative CT scan: ___ EMG: ___ Other: Negative bone scan

PSYCHOSOCIAL FACTORS

Living situation:	Patient speaks English and German and lives with his single mother, who works full time. His grandparents drive him to his therapy appointments.
Behavior:	Elementary school participation is limited because he cannot write.
Occupation:	Student
Recreation and leisure:	Has stopped all play
Functional disability:	Play and running are limited.
Concerns:	Patient is very protective of arm movements and cradles the arm when playing and running. He believes his hand is still broken, which is why it hurts so much when he moves it.

PROVISIONAL PAIN CLASSIFICATION (in order of dominance)

1. **Motor/autonomic pain mechanism**
2. **Central sensitization**
3. **Nociceptive:ischemia** from immobilized connective tissue

PAIN EDUCATION TOPICS

1. Interpreter services for all patient and caregiver education
2. Yellow flag: Negative effects of belief that fracture has not healed and need to dispel this belief
3. Good vs bad pain, no-worse concept
4. Use of elastic tubular bandage instead of sling for swelling, support, and pain relief
5. Strategies to activate the brain's pain control center (eg, mirror therapy to show the brain that the hand and arm are fine)
6. Strategies to improve meaningful function and improve limitation from pain (ie, get back to playing)
7. Nociceptive:ischemia musculoskeletal pain mechanism; need for increased blood flow

(continues on next page)

APPENDIX 8.C Orthopedic Outpatient, 10-Yr-Old Male *(continued from previous page)*

Physical Therapy/Occupational Therapy Objective Evaluation

OBJECTIVE FINDINGS
- No mechanical evaluation performed; patient refused to move his arm on observation and request
- Significant lymphedema in right hand and forearm up to mid humerus
- Purple color throughout hand and lower forearm
- Hypersensitivity to light touch throughout UE, upper trapezius, and cervical paraspinals on the right
- Positive two-point touch discrimination; loss on side of symptoms for right UE

PROVISIONAL MECHANICAL CLASSIFICATION

Other—Chronic regional pain syndrome (psychological screen)

Other—Restoration of function; possible mechanical examination at a later time

PROVISIONAL PAIN CLASSIFICATION

Motor/autonomic pain mechanism

TREATMENT

Treatment: Issued very light elastic tubular bandage for hand, wrist, and forearm up to elbow; patient was receptive to using this bandage, which is more protective of skin than the sling. Provided education comparing bones that are broken vs not broken with healed broken bones; radiologist showed patient his initial (ER) and follow-up films. Pain education included good vs bad pain. Began brain-down movement approach with mirror therapy (patient thought this was "cool") using the mirror to create image of hand and arm moving and touching different parts of his body; putting weight on hand aided in dispelling belief of nonhealed fracture; distraction play with lower extremity balance activities used to initiate reflex UE movements to catch balance. Slow progression to AROM using board games, balloon volleyball, and toss and catch off wall, all games he enjoyed.

Treatment summary: **12 visits over 24 wk:** 1×/wk for 2 wk

Goals:

	PSFS	
	Initial	Discharge
Return to writing in school	0	10
Return to playing catch recreationally with friends	0	10
Pain limitation to function (unable to assess)		
Pain intensity rating—Faces scale	Severe	Minimal-none

Abbreviations: AROM = active range of motion; CT = computed tomography; EMG = electromyography; ER = emergency room; MRI = magnetic resonance imaging; PSFS = Patient-Specific Functional Scale; R = right; UE = upper extremity.

APPENDIX 8.D Orthopedic Outpatient, 32-Yr-Old Female

Physical Therapy/Occupational Therapy Initial Evaluation

SUBJECTIVE FINDINGS

Chief complaint:	Low back, bilateral buttock, R thigh, R calf pain; foot pain, plantar surface and all toes, especially 1st digit
Descriptors:	Burning, stabbing, numbness, tingling, cramping
Onset:	Chronic R L5 radiculitis with 7-yr history of episodic R lower extremity pain. Initially diagnosed with R femoral and lateral femoral cutaneous pain after vaginal delivery 5 yr ago. Intermittent feelings of weakness. Recent exacerbation 8 mo ago.
Frequency:	Constant in R calf, intermittent in thigh and low back
24-hr behavior:	Always worse at end of day
Subjective pain:	Likert / Faces scale: Other: Oswestry 42/100; numeric pain rating scale 7-8/10
Aggravating factors:	Sitting and driving, walking excessively / elliptical / working out
Relieving factors:	Standing temporarily, lying temporarily

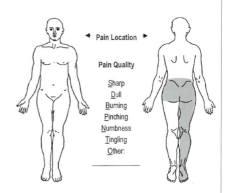

Pain Location

Pain Quality
Sharp
Dull
Burning
Pinching
Numbness
Tingling
Other:

PATIENT EDUCATION CONSIDERATIONS

Readiness to learn:	Ready and self-motivated Extrinsically motivated Limitations (see below)
Limitations to learning:	Cognitive Physical Language Financial Cultural Other: None
Teaching method preferred:	Handout Verbal Demonstration Practice Other:
Explain:	

(continues on next page)

APPENDIX 8.D Orthopedic Outpatient, 32-Yr-Old Female *(continued from previous page)*

MEDICAL HISTORY

Past medical history:	Unremarkable other than chronic back pain history
Family history:	No significant family history
Surgery and invasive procedures:	3 epidural steroid injections at 2 different pain clinics—not helpful, worsened symptoms
Medications:	Ambien 5 mg for sleep, ibuprofen 800 mg 3×/day—no major relief Allergies: Penicillin
Previous treatments:	Physical therapy (4 trials over 7 yr, modalities and strengthening; mechanical diagnosis and therapy, no directional preference reported), acupuncture (intermittent relief), chiropractor (manipulations and modalities—worse)

Diagnostic tests:

X-ray:	MRI:	CT scan:	EMG:	Other:
	Mild degenerative changes throughout L spine, L4-5 bulge with annular tear, L3-4 annular tear, patchy bone marrow edema bilateral inferior sacral ala consistent with persistent stress response		R superficial peroneal neuropathy	Negative bone scan

PSYCHOSOCIAL FACTORS

Living situation:	Lives with husband, 2 children 5 and 2 yr old. Husband works full time. Patient is happily married.
Behavior:	Patient is frustrated but cooperative and reports being depressed at times. Husband is supportive and helpful at home and with children.
Occupation:	Choir director; stands all day without significant opportunities to sit
Recreation and leisure:	Enjoys working out and is motivated to do so; likes weight-training classes, elliptical use, running, and walking, but all limited in past year
Functional disability:	Is limited in lifting weight >5 lb, is unable to do cardio >10 min without worsening calf and leg symptoms, is unable to sit or drive for prolonged periods, continues to maintain an active life but is getting depressed and negative about her situation
Concerns:	4 rounds of physical therapy and 3 epidural steroid injections brought no major relief; trials of gabapentin and pregabalin brought no relief and were not tolerated (caused constipation and mental sluggishness); patient must stand for work as choir director

PROVISIONAL PAIN CLASSIFICATION (in order of dominance)
1. **Motor/autonomic pain mechanism**
2. **Central sensitization pain mechanism**
3. **Peripheral neurogenic pain mechanism**—remodeling phase

PAIN EDUCATION TOPICS
1. Good vs bad pain, pain–brain connection
2. Strategies to activate the brain's pain control center: Deep breathing
3. Strategies to improve meaningful function and improve limitation from pain
4. Effects of life-changing events on pain, pain psychology and coping, reasons pain worsened with birth of 1st child
5. Nociceptive:ischemia musculoskeletal pain mechanism: Need for increased blood flow using movement and prolonged low-level heat
6. Connective tissue healing and remodeling guidelines: Need for regular progressive movement, no-worse concept as indicator of safe progression
7. Musculoskeletal nerve pain and need for regular movement: No-worse concept as indication of safety in movements and activities
8. Posture and body mechanics strategies for home activities including shopping, laundry, and driving; pacing by adding 5 min of activity per day
9. Desensitization program

Provisional pain classification supporting information:
- Motor/autonomic pain indicated by mild initiation of multisystem involvement (ie, constipation and mild gastrointestinal distress at times, mild depression, mild hormonal period imbalances)
- Location, description, and aggravating and alleviating factors indicate central sensitization and peripheral neurogenic pain mechanisms
- Mechanically inconclusive classification based on limited directional preference
- Referral to rheumatology with discussion based on inconclusive spinal examination from initial evaluation

(continues on next page)

APPENDIX 8.D Orthopedic Outpatient, 32-Yr-Old Female *(continued from previous page)*

Physical Therapy/Occupational Therapy Objective Evaluation

OBJECTIVE FINDINGS

Visits 1 and 2:	• Mechanical evaluation performed and inconclusive findings reassessed • Allodynia with light touch in areas of pain on R lower extremity • Oswestry 42/100 • PHQ-9 score of 5/10 (low end of mild depression) • Readiness to change stage—action • Begin pain education, set movement guidelines for tolerance of walking and elliptical use • Core and cardiovascular aquatic therapy program initiated based on patient-reported enjoyment of water • Distal intermittent soft tissue "wringing" with intermittent relief reported for nerve sensitivity • Neural flossing and tensioning both irritating to lower extremity symptoms so discontinued • Scrubbing weightbearing program initiated with 30-sec increments increased pain but no worse as a result
Posture:	Limited R lower extremity weightbearing, decreased lordosis
Active range of motion:	Severe loss of flexion, extension, and R side glide in standing; moderate loss of L side glide in standing
Repeated test movements:	Loaded flexion, extension, and side glide all increased and worsened pain in distal symptoms. Unloaded examination was unremarkable for any relieving positions. L side lying decreased pain, no better as a result; on return to standing, symptoms returned. Patient required rest breaks from standing.
Neurological examination:	Normal motor L2-S1, hypersensitivity R calf and thigh, reflexes within functional limits in patella and gastrocnemius; decreased two-point touch discrimination at site of symptoms
Neurodynamic test:	Positive straight leg raise R and L, positive slump R and L, repeated movement with ankle dorsiflexion, increased pain but no worse as a result

PROVISIONAL MECHANICAL CLASSIFICATION

Visit 3
Mechanically inconclusive
Seronegative spondyloarthopathy confirmed from rheumatologist via +HLA-B27. Patient prescribed etanercept with 20% relief reported over 2 wk.

PROVISIONAL PAIN CLASSIFICATION (in order of dominance)

Visit 3
1. **Motor/autonomic pain mechanism**
2. **Central sensitization pain mechanism**
3. **Peripheral neurogenic pain mechanism**—ischemic, neural dependent, remodeling phase

Intervention Visits 1–5

• Left–right discrimination 90% in both extremities, 1.7 sec average bilaterally

TREATMENT

Treatment:
- Begin pain education: Baseline Activity Tolerance tool, central nervous system, nerve pain
- Relaxation, breathing patient education handouts
- Initiate Activity Pyramid baseline finding and charting for activities of daily living and low aerobic exercise
- Initiate scrubbing program; husband to initiate lower extremity desensitization through tactile stimulation with increasing levels of massage and pressure
- Provide posture strategies for picking up children to encourage use of lordosis, provide lumbar roll for driving; review body mechanics strategies of unweighting the R lower extremity for work-related standing as a choir director, but minimizing asymmetrical postures. Reinforce moving strategies during day for mechanical ischemic nerve pain and other symptoms.
- Reinforce breathing and relaxation; redirect interpretation of emotional vs mechanical pain.
- Initiate scrubbing and stress loading program; train husband to do soft tissue work initially for visits 1-5, then as nerve irritation diminishes, perform work 80% less frequently and progress to neural mobilization and active strengthening.
- Progress restoration of cardio fitness through swimming laps and core strengthening program in the pool; transfer improvements in ability to recruit abdominals and glutes in the pool to land program.
- Promote upper extremity strengthening for improvements in household chores (eg, grocery shopping, laundry).
- Provide upgraded gym program: Improve postural awareness of lordosis and forward head using physio ball and alternating arm movements and resisted push, pull, and waist to overhead upper extremity functional patterns.

Treatment summary: **10 visits over 15 wk:** Strengthening program 1×/week for 5 wk, then progress to every 2 wk. Initial need to treat the dominating motor/autonomic mechanism first because of peripheral nerve allodynia and lack of success with multiple other therapy interventions. Patient initially presented as active with no major psychosocial flags, yet she was progressively worsening. Her cortical screenings were within normal limits and inconclusive for any mechanical findings. As this patient progressed with central nervous system pain interventions, her nerve sensitivity diminished, and she was able to progress to functional independence. The patient significantly improved with scrubbing and her husband's desensitization using both compression and traction with progression from light touch to deep manual massage of the R lower extremity. As nerve irritation diminished, a directional preference for extension presented, and patient was able to find relief in prone lying and prone on elbows when with the children.

(continues on next page)

APPENDIX 8.D Orthopedic Outpatient, 32-Yr-Old Female *(continued from previous page)*

		PSFS	
		Initial	Discharge
Goals:	Stand through a choir concert 1-2 hr	2	9
	Perform regular household tasks of laundry, grocery shopping, and intermittent child lifting	0	8
	Return to a 3-4 day/wk cardio program	0	8
	Pain limitation to function	7	10
	Pain intensity rating	7	0-1
		PHQ-9	
		5 (mild depression)	0 (no depression)
		Oswestry	
		42/100	10/100

Abbreviations: CT = computed tomography; EMG = electromyography; L = left; MRI = magnetic resonance imaging; PHQ-9 = Patient Health Questionnaire; PSFS = Patient-Specific Functional Scale; R = right.

APPENDIX 8.E Outpatient, 29-Yr-Old Female

Physical Therapy/Occupational Therapy Initial Evaluation

SUBJECTIVE FINDINGS

Chief complaint:	Chronic pelvic and back pain
Descriptors:	Dull, cramping, spasms; bladder and pelvic floor spasms, pulling, tightness, chronic sense of urgency
Onset:	1 yr, 2 mo ago, patient was sitting at work and noted urinary urgency and pelvic pain not relieved with voiding; has worsened since then
Frequency:	Intermittent lower back and pelvic pain, both constant when sitting
24-hr behavior:	No pattern
Subjective pain:	Likert / (Faces) scale: 7-10
Aggravating factors:	No pattern
Relieving factors:	Walking, heat, massage, cyclobenzaprine

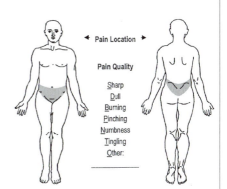

Pain Location

Pain Quality
- Sharp
- Dull
- Burning
- Pinching
- Numbness
- Tingling
- Other: _____

PATIENT EDUCATION CONSIDERATIONS

Readiness to learn:	(Ready and self-motivated) Extrinsically motivated Limitations (see below)
Limitations to learning:	Cognitive Physical Language Financial Cultural (Other:) Tearful over multiple interventions attempted
Teaching method preferred:	(Handout) (Verbal) (Demonstration) (Practice) Other: _____
Explain:	

(continues on next page)

> **APPENDIX 8.E Outpatient, 29-Yr-Old Female** *(continued from previous page)*

MEDICAL HISTORY

Past medical history:	Endometriosis (gynecologist feels not related), rosacea, urinary urgency only with flare-ups, positive antinuclear antibody test but rheumatic workup negative for autoimmune or connective tissue disorder, hypothyroid, irritable bowel syndrome
Family history:	Mother has a history of uterine cancer
Surgery and invasive procedures:	Abdominal laparoscopy in 2005 due to endometriosis; epidural steroid injection for herniated nucleus pulposus L5/S1 brought no relief
Medications:	Antiseizure medication, muscle relaxants, ibuprofen all help in some way; levothyroxine 50 mg Allergies: None
Previous treatments:	PT x 2 trials (1st with core strengthening), 2nd recent internal pelvic floor therapy for 8 months with improvements in ability to relax and contract pelvic floor

Diagnostic tests:	X-ray:	MRI: L5-S1 herniated nucleus pulposus	CT scan:	EMG:	Other:

PSYCHOSOCIAL FACTORS

Living situation:	Lives alone; works as a government analyst; has a good family and support system; currently enrolled in a master's program at night
Behavior:	Is tearful and anxious about recurrent condition, which started for no apparent reason, and its cause; had prior negative experience with physical therapy so is pessimistic about treatment; had recent pelvic floor internal physical therapy for 8 mo with no relief except for improvements in relaxation and contraction of pelvic floor
Occupation:	Full-time analyst and part-time student
Recreation and leisure:	Has stopped all physical activity but is receptive to a walking program
Functional disability:	Cardio and running are limited; is unable to sit upright with any lordosis without pelvic pain or sense of urgency
Concerns:	Very protective of spinal movements; negative about posture correction discussions; doesn't want to have this pain for the rest of her life

PROVISIONAL PAIN CLASSIFICATION (in order of dominance)

1. **Motor/autonomic pain mechanism**—dominating mechanism
2. **Affective** (anxiety)
3. **Central sensitization**
4. **Peripheral neurogenic pain mechanism**—container dependent

PAIN EDUCATION TOPICS

1. Walking program for overall fitness and initiation of movement that is somewhat enjoyable
2. Heat vs ice for low back flare-ups and anxiety surrounding spasms
3. Good vs bad pain, no-worse concept
4. Posture support with donut pillow because of tactile discomfort with lumbar support close to her spine and inability to correct posture without a negative connotation
5. Relaxation strategies to activate the brain's pain control center: Diaphragm breathing and relaxation training
6. Cognitive–behavioral therapy with pain psychologist for coping with anxiety regarding condition and length of treatment with no benefit
7. Brain-down movement training: Build representation of symptom area in brain (ie, the "virtual part" has symptoms, too)
8. Discussion of traumatic physical therapy experience and manipulation of her back and fear of manual intervention (other than internal pelvic floor work)
9. Nociceptive:ischemia musculoskeletal pain mechanism: Need for increased blood flow and conditioning
10. Discussion of directional preference in history for extension bias and reinforcement of a gradual introduction of flexion as she improves

PSYCHOSOCIAL YELLOW FLAGS

Check all that apply.

Attitudes and beliefs about pain	✔	Belief that pain is harmful or disabling, resulting in avoidance behaviors (eg, guarding, fear of movement)
		Belief that all pain must be abolished before attempting to return to work or normal activity
	✔	Expectation of increased pain with activity or work; lack of ability to predict capability
	✔	Catastrophizing, thinking the worst, misinterpreting bodily symptoms
	✔	Belief that pain is uncontrollable
		Passive attitude toward rehabilitation
Behaviors		Use of extended rest, disproportionate downtime
	✔	Reduced activity level, with significant withdrawal from activities; boom-bust cycle of activity
	✔	Avoidance of normal activity, progressive substitution of lifestyle away from productive activity
		Report of extremely high intensity of pain (eg, "above 10" on a 0-10 scale)
		Excessive reliance on use of aids or appliances
	✔	Reduction in sleep quality since onset of pain
		High intake of alcohol or other substances (possibly as self-medication), with an increase since onset of pain
		Smoking

(continues on next page)

APPENDIX 8.E Outpatient, 29-Yr-Old Female *(continued from previous page)*

Compensation issues	Lack of financial incentive to return to work
	Delay in accessing income support and treatment cost, disputes over eligibility
	History of claims due to other injuries or pain problems
	History of extended time off work due to injury or other pain problems (eg, >12 weeks)
	✔ Previous experience of ineffective case management (eg, absence of interest, perception of being treated punitively)
Diagnosis and treatment	✔ Experience with a health professional who sanctioned disability or did not provide interventions to improve function
	✔ Experience of conflicting diagnoses or explanations for pain, resulting in confusion
	✔ Catastrophizing and fear (eg, of "ending up in a wheelchair") caused by diagnostic language
	✔ Dramatization of pain by a health professional resulting in dependency on treatments and continuation of passive treatment
	✔ Frequent visits to a health professional in the past year (excluding the present episode of pain)
	Expectation of a "techno-fix" (eg, view of body as a machine)
	✔ Lack of satisfaction with previous treatment for pain
	Acceptance of advice to withdraw from job
Emotions	✔ Fear of increased pain with activity or work
	✔ Depression, especially long-term low mood, loss of sense of enjoyment
	Increased irritability
	✔ Anxiety about heightened awareness of body sensations, including sympathetic nervous system arousal
	✔ Feeling of being under stress and unable to maintain a sense of control
	✔ Presence of social anxiety or disinterest in social activity
	✔ Feeling of being useless and not needed
Family	Overprotective partner or spouse (usually well intentioned) who emphasizes fear of harm or catastrophizes
	Solicitous behaviors from spouse (eg, taking over tasks)
	Socially punitive responses from spouse (eg, ignoring, expressing frustration)
	Lack of support by family members for an attempt to return to work
	✔ Lack of available support person with whom to talk about problems
Work	History of manual work in industries such as fishing, forestry, farming, construction, nursing, trucking, migrant or contract labor
	✔ Pattern of frequent job changes, experience of stress at work, job dissatisfaction, poor relationships with peers or supervisors, lack of vocational direction
	Belief that work is harmful, will do damage, or is dangerous
	✔ Unsupportive current work environment
	Low educational background, low socioeconomic status
	✔ Job that involves significant biomechanical demands such as lifting; manual handling of heavy items; extended sitting, standing, driving, or vibration; maintenance of sustained postures or movements; inflexible work schedule without breaks
	Minimal availability of selected duties and graduated return-to-work pathways with poor implementation
	✔ Absence of interest of supervisor, peers, employer

Physical Therapy/Occupational Therapy Objective Evaluation

OBJECTIVE FINDINGS

Visit 1:
- Mechanical evaluation performed: directional preference for extension indicated; need for overpressure, which reproduced pelvic pain from lumbar spine; patient tearful and concerned with anyone touching her back based on a poor previous manipulation by a physical therapist with increased pain as a result
- Education regarding steps program and monitoring basic level of ambulation and function
- PASS score 63/100 (high end of moderate pain-related anxiety)
- Oswestry score = 25/50 (severe disability)
- Readiness to change stage: preparation, ready to take action with direction
- Set baseline walking and sitting goals based on Oswestry and PSFS scores and steps program average
- Initiate pain education

Posture:	Decreased lordosis
Active range of motion:	Flexion minimum loss, extension moderate loss, right and left side glide nil loss
Repeated test movements:	Repeated flexion in lying increased vaginal, abdominal, and pelvic pain; repeated extension in standing had no effect; repeated extension in lying produced pelvic pain but no worse as a result, anxiety, decreased buttocks and back pain
Neurological examination:	Within functional limits; weakness in bilateral gluteus medius 3+/5, extensors 3+/5; unable to perform core endurance plank test 10 sec on front or on side due to pain

PROVISIONAL MECHANICAL CLASSIFICATION

Visit 1
Lumbar derangement, unilateral/asymmetrical above knees—partial centralization
Other behavioral—psychological screen for cognitive anxiety

PROVISIONAL PAIN CLASSIFICATION (in order of dominance)

Visit 1
1. **Motor/autonomic pain mechanism**—multisystemic (gastrointestinal, genitourinary, dermatological, musculoskeletal, endocrine), dominating initially
2. **Affective pain mechanism**—pain-related anxiety
3. **Central sensitization**
4. **Peripheral neurogenic pain mechanism**—container related, lumbar spine disc producing pelvic pain
5. **Nociceptive:ischemia pain mechanism**—lumbar spine, remodeling phase

Intervention Visit 1:
- Provide anxiety management strategies; outpatient psychology evaluation in process from referring physician same day as physical therapy evaluation
- Begin walking program and baseline assessment of function
- Take baseline measurements—Oswestry, PSFS, PASS

(continues on next page)

APPENDIX 8.E Outpatient, 29-Yr-Old Female *(continued from previous page)*

- Review pain education and prior physical therapy experiences; ascertain potential lumbar spine referral pattern for pelvic pain she has been experiencing
- Provide education on posture in sitting and determine a strategy that will work for her in class (eg, pillow support, discreet standing in back)
- Train in extension with patient overpressure, 10x, 5-6x/day

Intervention Visit 6:

- Low back function is improving (40% better), but patient reports still not being aware of her back and pelvis region and finds it difficult to correct her posture or know where she is in space.
- Sitting tolerance has doubled with donut pillow.
- Strengthening program limited to 3 repetitions of clam, plank, and sit-to-stand exercises secondary to anxiety with progression of exercise and flare-ups that cause her to regress.
- Patient easily met the 10,000 steps/day program and was ready to progress to elliptical use but fearful.
- Localization evaluation: Precision testing with only 20% accuracy on R side of spine and 40% on L side for 6-point touch testing. Extension ROM within functional limits now, but continued pelvic and lumbar spine pain despite overpressure and therapist mobilization mechanically.
- Initiated patient in localization of touch to her lumbar spine with visual feedback and then 3x/wk sensory retraining when support system available with 6-point touch testing.
- Used flash cards for lumbar spinal motions.

PROVISIONAL MECHANICAL CLASSIFICATION

Visit 6
Other chronic pain—psychological screen health-related anxiety progressing with anxiety strategies and psychologist 1x/wk
Mechanical—directional preference for extension

PROVISIONAL PAIN CLASSIFICATION

Visit 6
Motor/autonomic pain mechanism—sensorimotor approach

Intervention Visits 7-12:

- Continued psychotherapy for anxiety management
- Patient realized she wants to seek other employment for a more positive work experience based on her negative perceptions of her supervisor and lack of ability to progress in her current work environment.
- Initiated formal biofeedback training in sitting positions primarily
- Provided instruction in deep breathing
- Provided sensorimotor cortical retraining for low back pain: Stage 1, sensory localization (determine site of stimulus) and motor laterality recognition; Stage 2, sensory localization and stimulus type (determine site and size of probe) and imagined movements using videotaped model performing motions patient was fearful of, with graded exposure with anxiety symptoms; Stage 3, graphesthesia training (determine letters and numbers of varying size and orientation) and local stabilization training (diaphragm breathing with pelvic floor and postural bracing, plank, sideplank, lower extremity strengthening); Stage 4, graphesthesia training (determine three-letter words of varying size and orientation and overlap) and full-range movements forward and backward side glide, left and right, integrated with upper and lower body, triplanar core exercise on discharge
- Provided education regarding tissue remodeling and effective remodeling and progression of sitting tolerance with restoration of function program
- Progressed full centralization of lumbar derangement with extension procedures and posture education

TREATMENT

Treatment:
- Provide posture strategies for sitting to encourage neutral spine mechanics with extension bias. Donut pillow with progression to lumbar support as back sensitivity is abolished and improved with sensory retraining.
- Reinforce get up and move sitting strategies or stretching during day for mechanical pain. Slow progression with 5% vs 10% progression for core and lower extremity strengthening program.
- Reinforce deep breathing, imagery, and relaxation to redirect interpretation of emotional vs mechanical pain.
- Recommend baths for pain when cyclobenzaprine is not available or as a substitute.
- Progress and pace full restoration of lumbar ROM and strength.
- Progress to full cardio program 3-4x/wk for 30-40 min on treadmill or elliptical. Patient continued to use her pedometer as she felt it gave her an idea of her mobility when she was working all day.
- Upgrade gym program for lower body for full functional strength on manual muscle testing.
- Progress core stability and cardiovascular exercises and high-intensity interval training after completion of sensorimotor training program.

Treatment summary: **12 total visits over 24 wk, psychotherapy 1x/wk for total of 16 sessions.** This case demonstrates the value of pain mechanism classification. Central nervous system pain mechanism classification prompted clinical reasoning to initiate a brain-down approach that included reassessment of and a focus on dominating central pain mechanisms. The patient presented with all pain mechanisms; her condition was multisystemic, and she had significant cortical smudging and lack of sensory awareness of her spine. Patient education focused on pain mechanisms, graded exposure to function, psychology intervention, and cortical sensorimotor remodeling. Her case was finalized with a body-up approach and assurance of an accurate mechanical diagnosis of symptoms related to the lumbar spine. Through use of her directional preference in extension and sensorimotor retraining, the patient was able to regain her body awareness and gradually progress function with a graded strengthening and gym program. Fear exposure and psychological interventions in conjunction with active care helped her progress through her fear of movement and catastrophic thinking regarding chronic disability.

Goals:

	PSFS	
	Initial	Discharge
Tolerate prolonged sitting through coursework (3 hr) with scheduled rest breaks (lumbar)	0	9
Perform regular cardiovascular program on elliptical or treadmill 30-40 min, 3-4 days/wk	1	10
Pain limitation to function	3	10
Pain intensity rating	Lumbar 7/10, pelvis 5/10 and need to urinate	1/10, intermittent at discharge; no symptoms in pelvic region
PASS	63/100	12/100
Oswestry	50 (severe disability)	8 (minimal disability)

Abbreviations: CT = computed tomography; EMG = electromyography; MRI = magnetic resonance imaging; PASS = Pain Anxiety Symptom Scale; PSFS = Patient-Specific Functional Scale; ROM = range of motion.

APPENDIX 8.F Clinical Reasoning for CNS Pain Intervention

Central Nervous System Pain Mechanisms: Intervention		
Central Sensitization	**Affective Pain Mechanism Conscious (C) vs Unconscious (U)**	**Autonomic/Motor Pain Mechanism**
Education: • Explanation of the nondamaging nature of pain: hurt vs harm; interpretation of inputs • Pain mechanism education • Discussion of the role of negative emotions, thoughts, and beliefs; review pain journal • Training in coping strategies for fear of motion or activity; use relaxation, diaphragm breathing training • Explanation of the Activity Pyramid: Green, yellow, and red lights, flare-up management • Identification of the activity baseline and explanation of the no-worse concept; return control to patient **Activity:** • Graded exposure to patient-identified fearful/harmful activity; build low aerobic activity, HR at 55%-75% max, for 2-5 hr/wk • Weight training to build upper and lower extremity strength; start with isolated movements and progress to function at HR 55%-75% of maximum, 2x/wk • Deep muscle training for spine postural stabilization; progress to function, 2x/wk • High-intensity interval training (HIIT); progress to 10-20 min intervals, HR >75% of max, 1-2x/wk • Mechanical exam	Same as central sensitization **(C) Education:** • Regarding readiness stage • Negative emotions' contribution to pain • Focused discussion based on psychometric tools (PHQ-9, PASS, Yellow Flag Risk Form) • Interdisciplinary cognitive–behavioral therapy program, if Yellow Flag Risk Form score >55 **(U) Education:** Tension myositis syndrome; discuss treatment progression: • Understand mechanism; brain's efforts to protect are causing tissue ischemia • Acknowledge activation of mechanism related to unconscious repressed, negative emotions • Refer to investigative psychologist if unable to self-treat with John Sarno's books (*The Mindbody Prescription: Healing the Body, Healing the Pain; Healing Back Pain: The Mind-Body Connection; The Divided Mind: The Epidemic of Mindbody Disorders*) Patients must have **psychological evaluation**, if this mechanism is classified as dominating.	Education and activity same as central sensitization **Treatment for output systems with symptoms:** Lymphedema: Lymph massage, compression stockings Tone and spasticity: Facilitatory and inhibitory techniques Immune system and metabolic disorders: Build low aerobic activity, HR 55%-75% of maximum, 2-5 hr/wk; progress to 10-20 min HIIT, HR >75% of maximum, 1-2x/wk **Treatment for cortical disinhibition:** Sensorimotor retraining approach: 5 stages to progress, 3x/day *Sensory retraining:* (1) localization training, (2) localization and precision stimulus type, (3) graphesthesia with letters & numbers, (4) graphesthesia with 3-letter words, (5) graphesthesia with simple calculations • Progress visualization, size, orientation, speed, overlapping • Progress to next stage when accuracy is 80% *Motor retraining:* (1) left–right discrimination, (2) imagined movements, (3) reflective movements, (4) local isometric bracing, (5) small-range movements with feedback, (6) full-range movements with feedback (mirrors, palpation, elastic tape, watching, imagining) • Progress therapy as patient masters exercise

Melissa C. Kolski, PT, OCS, Dip MDT, has over 15 years of clinical experience with a specialty interest in spine care and treatment of patients with musculoskeletal pain and dysfunction. She is a board-certified orthopedic specialist and diplomate in mechanical diagnosis and therapy. Melissa is an education program manager and practicing clinician at the Rehabilitation Institute of Chicago and teaches nationally. She is a member of American Physical Therapy Association in the orthopedic section, pain management and foot and ankle special interest groups, and McKenzie Institute. She is a member of the Specialization Academy of Content Experts for Orthopedic Clinical Specialists in the American Board of Physical Therapy Specialties.

Annie O'Connor, PT, OCS, Cert. MDT, is Corporate Director of the Musculoskeletal Practice and Clinical Manager of the River Forest Spine and Sport Center at the Rehabilitation Institute of Chicago. She lectures nationally and internationally on musculoskeletal pain classification and intervention, neurodynamic evaluation and treatment, mechanical diagnosis and therapy of spine and extremities, kinetic chain evaluation, and functional manual therapy and exercise prescription. She was instrumental in establishing the allied health's clinical diagnostic approach for musculoskeletal pain at the Rehabilitation Institute of Chicago. She is a member of American Physical Therapy Association in both the orthopedic section and canine special interest group, the North American Spine Society, and McKenzie Institute. She continues to treat orthopedic, neurological patients, and canines with musculoskeletal pain to achieve the best life possible.